GASTROENTEROLOGY AND HEPATOLOGY

PEARLS OF WISDOM

John K. DiBaise, M.D.

NOTE

The intent of GI Pearls of Wisdom is to serve as a study aid to improve performance on a standardized examination. It is not intended to be a source text of the knowledge base of medicine or to serve as a reference in any way for the practice of clinical medicine. Neither Boston Medical Publishing Corporation nor the editors warrant that the information in this text is complete or accurate. The reader is encouraged to verify each answer in several references. All drug use indications and dosages must be verified by the reader before administration of any compound.

DEDICATION

To the loves of my life –

Michelle, Samantha, Maximillian and Rachel

EDITOR-IN-CHIEF:

John K. DiBaise, M.D.
Assistant Professor of Internal Medicine
Section of Gastroenterology and Hepatology
University of Nebraska Medical Center
Omaha, NE

CONTRIBUTING AUTHORS:

James L. Achord, M.D., MACG, FACP
Professor Emeritus
University of Mississippi Medical Center
Jackson, MS
Gastrointestinal Bleeding

Michael Ahn, M.D.
Gastroenterology Fellow
University of California at San Diego
San Diego, CA
**Large Intestine, Congenital and
  Structural Abnormalities**

Tariq Akbar, M.D.
Gastroenterology Fellow
Clinical Instructor of Medicine
University of Vermont
Burlington, VT
**Liver, Infections and Granulomatous
  Diseases**

Bhupinderjit S. Anand, M.D., Ph.D.
Professor of Medicine
Baylor College of Medicine
Gastroenterology Section
Houston, TX
Liver, Cirrhosis and its Complications

Frank A. Anania, M.D., FACP
University of Maryland Medical Center
Baltimore, MD
**Liver, Alcoholic Liver Disease and Non-
  Alcoholic Steatohepatitis**
Liver, Metabolic Disorders

Mohammed R. Annes, M.D.
Gastroenterology Fellow
Clinical Instructor of Medicine
University of Vermont
Burlington, VT
Liver, Vascular Disorders

Gowri Balachandar, M.D.
Gastroenterology Fellow
Texas Tech University Health Science Center
Lubbock, TX
**Gallbladder and Biliary, Surgical
  Therapy of Gallstones and Postoperative
  Complications**
Small Intestine, Infections and Tumors

Jamie S. Barkin, M.D., MACG
Professor of Medicine
Chief, Division of Gastroenterology
Mount Sinai Medical Center
Miami Beach, FL
**Pancreas, Acute and Chronic
  Pancreatitis**

Randall E. Brand, M.D.
Assistant Professor of Internal Medicine
Section of Gastroenterology and Hepatology
University of Nebraska Medical Center
Omaha, NE
  Pancreas, Tumors

John M. Carethers, M.D.
Assistant Professor of Medicine
University of California at San Diego
La Jolla, CA
**Small Intestine, Congenital and
  Structural Abnormalities**
**Large Intestine, Congenital and
  Structural Abnormalities**

Maurice A. Cerulli, M.D.
Chief, Division of Gastroenterology
The Brooklyn Hospital Center
Clinical Associate Professor of Medicine
New York University School of Medicine
Brooklyn, NY
Gastrointestinal Bleeding

Deborah Cohen, MMSc, RD, CNSD
Sinai Hospital
Baltimore, MD
**Nutrition, Enteral and Parenteral
  Feeding and Deficiency Syndromes**

Darwin L. Conwell, M.D.
The Cleveland Clinic Foundation
Division of Gastroenterology
Cleveland, OH
**Pancreas, Congenital and Structural
  Abnormalities**

Joseph Cullen, M.D.
Associate Professor of Surgery
University of Iowa Hospital and Clinics
Iowa City, IA
**Stomach, Ulcer-Associated Conditions,
  Ulcer Surgery and Post-Gastric Surgery
  Syndromes**

Istvan Danko, M.D., Ph.D.
Pediatric Gastroenterology Fellow
University of Wisconsin
Waisman Center
Madison, WI
**Liver, Congenital and Structural
  Abnormalities and Pediatric Diseases**

Themistodes Dasopoulos, M.D.
Instructor of Clinical Medicine
The University of Chicago Hospital
Department of Gastroenterology
Chicago, IL
**Small Intestine, Maldigestive and
  Malabsorptive Diseases**
**Miscellaneous, Gastrointestinal
  Complications of AIDS**

John K. DiBaise, M.D.
Assistant Professor of Internal Medicine
Section of Gastroenterology and Hepatology
University of Nebraska Medical Center
Omaha, NE
Stomach, Infections and Tumors

Michelle O. DiBaise, PA-C, MPAS
Department of Internal Medicine
Section of Dermatology
Omaha, NE
**Miscellaneous, Gastrointestinal
  Dermatoses**

Anthony J. DiMarino, Jr., M.D.
Chief, Division of Gastroenterology and
Hepatology
Thomas Jefferson University
Jefferson Medical College
Philadelphia, PA
**Miscellaneous, Short Bowel Syndrome
  and its Complications**

Douglas A. Drossman, M.D.
Professor of Medicine and Psychiatry
Division of Digestive Diseases
University of North Carolina at Chapel Hill
Chapel Hill, NC
**Miscellaneous, Obesity and Eating
  Disorders**

Eli D. Ehrenpreis, M.D.
Assistant Professor of Clinical Medicine
The University of Chicago Hospital
Department of Gastroenterology
Chicago, IL
**Small Intestine, Maldigestive and
  Malabsorptive Diseases**
**Miscellaneous, Gastrointestinal
  Complications of AIDS**

Atilla Ertan, M.D.
Professor of Medicine
Associate Chief, Gastroenterology Division
Baylor College of Medicine
Chief, GI Section
The Methodist Hospital
Houston, TX
**Gallbladder and Biliary, Gallstone
  Disease and its Complications**

Ronnie Fass, M.D.
Assistant Professor of Medicine
University of Arizona Health Sciences Center
Director, GI Motility Laboratory
Southern Arizona VA Health Care Systems
Tucson, AZ
**Esophagus, Congenital and Structural
  Abnormalities**

Michael S. Fedotin, M.D.
Clinical Professor of Medicine
University of Missouri – Kansas City
Kansas City, MO
**Stomach, Gastric/Duodenal Ulcers and
  Complications**

Nicholas Ferrentino, M.D.
Assistant Professor of Medicine
Fellowship Program Director
Division of Gastroenterology and Hepatology
University of Vermont College of Medicine
Burlington, VT
Liver, Vascular Disorders
**Liver, Infections and Granulomatous
  Diseases**

Spencer T. Fung. M.D.
Gastroenterology Fellow
University of California at San Diego
San Diego, CA
**Small Intestine, Congenital and
  Structural Abnormalities**

John J. Gleysteen, M.D.
Professor of Surgery
University of Alabama at Birmingham
Chief, VA Surgical Service
Birmingham, AL
**Abdominal Cavity, Congenital
  Abnormalities, Abscesses and Fistulae**

Jeffrey Goldstein, M.D.
University of Rochester Medical Center
GI Unit
Rochester, NY
**Gallbladder and Biliary, Congenital and
  Structural Abnormalities**
**Stomach, Congenital and Structural
  Abnormalities**

Eric B. Goosenberg, M.D.
Clinical Assistant Professor of Medicine
Temple University School of Medicine
Associate Member and Attending
Gastroenterologist
Fox Chase Cancer Center
Philadelphia, PA
Esophagus, Infections and Tumors

Martin E. Gordon, M.D., FACP, FAAAS
Clinical Professor of Medicine
Yale School of Medicine
North Branford, CT
**Miscellaneous, Travel Matters in GI
  Diseases**

Glenn R. Gourley, M.D.
Professor
Department of Pediatrics
University of Wisconsin
Waisman Center
Madison, WI
**Liver, Congenital and Structural
  Abnormalities and Pediatric Diseases**

David S. Hodges, M.D.
Associate Professor of Internal Medicine
Texas Tech University Health Science Center
Lubbock, TX
Small Intestine, Infections and Tumors

Terrence Jackson, M.D.
Gastroenterology Fellow
University of Nebraska Medical Center
Omaha, NE
Pancreas, Tumors

David E. Johnston, M.D.
Associate Professor of Medicine
Department of Gastroenterology
University of New Mexico
Albuquerque, New Mexico
**Liver, Drug-Induced and Other
  Inflammatory Disorders**

Nyingi Kemmer, M.D.
Gastroenterology Fellow
University of Texas Medical Branch
Galveston, TX
**Gallbladder and Biliary, Motor
  Disorders**

Yvonne Renée Lee, M.D., FACP
Naval Medical Center
San Diego, CA
**Miscellaneous, Radiation and Ischemic
  GI Injury and Vascular Gut
  Abnormalities**

Elizabeth A. Lien, M.D.
Assistant Professor of Internal Medicine
Section of Infectious Diseases
University of Nebraska Medical Center
Omaha, NE
Large Intestine, Infections

Ramona Lim, M.D.
Gastroenterology Fellow
University of Miami School of Medicine
Miami, FL
**Pancreas, Acute and Chronic
  Pancreatitis**

Elizabeth Lyden, M.S.
Statistical Coordinator
Preventive and Societal Medicine
University of Nebraska Medical Center
Omaha, NE
**Miscellaneous, Biostatistics and
  Epidemiology**

James A. Lynch, Ph.D.
Assistant Professor
Preventive and Societal Medicine
University of Nebraska Medical Center
Omaha, NE
**Miscellaneous, Biostatistics and
  Epidemiology**

Mark E. Mailliard, M.D.
Associate Professor of Internal Medicine
Section of Gastroenterology and Hepatology
University of Nebraska Medical Center
Omaha, NE
Liver, Viral Hepatitis

John K. Marshall, M.D., FRCPC
Clinical Scholar in Gastroenterology
Department of Medicine
Division of Gastroenterology
McMaster University Medical Centre
Hamilton, Ontario, Canada
**Large Intestine, Non-IBD Colitides and
  Other Inflammatory Diseases**

Timothy McCashland, M.D.
Associate Professor of Internal Medicine
Section of Gastroenterology and Hepatology
University of Nebraska Medical Center
Omaha, NE
**Liver, Fulminant Failure and Liver
  Transplantation**

David McFadden, M.D.
Professor and Chief, Division of General
Surgery
UCLA Center for Health Sciences
Los Angeles. CA
**Pancreas, Inflammatory Diseases and
  Infections**

A. Steven McIntosh, M.D.
Gastroenterology Specialists, Inc.
Suffolk, VA
**Gallbladder and Biliary, Infections and
  Tumors**

Carolyn McIvor, M.B.B.S.
Assistant Professor of Internal Medicine
Section of Gastroenterology and Hepatology
University of Nebraska Medical Center
Omaha, NE
**Miscellaneous, Gastrointestinal and
  Hepatobiliary Disorders in Pregnancy**

Jane Meza, M.S.
Preventive and Societal Medicine
University of Nebraska Medical Center
Omaha, NE
**Miscellaneous, Biostatistics and
 Epidemiology**

Mohammed Mah'moud, M.D.
Assistant Professor of Medicine
Division of Gastroenterology and Hepatology
University of South Carolina School of
Medicine
Columbia, SC
**Miscellaneous, Foreign Bodies and
 Caustic Injury**

Bola Olusola, M.D.
Gastroenterology Fellow
University of Nebraska Medical Center
Omaha, NE
Stomach, Infections and Tumors

Isaac Raijman, M.D.
Gastroenterology and Liver Associates, PA
Clinical Assistant Professor
MD Andersen Cancer Center
Houston, TX
**Gallbladder and Biliary, Inflammatory
 Diseases**

Yehuda Ringel, M.D.
Division of Digestive Diseases
University of North Carolina at Chapel Hill
Chapel Hill, NC
**Large Intestine, Disorders of Pelvic
 Floor and Anorectum**

Tamar Ringel-Kulka, M.D.
Visiting Physician
Adolescent Health Section
Division of Community Pediatrics
Department of Pediatrics
University of North Carolina at Chapel Hill
Chapel Hill, NC
**Miscellaneous, Obesity and Eating
 Disorders**

Cory A. Roberts, M.D.
Assistant Professor
Department of Pathology and Microbiology
University of Nebraska Medical Center
Omaha, NE
Miscellaneous, GI and Liver Pathology

Robin D. Rothstein, M.D.
University of Pennsylvania Hospital
Division of Gastroenterology
Philadelphia, PA
**Small Intestine, Motor Disorders and
 their Complications**

Hemant K. Roy, M.D.
Assistant Professor of Internal Medicine
Section of Gastroenterology and Hepatology
University of Nebraska Medical Center
Omaha, NE
**Large Intestine, Tumors, Polyps and
 Associated Syndromes**

Thomas Schiano, M.D.
Assistant Professor of Medicine
The Mount Sinai Hospital Medical Center
Division of Liver Diseases
New York, NY
Liver, Tumors and Cysts

Ashok Shah, M.D.
University of Rochester Medical Center
GI Unit
Rochester, NY
**Gallbladder and Biliary, Congenital and
 Structural Abnormalities**
**Stomach, Congenital and Structural
 Abnormalities**

Edy E. Soffer, M.D.
The Cleveland Clinic Foundation
Division of Gastroenterology and Hepatology
Cleveland, OH
**Large Intestine, Constipation, Motor
 Disorders and IBS**

Roger D. Soloway, M.D.
Marie B. Gale Centennial
Professor of Medicine
Vice Chair, Department of Internal Medicine
for TDCJ Affairs
Galveston, TX
**Gallbladder and Biliary, Motor
 Disorders**

Eugene F. Tharalson, M.D.
Senior Resident
Department of Internal Medicine
University of Arizona Health Sciences Center
Tucson, AZ
**Esophagus, Congenital and Structural
 Abnormalities**

Gervais Tougas, M.D.
Associate Professor of Medicine
McMaster University Medical Centre
Hamilton, Ontario, Canada
Esophagus, Motor Disorders

Eugene A. Trowers. M.D., M.P.H.
Associate Professor of Internal Medicine
Division of Gastroenterology and Hepatology
Texas Tech University Health Science Center
Lubbock, TX
**Gallbladder and Biliary, Surgical
 Therapy of Gallstones and Postoperative
 Complications**

Jeffrey Tuvlin, M.D.
Gastroenterology Fellow
The University of Chicago Hospital
Chicago, IL
**Miscellaneous, GI Complications of
  AIDS**

Jon A. Vanderhoof, M.D.
Professor of Pediatrics
Director, Joint Section of Pediatric
Gastroenterology and Nuttrition
Omaha, NE
Miscellaneous, Pediatric GI Diseases

Rajeev Vasudeva, M.D., FACG
Professor of Medicine
Director, Division of Digestive Diseases and
Nutrition
University of South Carolina School of
Medicine
Columbia, SC
**Esophagus, GERD and Inflammatory
  Diseases**
**Miscellaneous, Foreign Bodies and
  Caustic Injury**

William E. Whitehead, Ph.D.
Professor of Medicine
University of North Carolina at Chapel Hill
Division of Digestive Diseases
Chapel Hill, NC
**Large Intestine, Disorders of Pelvic
  Floor and Anorectum**

Howard J. Worman, M.D.
Associate Professor of Medicine and Anatomy
and Cell Biology
Director, Division of Digestive and Liver
Diseases
College of Physicians and Surgeons
Columbia University
New York, NY
**Liver, Autoimmune and Overlap
  Conditions**

John M. Wright, M.D.
University of Vermont College of Medicine
Division of Gastroenterology and Hepatology
Burlington, VT
Liver, Vascular Disorders
**Liver, Infections and Granulomatous
  Diseases**

Richard A. Wright, M.D.
Professor of Medicine
Chief, Division of Gastroenterology and
Hepatology
University of Louisville Health Sciences
Center
Louisville, KY
**Stomach, Motor and Functional
  Disorders**

Renee L. Young, M.D.
Associate Professor of Internal Medicine
Section of Gastroenterology and Hepatology
University of Nebraska Medical Center
Omaha, NE
**Large Intestine, Inflammatory Bowel
  Disease and its Complications**

Saeed Zamani, M.D.
Gastroenterology Fellow
Thomas Jefferson University Hospital
Jefferson Medical College
Philadelphia, PA
**Miscellaneous, Short Bowel Syndrome
  and its Complications**

WE APPRECIATE YOUR COMMENTS!

We appreciate your opinion and encourage you to send us any suggestions or recommendations. Please let us know if you discover any errors, or if there is any way we can make Pearls of Wisdom more helpful to you. We are also interested in recruiting new authors and editors. Please call, write, fax, or e-mail. We look forward to hearing from you.

Send comments to:

Boston Medical Publishing Corporation
237 S. 70th Street, Suite 206, Lincoln, NE, 68510

888-MBOARDS (626-2737)
402-484-6118
Fax: 402-484-6552
E-mail: bmp@emedicine.com
www.emedicine.com

INTRODUCTION

Congratulations! Gastroenterology and Hepatology *Pearls of Wisdom* is designed to help you learn about gastrointestinal and liver diseases and prepare you for the Board Examination in Gastroenterology and Hepatology. This book is one in a series of *Pearls of Wisdom* texts which include all areas of medicine. Before you get started, a few words are appropriate discussing the intent, format, limitations and proper use of this book.

Since *Pearls* is primarily intended as a study aid, the text is structured in a question and answer format. Most of the questions are short with short answers. This is to facilitate moving through a large body of information. Such a format, while quite unlike the format used in the actual Board Examination, is useful to enable you to assess your strengths and weaknesses in a particular area. This allows you to concentrate further studies on areas of interest or weakness. Emphasis has been placed on distilling trivia and key facts that are easily overlooked, that are quickly forgotten, and that somehow seem to occur frequently on board examinations.

It must be emphasized that any question and answer book is most useful as a learning tool when used in conjuction with a subject-specific textbook. Truly assimilating *Pearls* facts into a framework of knowledge absolutely requires further reading on the surrounding concepts. The more active the learning process, the better the understanding. Use this book with your preferred source texts handy and open. When you encounter a question that you cannot recall the answer or that you find of particular interest, you are strongly encouraged to review the pertinent area in the textbook at hand.

The chapters are organized to include all aspects of gastroenterology and hepatology. Some areas are covered more thoroughly than others. The questions within each chapter are randomly arranged to simulate board examinations and the way questions arise in real life. There are several areas of redundancy. This is intentional – redundancy is a good thing when preparing for board examinations.

Pearls does have limitations. While great effort has been made to verify that the questions and answers are accurate, discrepancies and inaccuracies sometimes occur. Most often this is attributable to variance between original sources. We have tried to verify in several references the most accurate information. Keep in mind that some answers may not be the answers you would prefer. In addition, *Pearls* risks accuracy by aggressively pruning complex concepts down to the simplest level; the dynamic knowledge base and clinical practice of medicine is not like that. Furthermore, new research and practice occasionally deviates from that which likely represents the correct answer for test purposes. Remember, this book is designed to maximize your score on a test. Refer to your most current sources of information and mentors for direction in practice.

Each question is preceded by two boxes. This permits you to check off areas of interest, weakness or simply note that it has been read. This also allows for re-reading without having uncertainty about what was reviewed earlier.

We welcome your comments, suggestions and criticism. Please make us aware of any errors you find. We hope to make continuous improvements and would greatly appreciate any input with regard to format, organization, content, presentation, or about specific questions. We are also interested in recruiting new contributing authors and publishing new textbooks. For more information, contact our manager at Boston Medical Publishing, Terri Lair, at (toll free) 1-888-MBOARDS. We look forward to hearing from you!

Study hard and good luck on the Boards!

J.K.D.

TABLE OF CONTENTS

GASTROENTEROLOGY

ABDOMINAL CAVITY - CONGENITAL ABNORMALITIES, ABSCESSES AND FISTULAE

John J. Gleysteen, M.D.

❏❏ **How and where is particulate material in the peritoneal cavity normally cleared from the cavity?**

Through modified lymphatics located along the diaphragm undersurface, stomas of which open when the diaphragm relaxes creating negative intra-abdominal pressure. Diaphragmatic muscle contractions then force lymphatics cephalad, aided by one-way valves.

❏❏ **What is the therapeutic purpose of the "Semi-Fowler's position"?**

To minimize subphrenic infections and absorption of peritoneal toxins by reducing upward diaphragmatic excursion. It is this excursion that increases abdominal negative pressure, promotes migration of fluid upward to lie under the diaphragm and opens lymphatic stoma for systemic absorption.

❏❏ **The presence of rebound or percussive tenderness and guarding help to diagnose peritonitis in what way?**

They indicate extension to and irritation of the abdominal wall peritoneal surface, whereas localized inflammatory processes between visceral surfaces produce non-specific, dull aching pain that may be difficult to localize.

❏❏ **When is the most effective time to use antibiotics to treat peritoneal contamination?**

The estimated "grace period" is 4 to 6 hours after contamination.

❏❏ **Clinically significant *Candida* peritonitis, usually responsive to low-dose amphotericin B or fluconazole, is most likely to be found in what situations?**

In patients on long-term antibiotics or after gastric perforations.

❏❏ **T/F: The process of abscess formation and maturation is deterrent but not cidal to contained bacteria.**

True. While abscess formation and maturation initially retards bacterial escape and septicemia and decreases bacterial access to oxygen and glucose, it also creates a barrier to penetrating phagocytes and systemic antibiotics. Therefore, bacteria can persist as vegetative forms and can rejuvenate in a changed environment; ergo, the surgical principle that abscesses must be drained.

❐❐ **Although the overall incidence of intra-abdominal abscess has progressively declined, what is the most common cause?**

While formerly perforated appendicitis, colonic diverticulitis is now the most common cause as a result of more rapid diagnosis and treatment of appendicitis.

❐❐ **When searching for an intra-abdominal abscess, a high-resolution CT scan is the procedure of choice with two limitations. Name the limitations.**

1) Interloop abscesses and 2) Inability to differentiate sterile from contaminated fluid collections.

❐❐ **Percutaneous drainage of abscesses after CT scan identification should be avoided in what situations?**

1) Noninfected peripancreatic phlegmon.
2) Infected organized hematomas.
3) Abscess with enteric fistulae.
4) Fungal infections.
5) Abscess within necrotic tumors.

❐❐ **How often are abdominal x-ray findings of pneumoperitoneum in an unoperated patient associated with a perforated hollow viscus?**

Ninety percent of cases. These cases require urgent surgical intervention.

❐❐ **Aside from iatrogenic causes of non-surgical pneumoperitoneum, the second most common source of gas/air in the abdominal cavity is from where?**

Above the diaphragm. Ruptured alveoli can lead to pneumomediastinum which can: 1) rupture into the pleural space and then into the abdomen directly through the diaphragmatic hiatus or fenestrations, or 2) dissect into the retroperitoneum and then rupture through the mesentery.

❐❐ **T/F: In patients with significant abdominal distension who develop oliguria unresponsive to hemodynamic changes or corrections, increased intra-abdominal pressure (IAP or "compartment syndrome") should be considered.**

True. Follwing the diagnosis of IAP (intra-abdominal pressure above 20 mmHg) measured with a bladder catheter and manometer, appropriate efforts, including surgical exploration, directed at intra-abdominal decompression should be followed with diuresis expected afterwards.

❐❐ **An adolescent of Iranian or Jordanian ancestry develops episodic, non-radiating, diffuse abdominal pain with associated fever and without any post-episode sequelae. What inherited disorder may he have?**

Familial Mediteranean Fever.

❐❐ **Aerophagia may cause sudden localized or diffuse abdominal distention with normal bowel sounds and localized tympany and pain. Most often, the air collects in what two places?**

Stomach and splenic flexure of the colon.

❐❐ **Although the specific risk of postoperative abdominal adhesive complications may vary according to the acute need and location of the initial surgical procedure, what is the approximate overall risk of hospital readmission later for these complications?**

Studied over a ten-year follow-up interval, 4% of 30,000 initial procedures and 5.5% of hospital readmissions were directly attributable to postoperative adhesions.

❑❑ **A rectal shelf of Blumer is often associated with metastatic gastric or breast cancer. How is this distinguished from a rectal stricture?**

The Blumer shelf is an extrarectal mass indenting the anterior wall of the rectum, and is distinguished from a stricture by the fact that: 1) it doesn't encircle the circumference and 2) often the mucosa can be made to move over the shelf.

❑❑ **Carnett's Test is a physical examination means of differentiating an abdominal wall mass from an intra-abdominal mass (and abdominal wall pain from intra-abdominal pain). How is this test performed?**

The supine patient is asked to extend his legs and lift his/her feet up from the bed or table, thereby tensing the abdominal musculature. Alternatively, the patient can raise his/her head. An intra-peritoneal mass will nearly disappear when the abdominal muscles tighten, whereas an abdominal wall mass will persist. Likewise, pain from an intra-abdominal source will usually lessen, whereas abdominal wall pain will not.

❑❑ **Abdominal wall crepitance surrounding a postoperative incision but without wound discharge and odor or skin discoloration has what significance?**

It is innocuous. Termed "pseudo-gas gangrene," it occurs because air is entrapped in the subcutaneous tissue. It will soon be absorbed.

❑❑ **Acute development of a tender lump in the right lower quadrant after spasmodic coughing, about half-way between the umbilicus and pubic tubercle, may likely be due to what?**

Rectus muscle rupture or torn inferior epigastric artery. This may be differentiated from a strangulated Spigellian hernia by the absence of vomiting. Patients that are pregnant or on anticoagulant therapy are also at increased risk for this problem.

❑❑ **What four structures may remain patent rather than obliterate in the umbilicus at birth?**

1)   Umbilical vein.
2)   Omphalo-mesenteric duct (fecal).
3)   Hypogastric arteries.
4)   Bladder-urachal fistula (urine).

❑❑ **What is a likely cause of a sudden appearance of feculent discharge from the umbilicus in a middle-aged, unoperated patient?**

Colonic diverticulitis or colon carcinoma.

❑❑ **Acute mesenteric lymphadenitis is as common as acute appendicitis and can mimic this disease in children. After what age does the incidence drop and become exceedingly unlikely?**

Fifteen years of age.

❑❑ **Acute extra-abdominal conditions that are common and may mimic acute inflammatory intra-abdominal disease number at least three. Name them.**

1)   Coronary occlusion/myocardial infarction.
2)   Diaphragmatic pleurisy.
3)   Herpes zoster.

❑❑ **A psychogenic disease usually occurring in females, in which acute abdominal symptoms are out of proportion to physical findings and in which there are often several surgical scars on the abdomen is suggestive of what diagnosis?**

Münchausen's Syndrome.

☐☐ **What type of bowel fistulae frequently spontaneously close if surrounding active bacterial peritonitis is cleared?**

Lateral bowel fistulae, which permit normal progression of some intestinal contents beyond the fistula through normal bowel.

☐☐ **If a colonic fistula is present, whether cutaneous or internal, what is the problem with treatment by proximal loop colostomy or cecostomy?**

Neither procedure is totally diverting and thereby may cause persistent contamination.

☐☐ **The five major physical deterrents to spontaneous closure of an external bowel fistula are:**

1) End-fistula (discontinuous with bowel).
2) Gastrointestinal tract obstruction exists distal to the fistula.
3) Foreign body such as prosthetic mesh is in continuity with the fistula.
4) Gastrointestinal mucosa has extended through the fistula tract and fused with skin (epithelialization).
5) Active peritonitis or local abscess is present.

☐☐ **The two benefits of parenteral nutritional support for bowel fistula closure are:**

1) Increased proportion close without surgical intervention.
2) Reduced average time for closure.

☐☐ **T/F: All enterocutaneous fistula treatment is aided by the use of somatostatin or octreotide. What are theoretical reasons for use of these agents?**

False. Theoretical reasons for use include: 1) more rapid closure interval by reducing high volume secretory rates of pancreatic enzymes and 2) duration of parenteral nutrition and its inherent morbidity is reduced because of more rapid closure rate. The ultimate closure of low volume fistulas is not enhanced by use of these peptides.

☐☐ **A defect in what lining or layer through which any abdominal wall hernia - be it umbilical, hiatal, inguinal or incisional - must extrude is called:**

The "endoabdominal fascia." This is a continuous lining of the abdominal cavity that is given other names when it lies over various muscles such as transversalis (muscle) fascia, psoas (muscle) fascia and so on.

☐☐ **How does gastroschisis in newborns differ from omphalocele?**

1) Gastroschisis is a defect of abdominal wall lateral to umbilicus that results when the abdominal wall has failed to close, whereas omphalocele is a defect in closure of the umbilical ring.
2) No sac is found over the protruded intestines in gastroschisis, whereas an amniotic sac usually lies over the intestines in omphalocele.

☐☐ **Persons with cystic remnants or fibrous bands at the umbilical end of the omphalomesenteric duct are at risk for what problems:**

Acute volvulus and intestinal obstruction. Occasionally, an acute abdomen due to cyst infection may occur.

☐☐ **What is the persistence of the intestinal end of the omphalomesenteric duct called?**

Meckel's diverticulum. This is a true intestinal diverticulum with all intestinal wall layers represented.

❑❑ **Congenital abdominal hernias that are caused by abnormal rotation of the intestine and create obstructive symptoms in adults (usually) have what two anatomic descriptions.**

1) "Right mesocolic" with entrapment of proximal small bowel in mesentery under the right colon.
2) "Left mesocolic" with entrapment of rotated small bowel under the left/sigmoid colon.

ACUTE AND CHRONIC PANCREATITIS

Ramona Lim, M.D. and Jamie S. Barkin, M.D., MACG

❏❏ **What are the most common causes of acute pancreatitis?**

Gallstones and alcohol. Idiopathic acute pancreatitis accounts for 8% to 25% of cases; however, up to two-thirds of these patients may have microlithiasis or Sphincter of Oddi dysfunction identified by inspection of bile and Sphincter of Oddi manometry, respectively. Other causes include hypertriglyceridemia, hypercalcemia, trauma, pancreatic tumors, medications, vasculitis and certain viral and bacterial infections.

❏❏ **T/F: Patients with coexisting alcoholism and cholelithiasis should undergo prophylactic cholecystectomy in order to prevent an episode of acute pancreatitis.**

False. Cholecystectomy has not been shown to prevent recurrent episodes of pancreatitis in patients with coexisting alcoholism. The pancreatitis nearly always follows the course of alcohol-related pancreatitis.

❏❏ **What is the mortality rate of gallstone-associated pancreatitis?**

Twelve percent during the first attack. Mortality tends to decrease with subsequent attacks.

❏❏ **What etiology of acute pancreatitis should be suspected in patients without measurable elevation in serum amylase levels?**

Severe hypertriglyceridemia may result in false-negative serum values of amylase and lipase. While measured serum amylase activity is frequently normal, urinary amylase concentration is markedly elevated. Recurrences may be prevented by treatment aimed at avoiding elevations in serum triglycerides greater than 1000 mg/dL.

❏❏ **Which form of pancreatitis is more commonly associated with hyperparathyroidism, acute or chronic?**

Chronic pancreatitis. Acute pancreatitis accounts for one-third of cases.

❏❏ **T/F: Pregnancy is associated with an increased incidence of acute pancreatitis.**

True. Most episodes occur in the third trimester or the postpartum period. Coexisting cholelithiasis or microlithiasis is present in about 90% of cases. The overall prognosis is good.

❏❏ **What percentage of acute pancreatitis is drug-related?**

Five percent. Drugs that are definitely associated with acute pancreatitis include azathioprine, 6-mercaptopurine, sulfonamides, thiazide diuretics, furosemide, estrogens, tetracyclines, valproic acid, pentamidine, intravenous lipid infusion and L-asparaginase. Other drugs with a less certain association include chlorthalidone, ethacrynic acid, phenformin, nonsteroidal anti-inflammatory agents, nitrofurantoin, methyldopa, corticosteroids, didanosine, ACE inhibitors, 5-ASA compounds, cimetidine, ranitidine, acetaminophen, metronidazole and salicylates.

❏❏ **What compounds have a dose-related effect in drug- and poison-induced pancreatitis?**

Ethyl alcohol, organophosphorus insecticides and intravenous lipid infusions.

❑❑ **What etiologies must be considered in post-transplant patients with acute pancreatitis?**

Secondary hyperparathyroidism, hyperlipidemia, viral infections, vasculitis and immunosuppressive therapy, particularly corticosteroids, azathioprine and L-asparaginase.

❑❑ **What infections cause acute pancreatitis in immunocompetent hosts?**

Overall, infection-associated pancreatitis is uncommon; however, several viruses have been implicated and include mumps, coxsackie and Hepatitis A and B. Bacterial causes include *Mycoplasma*, *Salmonella*, and *Mycobacterium tuberculosis*. Intraductal parasitic infections, particularly ascaris, fasciola and clonorchis, have also been cited.

❑❑ **What are the two most common causes of acute pancreatitis in AIDS patients?**

Drugs and infections. Drugs commonly implicated in these patients include pentamidine, trimethoprim-sulfamethoxazole and didanosine. Cytomegalovirus accounts for the majority of infection-related cases. Other infectious agents implicated include *Cryptococcus neoformans*, *Mycobacterium tuberculosis,* and herpes simplex virus. Disseminated infections with *Mycobacterium avium* complex, *Toxoplasma gondii*, *Pneumocystis carinii, Leishmania* species, and *Candida* species may involve the pancreas but rarely cause clinical symptoms.

❑❑ **What type of trauma may cause acute pancreatitis?**

Blunt, rather than penetrating, trauma may induce pancreatitis and usually involves the body of the pancreas where it is compressed against the spine. In adults, this frequently results from seat belt injury. Trauma is the most common cause of acute pancreatitis in children, frequently resulting from bicycle handle bar injury. Sequela of trauma includes pancreatic duct strictures, which may result in recurrent and chronic pancreatitis.

❑❑ **T/F: A patient with so-called "idiopathic" acute pancreatitis should undergo pancreatic duct imaging.**

True. Approximately 35% to 40% of patients with idiopathic pancreatitis have surgically or endoscopically remediable abnormalities detected by endoscopic retrograde cholangiopancreatography (ERCP). Such conditions include ultrasound-negative choledocholithiasis and cholelithiasis (microlithiasis); choledochoceles; obstruction of pancreatic duct by calculi, strictures, small pseudocysts, annular pancreas or carcinoma; ampullary tumors; Sphincter of Oddi dysfunction; and (more controversial), pancreas divisum. Magnetic resonance cholangiopancreatography (MRCP) is a noninvasive imaging modality which also allows direct visualization of the pancreaticobiliary system without intra-pancreatic ductal contrast medium injection and thus avoids the most frequent complication of ERCP - acute pancreatitis. Preliminary evidence suggests that its diagnostic accuracy in centers with sufficient expertise rivals that of ERCP; however, additional randomized trials and greater experience at the local level are necessary before this noninvasive technique is employed routinely.

❑❑ **What clinical prognostic scoring criteria are used to assess the severity of patients with acute pancreatitis?**

Ranson's criteria and APACHE-II grading systems are used to assess the degree of severity of patients' pancreatitis. Ranson's criteria, used in assessing the severity of ethanol-associated pancreatitis, can only be applied at 48 hours. Fewer than 3 positive signs indicates mild disease with a mortality rate near zero. The mortality rate increases to 10-20% when three to five signs are present and is > 50% with six or more signs. A variant of these criteria is utilized to assess the severity of non-alcohol-related pancreatitis. The APACHE-II scoring system has the advantage of being calculated at the time of admission and is based on a point system depending upon the patient's age, chronic illness and various physiologic variables. It is, however, a cumbersome and clinically impractical system. A score > 8 suggests severe pancreatitis.

❑❑ **T/F: The magnitude of hyperamylasemia correlates with the severity of pancreatitis.**

False. The serum amylase level typically rises 2 to 12 hours after onset of symptoms and slowly declines over 3 to 5 days. Conversely, elevations of serum lipase levels tend to rise later and persist longer. The magnitude of hyperamylasemia has no prognostic value in acute pancreatitis; levels may remain normal in up to 10% of cases of fatal pancreatitis.

❏❏ **What are non-pancreatic sources of hyperamylasemia?**

Diseases of the salivary glands, lungs, fallopian tubes, ovarian cysts, gallbladder and small bowel may result in elevations of serum amylase. In addition, tumors of the colon, lung and ovary may cause hyperamylasemia. Any condition associated with increased small bowel permeability (perforation, infarction, obstruction) or diminished renal clearance of pancreatic enzymes may cause elevations in both amylase and lipase in the absence of clinical pancreatitis.

❏❏ **What is macroamylasemia?**

A condition in which amylase complexes with immunoglobulin A. These large molecules do not undergo glomerular filtration. Therefore, serum amylase activity is increased but urinary amylase levels and the amylase-creatinine clearance ratio are low. Similarly, macrolipasemia, in which lipase is complexed with immunoglobulin A, has also been documented in patients with cirrhosis and non-Hodgkin's lymphoma. Knowledge of these entities may prevent patients with elevated serum amylase or lipase secondary to macroamylasemia and/or macrolipasemia from unnecessary evaluation and treatment for pancreatic disease.

❏❏ **What percentage of patients with acute pancreatitis have pulmonary manifestations?**

Approximately 10% to 20%. Pleural effusions occur commonly, are usually left-sided and are exudative with high fluid amylase levels. Early arterial hypoxemia occurs due to right-to-left shunting from microthrombi of the pulmonary vasculature and adult respiratory distress syndrome occurs in up to 20% of patients with severe acute pancreatitis.

❏❏ **T/F: All acute fluid collections which develop in the course of acute pancreatitis should be drained.**

False. More than half of all peripancreatic fluid collections associated with acute pancreatitis will resolve spontaneously within six weeks. They may occur as a result of sympathetic effusion or extravasated pancreatic exocrine secretions secondary to duct rupture. Intervention may be considered when the collection persists beyond six weeks after the onset of pancreatitis and results in symptoms or complications resulting from mass effect or infection.

❏❏ **In what percentage of patients with acute pancreatitis do pancreatic pseudocysts develop?**

Approximately 15%. Pseudocysts do not have a true epithelial lining but are instead surrounded by granulation tissue and collagen. Eighty-five percent are located in the body or tail and 15% in the head of the pancreas.

❏❏ **T/F: A CT scan should always be obtained in a patient with acute pancreatitis.**

False. A CT scan with rapid bolus intravenous contrast should be obtained whenever severe pancreatitis is clinically suspected based upon: 1) failure of the patient to improve clinically, 2) presence of organ failure or 3) suspicion of infected necrosis with fever or leukocytosis. It is not possible to clinically distinguish sterile necrosis from infected necrosis.

❏❏ **What is the significance of pancreatic necrosis identified by an abdominal CT scan?**

The presence of pancreatic necrosis portends a more unfavorable outcome. Areas of pancreatic necrosis fail to enhance during CT scanning after rapid bolus injection of contrast material. The diagnosis of pancreatic necrosis is established when there are focal or diffuse zones of nonenhanced pancreatic parenchyma > 3 cm or involving > 30% of the pancreas. Patients with pancreatic necrosis have a 30% to 50% chance of developing infection of the necrosis; more necrosis worsens the prognosis. CT scan findings are generally not helpful in differentiating sterile from infected necrosis, although the presence of gas bubbles is suggestive of infected necrosis. CT-guided needle aspiration with Gram stain and culture of the aspirate allows diagnosis of suspected infected necrosis.

❑❑ What are causes of early mortality in acute pancreatitis?

Cardiovascular collapse mediated by circulating vasoactive kinins, adult respiratory distress syndrome, intraabdominal hemorrhage, acute renal failure and acute cholangitis account for early mortality in acute pancreatitis. When acute renal failure occurs in the setting of prolonged hypovolemia and shock, acute tubular necrosis ensues and the mortality rate approaches 50%.

❑❑ What are causes of late mortality in acute pancreatitis?

Septic complications, particularly infected pancreatic necrosis and abscess formation, and pneumonitis tend to occur after the first week of illness.

❑❑ What is the mortality rate of patients with pancreatitis who develop infected pancreatic necrosis?

Thirty-eight percent compared with 9% of patients with sterile necrosis. Blood cultures are neither sensitive for isolation of responsible microorganisms nor specific for site of infection. Sonographic or CT-guided percutaneous aspirates of suspected areas of necrosis are the procedures of choice when infected necrosis is suspected.

❑❑ What is the most common organism isolated in infected pancreatic necrosis?

E. coli is isolated in 51% of percutaneous aspirates. Gram stain or culture of these pancreatic aspirates may identify a single microorganism or a polymicrobial infection. Other common infections result from *Enterococcus* (19%), *Staphylococcus* (18%), *Proteus* (10%), *Klebsiella* (10%), *Pseudomonas* (10%), *Streptococcus faecalis* (7%), and *Bacteroides* (6%) species. These organisms likely reach the pancreas by translocation across the colonic wall followed by local lymphatic, rather than hematogenous, spread.

❑❑ T/F: There is a role for prophylactic antibiotics in acute pancreatitis.

True. While indiscriminate use of antibiotics is not advocated, there is evidence that empiric use of imipenem in patients with acute necrotizing pancreatitis may significantly reduce the incidence of septic events.

❑❑ What other organ system complications are associated with acute pancreatitis?

Polyserositis of articular synovium, pleura or pericardium may occur. Subcutaneous fat necrosis may cause a skin rash resembling erythema nodosum. Fat necrosis adjacent to synovium may result in arthritis revealing synovial fluid with many leukocytes and high lipase concentration. Evidence of distant fat necrosis, while clinically evident in only 1% of cases of acute pancreatitis, may be seen in up to 10% of patients on autopsy. Purtscher's retinopathy is a rare complication of acute pancreatitis and is manifested by sudden blindness due to occlusion of the posterior retinal artery with aggregated granulocytes.

❑❑ What complications of acute pancreatitis result in acute massive upper gastrointestinal bleeding?

Gastric variceal hemorrhage and hemosuccus pancreaticus. Isolated gastric varices resulting from splenic vein thrombosis may complicate acute pancreatitis. Splenectomy with gastric devascularization is curative. Hemosuccus pancreaticus, a rare event, refers to bleeding via the pancreatic duct into the duodenum. It arises from erosion of a pseudocyst into adjacent vasculature. Selective mesenteric arteriography during active bleeding distinguishes hemosuccus pancreaticus from hemobilia, identifies the source of arterial or venous bleeding and determines if the blood traverses a pancreatic pseudocyst or abscess prior to drainage into the pancreatic duct. Selective arterial embolization during angiography may also control bleeding.

❑❑ **What triad of clinical findings is suggestive of intra-pseudocyst hemorrhage?**

A sudden increase in the size of the pseudocyst, a localized bruit over the pseudocyst and a sudden decrease in hemoglobin and hematocrit without obvious external blood loss.

❑❑ **T/F: Pancreas divisum is associated with an increased incidence of acute recurrent pancreatitis.**

This is controversial. Pancreas divisum is a congenital failure of fusion of the ventral and dorsal pancreatic anlagen and is the most common congenital anatomic variant (5% to 10%) of the human pancreas. The majority of patients are not predisposed to develop pancreatitis. However, it is believed that the combination of pancreas divisum with a small accessory ampullary orifice may lead to pancreatitis.

❑❑ **What is the most common cause of chronic pancreatitis in adults?**

Chronic alcohol abuse accounts for 70% to 80%. The type of alcohol and pattern of drinking have no influence on the risk of developing chronic pancreatitis. It may be influenced by genetic predisposition in the host.

❑❑ **What is tropical pancreatitis?**

A nutritional pancreatitis seen in African and Asian countries resulting from severe protein-calorie malnutrition. It is characterized by hypoalbuminemia, marked emaciation, bilateral parotid gland enlargement and hair and skin changes resembling kwashiorkor. The pathophysiology of this form of chronic pancreatitis is felt to be due to nutritional antioxidant deficiencies (zinc, copper, selenium). Severe chronic calcific pancreatitis with large intraductal stones may develop and diabetes typically occurs several years after the onset of abdominal pain. Nutritional repletion may lead to a return to normal pancreatic exocrine function if instituted before extensive atrophy and fibrosis of the gland.

❑❑ **What genetic factors influence the development of chronic pancreatitis?**

Hereditary pancreatitis, inherited through an autosomal dominant gene of incomplete penetrance, has been described in different areas of the world (New Zealand, United States, Ireland, France). It affects both sexes equally and typically presents as episodes of acute pancreatitis in childhood by age 10 to 12. These patients progress from episodes of acute pancreatitis to chronic pancreatitis and have an increased incidence of pancreatic carcinoma. Mutations of the cystic fibrosis transmembrane conductance regulator (CFTR) gene and mutations in the cationic trypsinogen gene can lead to the development of chronic pancreatitis.

❑❑ **T/F: The diagnosis of chronic pancreatitis may be excluded in patients without abdominal pain.**

False. Although pain is the most common presenting symptom of patients with chronic pancreatitis, it may be absent in up to 15% of patients with alcohol-related chronic pancreatitis and in up to 23% of patients with non-alcoholic chronic pancreatitis.

❑❑ **What specialized test directly measures pancreatic exocrine function?**

In chronic pancreatitis, exocrine secretion is decreased. The secretin stimulation test measures the volume of secretion and the concentration of bicarbonate (collected via aspiration of duodenal contents) in response to injection of secretin. Bicarbonate levels < 50 mEq/L are consistent with the diagnosis of chronic pancreatitis. This test is invasive, requiring duodenal tube insertion for collection of secretions, and has a reported sensitivity of approximately 80% to 90%.

❑❑ **What conditions are associated with a false-positive secretin stimulation test?**

Diabetes mellitus, Billroth II gastrectomy and cirrhosis.

❑❑ **T/F: Steatorrhea is an early symptom of chronic pancreatitis.**

False. Ninety percent of exocrine function is lost before steatorrhea develops. A secretin test may be abnormal when sixty percent of the exocrine function is lost. Patients with so-called early chronic pancreatitis can have symptoms of bloating, abdominal discomfort, abdominal pain, or change in bowel habits when 60% to 90% of the pancreatic function is lost. Thus, early chronic pancreatitis can mimic a wide variety of gastrointestinal disorders.

❑❑ **What indirect tests of pancreatic secretory function are available?**

The bentiromide and pancreolauryl tests are both noninvasive methods of assessing pancreatic secretory function. They lack sensitivity except in patients with advanced chronic pancreatitis, when patients typically have already developed steatorrhea.

❑❑ **T/F: Plain abdominal radiographs are helpful in the diagnosis of chronic pancreatitis.**

True. While plain abdominal radiographs cannot exclude the diagnosis, the presence of focal or diffuse pancreatic calcification (seen in approximately 30% of cases) makes the diagnosis of advanced chronic pancreatitis almost certain and obviates the need for additional testing.

❑❑ **What osseous abnormalities are associated with chronic pancreatitis?**

Approximately 5% of patients demonstrate medullary infarcts or aseptic necrosis of the femoral or humeral head. The long bones of the hands and feet are affected most often. These abnormalities result from medullary fat necrosis during episodes of acute pancreatitis.

❑❑ **When is endoscopic retrograde cholangiopancreatography (ERCP) useful in the diagnosis of chronic pancreatitis?**

Changes of early chronic pancreatitis may not be seen on ERCP. ERCP assesses ductular changes, such as irregularity, dilatation, tortuosity, stenosis and ductal calculi, which occur in advanced chronic pancreatitis. ERCP is also useful in differentiating chronic pancreatitis from pancreatic cancer. Endoscopic ultrasound (EUS) is also capable of diagnosing chronic pancreatitis on the basis of both ductal and parenchymal changes and, thus, may be able to detect chronic pancreatitis earlier.

❑❑ **What is the most common complication of chronic pancreatitis?**

Pseudocysts occur in up to 25% of patients with chronic pancreatitis. In contrast with acute pseudocysts, chronic pseudocysts almost never resolve spontaneously. Hemorrhage into a pseudocyst with subsequent conversion into a pseudoaneurysm is potentially the most serious complication of chronic pancreatitis.

❑❑ **What is pancreatic ascites?**

Pancreatic ascites occurs as a consequence of persistent leakage of pancreatic fluid from a pseudocyst or a disrupted pancreatic duct. Its incidence in chronic pancreatitis is less than 1%, but may occur in up to 15% of patients with pseudocysts. It may be distinguished from ascites secondary to cirrhosis by the finding of high ascitic fluid amylase levels greater than serum levels and high fluid protein or albumin levels.

❑❑ **T/F: The presence of signs of fat-soluble vitamin deficiencies is highly suggestive of chronic pancreatitis.**

False. While the absorption of fat-soluble vitamins (A, D, E, and K) is diminished, marked deficiency is relatively uncommon. The clinical presence of easy bruisability, bone pain and decreased night vision, resulting from deficiencies of vitamins K, D, and A, respectively, is more suggestive of small intestinal disease with malabsorption.

❑❑ **T/F: Patients with chronic pancreatitis are predisposed to nephrolithiasis.**

True. Patients with untreated steatorrhea have high concentrations of long-chain fatty acids in the colon which bind intraluminal calcium and form insoluble calcium soaps. Consequently, less calcium is available to bind to and precipitate unabsorbed dietary oxalate as calcium oxalate and more free oxalate is absorbed and excreted in the urine. Hyperoxaluria and oxalate stone formation may then develop.

❏❏ How should hyperoxaluria be treated in patients with chronic pancreatitis?

Low dietary oxalate intake, low dietary long-chain triglycerides, pancreatic enzyme substitution and increased intake of either calcium (3 g/day) or aluminum in the form of antacids (3.5 g/day).

❏❏ T/F: Patients with chronic pancreatitis may have vitamin B_{12} malabsorption.

True. The probable mechanism is due to competitive binding of cobalamin by cobalamin-binding proteins (usually destroyed by pancreatic proteases). It is correctable with administration of pancreatic enzymes and occurs in 40% of patients with advanced chronic pancreatitis.

❏❏ T/F: Retinopathy may occur in patients with chronic pancreatitis.

True. Nondiabetic peripheral retinopathy may occur due to a deficiency of vitamin A and/or zinc. Diabetic retinopathy and other microvascular complications of diabetes are less common. However, the prevalence of diabetic retinopathy and neuropathy in patients with chronic pancreatitis is comparable to that of patients with idiopathic diabetes mellitus if corrected for the duration of diabetes.

❏❏ What nonsurgical modalities of pain control are available in chronic pancreatitis?

The following are utilized in an escalating order: cessation of alcohol intake, non-narcotic analgesics and celiac plexus block. Pancreatic enzyme supplementation should be utilized in all patients with chronic pancreatitis to correct exocrine insufficiency. Correctable causes of pain, such as the presence of a pseudocyst, duodenal or biliary narrowing and pancreatic ductal stricture/stone, should be sought. Surgery may offer longer-lasting pain control. Lateral pancreaticojejunostomy (modified Puestow) is preferred in patients with ductal obstruction in the head of the pancreas with distal duct dilatation, whereas partial pancreatic resection should be considered in patients without ductal dilatation, so-called small-duct disease or localized distal (tail) disease.

❏❏ How much lipase is necessary in the form of pancreatic enzyme supplementation for treatment of steatorrhea?

Malabsorption does not occur if more than 5% of normal maximal enzyme output is delivered to the duodenum. This requires 28,000 IU of lipase during a 4-hour postprandial period. Pancreatic enzymes are available in two forms: enteric and non-enteric-coated preparations. The advantage of enteric-coated compounds (e.g., Creon and Pancrease as opposed to Viokase) is that they do not dissolve in the stomach and are less susceptible to acid-pepsin inactivation. The non-enteric-coated preparation is preferable for treatment of the pain associated with chronic pancreatitis.

CHOLELITHIASIS AND ASSOCIATED CONDITIONS

Gowri Balachandar, M.D., Atilla Ertan, M.D., Isaac Raijman, M.D.,
and Eugene A. Trowers, M.D., M.P.H.

❑❑ **Seventy percent to 80% of gallbladder stones in the United States are composed of cholesterol. What is the composition of primary common bile duct stones?**

Brown pigment stones. Common bile duct stones are almost always associated with ascending cholangitis and colonization of the bile by enteric organisms.

❑❑ **What diseases are frequently associated with black pigment stone formation?**

Chronic hemolysis and cirrhosis.

❑❑ **What is the prevalence of gallstones in the United States?**

Approximately 10%. Gallstones are two to three times more common in women than men. Pima Indians are at highest risk of developing gallstones in the United States. A genetic influence is noted in gallstone formation. Pigment stones account for 10% to 25% of all gallstones in the United States.

❑❑ **Distal ileal diseases are recognized risk factors for the development of gallstones. What is the most common problem resulting in lithogenic bile in these diseases?**

The loss of specific bile acid receptors in the distal ileum results in excessive bile salt excretion and a diminished bile acid pool.

❑❑ **Ursodeoxycholic acid (UDCA) is a tertiary bile acid. What is the percentage of UDCA in the human bile acid pool?**

The percentage of UDCA in the human bile acid pool is 2% to 4%. The bile acid pool becomes enriched (up to 40%) with UDCA conjugates during UDCA treatment; however, there is little change in total bile acid secretion.

❑❑ **Describe the pathophysiogical mechanism(s) resulting in gallstone formation in the following groups: the elderly, the obese, the pregnant, those receiving clofibrate, and those receiving parenteral nutrition.**

Elderly – increased biliary cholesterol saturation.
Obese – increased 3-hydroxy-3-methyl glutaryl-CoA reductase activity.
Pregnant – increased biliary cholesterol saturation and impaired gallbladder motility.
Clofibrate therapy – decreased 7-alpha-hydroxylase activity with decreased bile salt production.
Parenteral nutrition – gallbladder stasis.

❑❑ **What are common conditions associated with the development of gallbladder sludge?**

Spinal cord injuries, prolonged parenteral nutrition and fasting and prolonged treatment with octreotide may cause gallbladder stasis-induced gallbladder sludge. Ceftriaxone may also result in the formation of sludge. Gallbladder sludge may cause acute cholecystitis and acute pancreatitis.

❑❑ **What is the rate of development of biliary pain per year in patients with previously asymptomatic gallstones?**

Two percent per year for five years in one study from Michigan. A recent Italian study reported rates of 12%, 17% and 20% at 2, 4 and 10 years, respectively. Therefore, prophylactic cholecystectomy is not indicated in an otherwise healthy person with asymptomatic gallstones.

❑❑ **What patients with asymptomatic gallstones would you recommend prophylactic cholecystectomy?**

Patients awaiting lung transplantation, patients with porcelain gallbladder and young women of American Indian ancestry. The last two conditions are associated with a high prevalence of gallbladder carcinoma.

❑❑ **What is the overall sensitivity of abdominal ultrasonography for the detection of gallstones?**

The overall sensitivity of abdominal ultrasonography is 95% for stones that are larger than 2 mm in diameter. In contrast, the sensitivity is only approximately 50% for common bile duct stones.

❑❑ **What is Mirizzi's syndrome?**

Mirizzi's syndrome is a rare complication of gallstones in which a stone becomes impacted in the neck of gallbladder or the cystic duct and extrinsically compresses the common bile duct resulting in jaundice. Preoperative diagnosis of this syndrome is important in order to avoid bile duct injury. This syndrome is rare, occurring in approximately 1% of all patients undergoing cholecystectomy.

❑❑ **What is the most common location of a bowel obstruction in patients with gallstone ileus?**

Characteristically, the obstruction occurs in the distal ileum where the lumen is the narrowest. The majority of patients with gallstone ileus are women and older than 70 years. Recurrent gallstone ileus may occur in approximately 5% of patients and a search should be made for an additional stone(s) during surgery.

❑❑ **Acalculous cholecystitis may occur in patients, especially the elderly and those with AIDS, with serious injury or illness and after major complicated surgeries. What is the cause of acalculous cholecystitis?**

The etiology of acalculous cholecystitis is unknown but possibilities include biliary/gallbladder stasis resulting from long-standing fasting, alterations in gallbladder flow, especially in elderly patients with peripheral vascular disease, prostaglandins and endotoxins. Gangrene, empyema and perforation of gallbladder more commonly complicate the course of acalculous cholecystitis than acute calculous cholecystitis.

❑❑ **When is cholecystectomy indicated in a patient with a gallbladder polyp?**

Polyps of 10 mm to 18 mm raise the question of cancer arising within an adenoma and should be removed as long as the patient is an acceptable surgical candidate. Open cholecystectomy and consideration of more radical surgery is indicated in patients with gallbladder polypoid lesion(s) larger than 18 mm.

❑❑ **A 56 year-old man presents for evaluation of jaundice. He had been well until three weeks ago when he noticed the onset of mild mid-epigastric pain which resolved spontaneously. His past medical and surgical histories were unremarkable. He reported an 8-pound weight loss which he blamed on a lack of appetite. Examination was notable only for jaundice and icteric conjunctivae. Laboratory tests revealed a total bilirubin of 8.6 mg/dl and an alkaline phosphatase of 565 IU/L. Aminotransferases were only slightly elevated. Amylase and lipase were normal. An abdominal ultrasound demonstrated dilated intra- and extra-hepatic bile ducts. What is the next most appropriate test?**

Endoscopic retrograde cholangiopancreatography. In this case, several gallstones were successfully removed after performing a sphincterotomy.

❑❑ **A 42 year-old man with no previous health problems presented to the hospital with a two day history of severe intermittent epigastric pain radiating to his back with associated nausea and** vomiting. He denied alcohol abuse, prior pancreatitis or gallstones. He had lost about 35 pounds over the last four months and attributed the weight loss to intentional dieting and exercise. On examination, he was febrile, jaundiced and tender to palpation over the epigastrium. Laboratory testing revealed a leukocyte count of 19,000 with a left shift, alkaline phosphatase of 650 IU/L, bilirubin of 4.8 mg/dl and amylase of 2,500 IU/L. An abdominal ultrasound showed some 'sludge' in the gallbladder but was otherwise normal. What is the most appropriate therapy for this patient?

Endoscopic retrograde cholangiography with sphincterotomy and stone extraction are most appropriate in the setting of acute gallstone-related cholangitis and severe pancreatitis. If he was hemodynamically unstable or had a concomitant coagulopathy, a nasobiliary stent could be placed to decrease the duration of the procedure and obviate the need for sphincterotomy, at least temporarily. Of course, intravenous antibiotics and other supportive measures are also necessary.

❑❑ **T/F: Prophylactic cholecystectomy is recommended in the management of asymptomatic cholelithiasis.**

False. Since almost all patients with cholelithiasis develop symptoms before they develop complications, there is no evidence to support prophylactic treatment in the management of asymptomatic gallstones. Two-thirds of patients with gallstones are asymptomatic. The annual rate of conversion from asymptomatic to symptomatic disease with biliary pain is only 1% to 4%. Patients with symptoms of gallstone disease have a 50% risk/year to reexperience biliary colic and their annual rate to develop biliary complications of 1% to 2%.

❑❑ **What are the exceptions to the above practice?**

Exceptions are a calcified gallbladder, children with gallstones, patients with sickle cell disease, the morbidly obese and American Indians. The risk of malignancy in calcified gallbladders exceeds 25%.

❑❑ **What ethnic group might benefit from prophylactic cholecystectomy for asymptomatic gallstones?**

American Indians appear to have rate of gallstone-associated gallbladder cancer that is sufficiently high to justify prophylactic cholecystectomy.

❑❑ **T/F: Prophylactic cholecystectomy is justified in diabetics.**

False. Diabetics seem to be prone to developing both gallstones and gallstone-related complications. It has been suggested that diabetics have a high morbidity and mortality when undergoing emergency operations for gallstones. However, these perceptions have not been borne out when confounding variables such as hyperlipidemia, obesity, cardiovascular disease and renal insufficiency are taken into account.

❑❑ **In the era of laparoscopic cholecystectomy, what are the indications for conventional open cholecystectomy?**

Open cholecystectomy should be reserved to patients with suspected cancer of the gallbladder, cases of severe acute or chronic inflammation, liver cirrhosis with portal hypertension, pregnancy, severe upper abdominal adhesions following previous surgery and in patients with biliary disease.

❑❑ **What are absolute contraindications to laparoscopic cholecystectomy?**

Inability to tolerate general anesthesia, uncontrolled coagulopathy, suspected cancer of the gallbladder, liver cirrhosis with portal hypertension and cholecystoenteric fistulas.

❑❑ **What are some relative contraindications to laparoscopic cholecystectomy?**

Morbid obesity, cardiopulmonary diseases, Mirizzi's syndrome, empyema of the gallbladder, a contracted gallbladder, pregnancy, severe acute or chronic inflammation of the gallbladder and patients who have previously undergone upper abdominal surgery.

❑❑ What is the role of percutaneous cholecystolithotomy?

This technique is being increasingly used in elderly and high-risk patients unsuitable for laparoscopic cholecystectomy. It is successful in achieving stone clearance but is associated with a high incidence of recurrent stone formation.

❑❑ If at laparoscopy, one unexpectedly encounters an acutely inflamed pus-filled gallbladder with multiple adhesions such that the anatomy around the porta hepatis is obscured and cholecystectomy is deemed unsafe, what therapeutic laparoscopic procedure could be done?

The fundus of the gallbladder is exposed, a trocar is inserted into the gallbladder and the contents aspirated. A drainage catheter can then be inserted into the gallbladder and the operation concluded.

❑❑ Hepatic cirrhosis is a major risk factor of morbidity and mortality in patients undergoing elective cholecystectomy. What are the major peri-operative causes of death associated with this condition?

The two major causes of death associated with this condition are intra-operative bleeding and post-operative hepatic failure.

❑❑ What conditions justify cholecystectomy in cirrhotics?

Symptoms are severe or the cirrhosis is well-compensated.

❑❑ What is the most common cause of death after cholecystectomy?

Most death occurring after cholecystectomy is related to cardiac disease, particularly myocardial infarction.

❑❑ T/F: The presence of acute cholecystitis is a contraindication to laparoscopic cholecystectomy.

False.

❑❑ What are the complications of laparoscopic cholecystectomy performed for acute cholecystitis?

The main intraoperative complications are perforation of the gallbladder, bleeding from the liver bed or cystic artery and iatrogenic injuries to the bowel or vessels due to unclear anatomy. The main postoperative complications are local wound hematoma or infection and systemic hematoma.

❑❑ What are sites of bile duct leaks after cholecystectomy?

Bile leaks can occur from the main duct, the cystic duct remnant (most common), a gallbladder leak due to trauma to a duct during dissection of the gallbladder from the liver, clipping of the right hepatic duct proximally leaving the hepatic end free to drain and damage to the duct of Luschka.

❑❑ Some patients undergoing laparoscopic cholecystectomy may have common bile duct (CBD) stones that may not be suspected at the time of the procedure. What is the natural history of these unsuspected CBD stones?

Unsuspected common bile duct stones are detected in 1.2% to 14% of patients undergoing cholecystectomy. A number of reports have documented the spontaneous passage of CBD stones into the duodenum. Only 0.5% to 0.8% of patients undergoing laparoscopic cholecystectomy will subsequently return with problems due to unsuspected CBD stones. These patients can easily be managed by endoscopic retrograde cholangiography.

❑❑ In a patient with a recent bile duct injury, what is the role of abdominal ultrasound?

Abdominal ultrasonography may demonstrate dilated intra/extrahepatic ducts, fluid collections or abscesses in the perihepatic region. It may also be helpful in suggesting changes of cirrhosis, splenomegaly and portal hypertension, which are particularly important considerations in planning an intervention in any such patient.

□□ What are situations in which the bile duct size is normal in a patient with bile duct injury?

Presence of a biliary fistula, long-standing partial obstruction with biliary fibrosis and cirrhosis.

□□ What is the most important cause of bile duct injury during laparoscopic cholecystectomy?

The most important cause of bile duct injury during laparoscopic cholecystectomy is aberrant biliary anatomy found in about 3% of patients.

□□ Where do biliary fistulae commonly arise after laparoscopic cholecystectomy?

The cystic duct stump.

□□ In some patients, bile duct injury with stricture formation may appear several months after laparoscopic cholecystectomy. What is the management at this time?

Prompt endoscopic dilatation of such strictures may lead to resolution without the need for surgical intervention.

□□ What is the significance of cholecystohepatic ducts?

Cholecystohepatic ducts (duct of Luschka), present in 3% to 5% of cadavers, may be transected during laparoscopic cholecystectomy and are another source of biliary leakage.

□□ What factors prevent spontaneous closure of postoperative biliary leaks?

Most postoperative biliary leaks heal spontaneously. The presence of distal biliary obstruction secondary to a stone or stricture contributes to the formation of leaks and bilomas and prevents spontaneous closure.

□□ T/F: Endoscopic retrograde cholangiography (ERC) should be performed routinely prior to laparoscopic cholecystectomy.

False. When comparing the low yield of detecting anatomic variants (3%) and clinically unsuspected stones (3.9%) versus a generally accepted 3% to 7% complication rate of ERC, the routine use of ERC prior to laparoscopic cholecystectomy is not necessary.

□□ In what situations should preoperative ERC be considered prior to cholecystectomy?

ERC should be considered preoperatively in patients with severe gallstone pancreatitis or acute cholangitis, in those having a high probability of having common bile duct stones or when there is a significant possibility of other pathology.

□□ What is the false positive rate of detecting common bile duct (CBD) stones with intraoperative cholangiogram?

3% to 4%.

□□ What factors predict the presence of CBD stones?

Four independent predictors of common bile duct stones are 1) Age greater than 55 years, 2) Elevated bilirubin over 1.7mg/dl, 3) Dilated CBD (> 6 mm) on ultrasonography, and 4) Suspected or detected common bile duct stone on ultrasonography.

□□ What is the probability of finding common bile duct stones using this four-predictor model?

The probability of finding a common bile duct stone using this four-predictor model ranges from 18% (no predictors present) to 94% (all four predictors present). When tested prospectively in patients suspected of having common bile duct stones, this model demonstrated that CBD stones were present in only 8% with none of the four predictors compared to 66% with two or more.

❏❏ **As independent parameters, which of these predictors has the highest positive predictive value?**

As independent parameters, increased bile duct diameter or presence of stones on ultrasonography had the highest positive predictive value for detecting a common bile duct stone (64% and 78%, respectively).

❏❏ **T/F: A recent history of pancreatitis correlates strongly with the presence of common bile duct stones.**

False. Except in cases of severe or persistent pancreatitis. In a recent study, common bile duct stones were present more frequently in groups with severe (63%) pancreatitis compared to the mild group (26%).

❏❏ **What is the best approach to take in patients with severe gallstone pancreatitis?**

Early cholecystectomy with common bile duct exploration is not the best approach in the setting of severe gallstone pancreatitis due to high morbidity and mortality. ERCP with sphincterotomy is the therapy of choice in this situation.

❏❏ **In a patient who has gallstone pancreatitis, when should cholecystectomy be performed?**

Cholecystecomy may be performed during the same hospitalization once the clinical signs of pancreatitis have resolved.

❏❏ **What should be done if small, unsuspected stones are visualized in the common bile duct during intraoperative cholangiography?**

Nothing. It is believed that most small stones will pass spontaneously without symptoms or complications. It is estimated that only 10% of small, unsuspected stones will become symptomatic. If they become symptomatic, ERC and endoscopic sphincterotomy with stone extraction can be performed.

❏❏ **T/F: An endoscopic approach is most useful to treat biliary fistulae.**

True. A 90% to 100% success rate is reported in treating biliary leaks with endoscopic management. Sphincterotomy alone, stent/nasobiliary catheter placement or the combination of sphincterotomy and stent placement have been used successfully to reduce the intrabiliary pressure and allow fistula healing.

❏❏ **T/F: The finding of a localized fluid collection or ascites in a patient who has recently undergone a laparoscopic cholecystectomy requires immediate surgical intervention.**

False. Postoperative ascites and edema of the gallbladder fossa on CT scan or ultrasonography is a normal postoperative change and has been reported in 19% and 22% of patients, respectively.

❏❏ **What non-invasive test is most useful in detecting post-cholecystectomy bile leaks?**

Hepatobiliary scintigraphy is highly sensitive and specific.

❏❏ **What confirmatory test(s) should be performed if a biliary leak is found on scintigraphy?**

Cholangiography, via an endoscopic or percutaneous approach, will usually confirm the presence of a leak, detect coexistent biliary strictures or retained stones and allow for the appropriate therapeutic procedure.

❏❏ **T/F: A CT scan can differentiate between the various types of fluid collections.**

False. CT scans have limited ability to differentiate bile from blood, ascites, pus or lymph.

❑❑ **What is the best approach to take in a patient who has a postcholecystectomy bile duct injury and presents with biliary peritonitis?**

This is usually caused by infected bile. External percutaneous drainage is the best initial approach. Definitive repair of the lesion can be done after the infection has been treated.

❑❑ **What is the first-line of investigation in a patient who presents early after laparoscopic cholecystectomy with jaundice?**

Endoscopic retrograde cholangiography.

❑❑ **In a patient with a bile duct injury following cholecystectomy, what is the procedure of choice if the distal CBD is found to be occluded by ERCP?**

If the distal duct is found to be occluded or transected and continuity to the proximal duct is lost, percutaneous transhepatic cholangiography (PTC) is necessary to outline the proximal ducts and to provide external biliary drainage. Surgery will eventually be necessary.

❑❑ **What is the classification of bile duct injuries?**

Type A - Injuries to minor ducts without loss of continuity of biliary tree
Type B - Injuries to aberrant right hepatic bile duct with duct occlusion
Type C - Injuries to aberrant right hepatic bile duct with transection
Type D - Lateral injuries that involve the main ducts and can progress to Type E injuries
Type E - Injuries to the main duct with complete obstruction

❑❑ **What are presenting symptoms in patients who have Type A injuries?**

Sixty-six percent of these patients present with a symptom complex of pain and fever. In about 33% of these cases, the presentation is that of an external bile fistula. Patients with Type A injuries are almost never jaundiced.

❑❑ **What is the optimal approach to take in patients who present in the early post-cholecystectomy period with abdominal distension suspicious of biliary leak?**

A CT scan or ultrasonography of the abdomen is used to search for intraperitoneal fluid. If a bile collection is present, it may be drained percutaneously. Biliary scintigraphy is then done to determine if a leak persists followed by therapeutic ERC if a leak is found.

❑❑ **What is the treatment of choice for Type E injuries?**

Roux-en-Y hepaticojejunostomy.

❑❑ **In a patient with suspected gallstones but atypical symptoms, what are the most appropriate initial investigative procedures?**

Endoscopy and/or UGI contrast radiography is performed to exclude disorders such as esophagitis or peptic ulcer disease.

❑❑ **Patients may have a variety of postoperative symptoms following cholecystectomy. In what group is investigation most likely to reveal a cause?**

Common postoperative symptoms include flatulence, bloating and right upper quadrant and epigastric pain. A small percentage present with severe abdominal pain, jaundice or emesis. Investigation in the latter group is more likely to reveal a distinct treatable cause.

❑❑ **What are the common clinical presentations of gallstone disease during pregnancy?**

Worsening biliary colic and acute cholecystitis are the most common clinical presentations. Jaundice and acute pancreatitis as a result of choledocholithiasis are rare.

❐❐ **T/F: Pregnancy is a contraindication to laparoscopic cholecystectomy.**

False. Improvements in anesthesia and tocolytic agents have made cholecystectomy safer during pregnancy. Complications such as spontaneous abortion and preterm labor are more common in operated women in the first and third trimesters of gestation, respectively. Laparoscopic cholecystectomy can be performed safely in a carefully controlled clinical setting.

❐❐ **What are the two types of Mirizzi's syndrome?**

Type I - The hepatic duct is compressed by a large stone that has become impacted in the cystic duct or Hartmann's pouch. Associated inflammation may contribute to the stricture.
Type II - The calculus has eroded into the hepatic duct, producing a cholecystocholedochal fistula.

❐❐ **What is the importance of recognition of the presence of Mirizzi's syndrome?**

Recognition of this syndrome is important during difficult cholecystectomy to reduce the likelihood of hepatic duct injury.

❐❐ **What is the ultrasound picture in Mirizzi's syndrome?**

Ultrasound reveals gallstones with a contracted gallbladder and moderate intrahepatic ductal dilatation.

❐❐ **What are the x-ray findings in gallstone ileus?**

An intestinal gas pattern compatible with intestinal obstruction in most patients; pneumobilia in half of all patients; and, a visible aberrant gallstone in a minority.

❐❐ **What is the size of the gallstone that causes gallstone ileus?**

Usually > 2.5 cm in diameter.

❐❐ **How does gallstone ileus present?**

Gallstone ileus should always be considered in an older patient with intestinal obstruction. It sometimes has a prior history of acute cholecystitis, but most of the stones erode slowly through the gallbladder and the symptoms may be minimal, especially in the elderly.

❐❐ **What are the characteristics of small bowel obstruction in gallstone ileus?**

As the gallstone progresses down the length of the gut, it intermittently obstructs the lumen. Characteristically, complete obstruction occurs in the ileum, where the lumen is the narrowest.

❐❐ **What happens when the gallbladder perforates into the adjacent intestine during an acute attack of cholecystitis?**

The acute attack often subsides as the inflamed organ is decompressed. If the gallstones are completely discharged and are small enough to pass rectally, an uncomplicated cholecystoenteric fistula results. However, if stones are still present in the gallbladder or common bile duct, chronic symptoms may arise.

❐❐ **What are the most common sites of cholecystoenteric fistula?**

In descending order of frequency, the duodenum, hepatic flexure of the colon, stomach and jejunum.

❐❐ **What investigations are useful for diagnosing cholecystoenteric fistula?**

Plain abdominal x-rays may show air in the biliary tree. Barium studies often reveal the site of communication. The gallbladder does not opacify on oral cholecystography. Ultrasonography of the gallbladder can detect air in the biliary tree but not the site of the fistula. CT scans are less useful in detecting gallstones and fistulae; although, they may show air in the biliary tree.

❒❒ **What problems can be caused by a cystic duct remnant in a patient who has undergone cholecystectomy?**

In some patients, the cause of postcholecystectomy symptoms has been attributed to pathology in the cystic duct remnant. The described abnormalities include cystic duct stones, fistulae, granulomas or neuromas. ERC is useful in delineating biliary anatomy in patients with suspected cystic duct remnant pathology. Treatment is cystic duct excision.

❒❒ **What tests should be performed in a patient with postcholecystectomy symptoms?**

Common bile duct stones are the most common cause of postcholecystectomy symptoms. Liver function tests, particularly alkaline phosphatase, may be elevated. Ultrasonography may reveal indirect signs, such as a dilated bile duct, but direct visualization of the stone is uncommon. ERC is an important diagnostic tool with which to confirm the presence of ductal stones and exclude the presence of bile duct stricture or tumor.

❒❒ **What other biliary cause of postcholecystectomy symptoms should be considered when common bile duct stones and cystic duct pathology have been ruled out?**

Sphincter of Oddi dysfunction.

❒❒ **Name three patterns of presentation in bile duct injury?**

Complete occlusion of the bile duct with rapid development of jaundice in the postoperative period; bile peritonitis; and, partial duct obstruction with intermittent episodes of pain, jaundice or cholangitis usually within 2 years of the cholecystectomy

❒❒ **What is the differential diagnoses of cholangitis in a patient with a history of cholecystectomy?**

Bile duct stricture and choledocholithiasis.

❒❒ **When is surgery recommended for benign biliary strictures?**

Complete ductal transection, failed previous repair and failure of endoscopic therapy.

❒❒ **T/F: It is possible to differentiate between choledocholithiasis and bile duct stricture on the basis of symptoms.**

False.

❒❒ **What radiologic evaluations should be considered in a patient with a suspected bile duct stricture?**

The evaluation should begin with ultrasonography to identify dilated ducts and/or a subhepatic fluid collection. In the early postoperative period, a ^{99m}Tc-labeled radionuclide scan may expeditiously and noninvasively demonstrate patency of the biliary tree and exclude bile leak. If these studies suggest bile duct injury, ERC is indicated to define and possibly treat the lesion.

❒❒ **If laparoscopic bile duct injury is suspected, what is the earliest time when an ERCP can be done?**

If a biliary fistula is suspected immediately following laparoscopic cholecystectomy, diagnostic and therapeutic ERC can be performed as little as 6 hours postoperatively.

❑❑ **How is an intrahepatic bile leak treated?**

These can be treated with short stents positioned below the leak.

❑❑ **What are characteristics of biliary type pain?**

Biliary pain is not colicky but rather a steady right upper quadrant or epigastric pain. The duration of pain is commonly 1 to 5 hours and is usually nocturnal. A postprandial association is also uncommon. Biliary pain is usually relieved by narcotics and the majority of patients experience pain at a clock-time that is characteristic for each patient.

❑❑ **What are consequences of stricture development following injury to the bile duct due to laparoscopic cholecystectomy?**

Cholangitis, biliary cirrhosis and eventual liver transplantation.

❑❑ **What options are available for removal of common bile duct stones if preoperative ERC fails?**

If the stones are small and the laparoscopic surgeon is skilled in laparoscopic bile duct exploration, an attempt at this treatment procedure is made. If it is not successful or large stones are found, an open bile duct exploration is the treatment of choice.

❑❑ **What is the approach to a patient with acute suppurative cholangitis?**

These patients have a very high mortality rate (10% to 50%) when operated on emergently. Emergency endoscopic decompression has a lower morbidity and mortality than either emergent percutaneous or surgical decompression. The decision to perform endoscopic sphincterotomy or place a stent or nasobiliary drain depends on the severity of the patients clinical condition at the time of the procedure.

❑❑ **What aberrant anatomy of the hepatic duct can lead to its misidentification as the cystic duct?**

In 20% of cases, the right anterior and right posterior hepatic ducts do not join to form the right hepatic duct (RHD). Instead, the right posterior hepatic duct (RPHD) joins the left hepatic duct proximally, and the right anterior hepatic duct (RAHD) joins it distally. In this situation, the RPHD is misinterpreted as the RHD and the RAHD as an accessory duct. In addition, the RAHD can also be confused with the cystic duct and divided during cholecystectomy.

❑❑ **In cases of laparoscopic bile duct injuries, what factor is associated with the best long-term results?**

Immediate identification with immediate repair is associated with the best long-term results. Unfortunately, in one recent study, only 10% of ductal injuries were discovered and operated on in the first week. The vast majority (70%) were diagnosed within the first 6 months.

❑❑ **What is the best initial approach to take in patients with bile duct injuries and biliary peritonitis?**

Biliary peritonitis is usually caused by infected bile. Percutaneous drainage is the best initial strategy. Definitive repair of the lesion can be done when the infection is treated.

❑❑ **What conditions make endoscopic removal of common bile duct stones difficult or impossible?**

Anatomical considerations such as previous upper gastrointestinal surgery or a large-sized calculus reduce the success of endoscopic extraction by most endoscopists.

❑❑ **T/F: Management of an elderly frail patient with ductal calculi and severe gallstone pancreatitis differs from a young healthy patient.**

False. ERCP and sphincterotomy can be safely performed in the elderly. However, following sphincterotomy and successful stone extraction, some reports suggest that frail elderly patients can be successfully managed without a cholecystectomy.

❐❐ In a patient with a recurrent bile duct stricture in whom a repeat attempt at operative bypass has failed or seems unwise, what option is available?

Consideration may be given to balloon dilation or possibly placement of metal stent across the stricture.

❐❐ How long should a stent remain in place in a patient with a biliary fistula and concomitant stricture?

Biliary fistulas associated with bile duct strictures will require long-term stenting, preferably with large bore stents (10- or 11.5-French stents). These patients will need one or two 10-Fr stents placed with interval changes every 3 months for a mean of 10 months.

❐❐ If a patient has an external biliary fistula, what test should be done first?

Fistulogram.

❐❐ In what situation is the best result achieved when stenting a biliary stricture?

If the stenotic segment is short (less than 1 cm) or if the stenosis is partial.

❐❐ What is the usual closure time of biliary leaks in the absence of stricture?

The majority of biliary leaks (not associated with stricture) close within 7 to 10 days after ablation of the biliary sphincter or stent placement.

❐❐ What are advantages and disadvantages of nasobiliary drainage?

Advantages include the ability to repeat cholangiography and to remove it without the need of a second ERCP. The risk of infection when improperly cared for, poor patient acceptance and discomfort and potential for electrolyte disturbances from external drainage of bile have been cited as disadvantages of this approach.

❐❐ What is the sump syndrome?

The sump syndrome is a complication of choledochoduodenostomy in which food debris accumulates in the bypassed segment of the native biliary tree. Recurrent episodes of pain or cholangitis may occur. These episodes may effectively be treated by endoscopic sphincterotomy of the native ampulla with removal of the debris.

❐❐ Name three possible mechanisms of benign obstruction at the level of the ampulla?

Inflammation, fibrosis or muscular hypertonicity.

❐❐ T/F: Biliary obstruction due to duodenal diverticula is a common occurrence.

False. One should be wary of attributing biliary obstruction to a duodenal diverticulum. It is much more likely that the diverticulum is innocent and that the jaundice is due to a more usual cause, particularly gallstones.

❐❐ Name two reasons that the common duct is rarely injured by penetrating duodenal ulcers.

1) The pancreas, which intervenes between most of the lower common duct and the duodenum, acts as a protective barrier and 2) Most duodenal ulcers occur within 2 to 3 cm of the pylorus, whereas the common duct meets the duodenum beyond this vulnerable area.

❑❑ **Name the most common benign polyp arising from the mucosa in the periampullary region.**

Mucosal polyp or papillary (villous) adenoma. The tumor is often multilobular or even multicentric and it may be difficult to distinguish from a low-grade carcinoma, even on frozen section examination.

❑❑ **Name five causes of secondary sclerosing cholangitis.**

Operative trauma and ischemia, chronic choledocholithiasis, cholangiocarcinoma, chronic pancreatitis and toxins such as absolute alcohol and formaldehyde.

❑❑ **Besides inflammatory bowel disease, name five chronic systemic diseases associated with sclerosing cholangitis.**

Recurrent pancreatitis, diabetes mellitus, celiac disease, rheumatoid arthritis and sarcoidosis.

❑❑ **In primary sclerosing cholangitis, how often is the pancreatic duct involved?**

10% to 15%.

❑❑ **Name two conditions that can mimic primary sclerosing cholangitis.**

Extrahepatic portal venous obstruction and metastatic cancer of the liver.

❑❑ **T/F: Surgery is indicated for patients with chronic pancreatitis and associated biliary strictures which produce chronic cholestasis.**

True. Surgery is indicated whenever a biliary stricture has produced chronic cholestasis or its complications. Persistent elevation of alkaline phosphastase levels, even with normal bilirubin levels, is a sufficient indication for surgery. If cholestasis is not relieved in this situation, secondary biliary cirrhosis may result.

❑❑ **Describe two possible causes of obstructive jaundice in a patient with annular pancreas.**

1) Recurrent pancreatitis in the head of the gland, causing edema or fibrosis that constricts the bile duct within the pancreas and 2) Fibrosis of the duodenal wall, through which the terminal portion of the bile duct passes.

❑❑ **How frequently do patients with hepatic artery aneurysms present with jaundice?**

Hepatic artery aneurysms, which are situated close to the bile ducts, present with jaundice in 50% of cases.

❑❑ **Jaundice occurs in what percentage of patients with acute cholecystitis without evidence of cystic duct or common bile duct obstruction?**

15%. This may be due to inflammation and swelling of the cystic duct.

❑❑ **What percentage of patients have concomitant gallstones in the gallbladder and the common bile duct?**

15%.

❑❑ **Cholangitis is found in what percentage of patients with malignant strictures?**

10% to 15%.

❑❑ **What is the average time for choledocholithiasis to result in secondary biliary cirrhosis?**

Five years.

❑❑ **What is the appropriate treatment for patients with polycystic liver disease who have cysts near the hilum of the liver causing compression of the bile ducts?**

Decompression or excision of the cysts and removal of any intraluminal debris.

❑❑ **Acalculous cholecystitis accounts for what percentage of gallbladder perforations?**

40%.

❑❑ **Name two anatomic variants leading to the development of common bile duct stones.**

Juxtapapillary diverticula and entry of the cystic duct to the distal CBD.

❑❑ **List three outcomes of gallbladder perforation.**

Localized perforation is most common and leads to a pericholecystic abscess. Next, is free peritonitis followed by cholecystoduodenal or cholecystoenteric fistulae.

❑❑ **What is the preferred treatment for lymphoma patients who present with obstructive jaundice?**

Chemotherapy is the preferred treatment. Local irradiation of the hilus of the liver may be used adjunctively.

❑❑ **When is gallstone dissolution with ursodeoxycholic acid indicated?**

Ursodeoxycholic acid is a naturally occurring bile acid and is occasionally used for dissolution of radiolucent, non-calcific cholesterol gallstones. The stones must not exceed 2 cm in diameter.

❑❑ **What is the recurrence rate of gallstones in patients treated with ursodeoxycholic acid?**

Recurrence is common – approximately 50% recur within a 5-year period. Patients should be monitored for gallstone recurrence by performing ultrasonography every 6 months for the first year. If all stones disappear, the treatment should be discontinued for 1 to 3 months. For recurrences, a second course may be effective.

❑❑ **When is cholecystectomy indicated for patients who fail gallstone dissolution with ursodeoxycholic acid?**

Cholecystectomy is recommended after the second failure.

❑❑ **T/F: Nonvisualization of the gallbladder on hepatic scintigraphy does not indicate pathology.**

False. Most often, nonvisualization of the gallbladder implies the existence of mechanical obstruction related to cholecystitis, cholelithiasis and, less commonly, carcinoma of the gallbladder.

❑❑ **Name the most common cause of ampullary obstruction.**

Stone or stones in the common bile duct.

❑❑ **T/F: A pancreatogram may, on occasion, show obstruction of the bile duct and the pancreatic duct at the same level. This double duct sign is usually due to biliary tract stones.**

False. The double duct sign usually suggests invasive carcinoma.

❑❑ **Name the three main indications for ERCP and sphincterotomy.**

1)   Postoperative residual stone in the common bile duct
2)   Complicated choledocholithatiasis
3)   Sphincter of Oddi dysfunction

❏❏ Name the four most common sites of trauma to the extrahepatic bile ducts.

1) Common bile duct (58.3%)
2) Common hepatic duct (23.6%)
3) Right hepatic duct (5.5%)
4) Left hepatic duct (2.8%)

❏❏ Name the most common presentation and treatment approach for complete blowout rupture of the fundus of the gallbladder.

Progressive early bile ascites requires early laparotomy while laparotomy can be delayed for an early seal of the perforation with delayed rupture.

❏❏ Name the most common presentation and treatment approach for avulsion of the gallbladder from the hepatic fossa.

This usually results in hemoperitoneum requiring an early laparotomy.

❏❏ Name the most common presentation and treatment approach for contusion or incomplete blowout of the gallbladder.

In general, minimal early symptoms occur. Late rupture of an ischemia-weakened fundus should be treated by laparotomy.

CONGENITAL AND STRUCTURAL ABNORMALITIES

John M. Carethers, M.D., Ronnie Fass, M.D., Spencer T. Fung, M.D., Jeffrey Goldstein, M.D., Ashok Shah, M.D. and Eugene F. Tharalson, M.D.

❏❏ **What type of fistula is the most common embryologic developmental anomaly?**

Tracheoesophageal fistula (85% - 90%). In the most common subtype, the upper part of the esophagus ends as a blind sac while the lower part is connected posteriorly to the trachea.

❏❏ **What is the H-type fistula?**

This occurs when the esophagus and the trachea are attached by a short connection, creating an H-type fistula.

❏❏ **What is the most common congenital abnormality associated with esophageal atresia?**

Cardiac abnormality, most commonly patent ductus arteriosus and septal defects.

❏❏ **When considering an operation for congenital tracheoesophageal fistula, what is the most important anatomic information the surgeons need?**

The type of fistula and whether the distance between the upper and lower ends of the esophagus is long (long gap) or closely approximated (short gap).

❏❏ **What is the most common anatomic presentation of esophageal duplication?**

In up to 80% of the cases, it presents as a cyst without luminal connection.

❏❏ **Where in the esophagus are duplication cysts most commonly encountered?**

The most common location is the distal third (60%) followed by the proximal third (23%).

❏❏ **At what age do vascular rings usually become symptomatic?**

Most commonly during infancy and early childhood; although, they may present at any age.

❏❏ **What are the most common vascular rings encountered in the pediatric population?**

Double aortic arches and right sided aortic arch with either patent ductus arteriosus or ligamentum arteriosum.

❏❏ **With what lesion is dysphagia lusoria commonly associated?**

Aberrant right subclavian artery. The artery arises from the left side of the aortic arch and on its course to the right arm compresses the esophagus posteriorly.

❏❏ **How common is an aberrant right subclavian artery in the general population?**

It has been estimated to occur in up to 1% of the population. The vast majority (90%) are asymptomatic.

❏❏ **What are the esophageal A-ring, B-ring and C-ring?**

These are radiographic terms. An A-ring is usually asymptomatic and involves hypertrophied muscle typically 1.5 – 2 cm above the squamocolumnar junction. The B-ring is synonomous with Schatzki's ring and involves only mucosa. A C-ring refers to the indentation on the esophagus created by the diaphragmatic crura.

❑❑ **How common is a Schatzki's ring?**

Unknown, because most of Schatzki's rings are asymptomatic. They are found in up to 14% of routine esophageal barium studies.

❑❑ **What is the relationship between luminal diameter of Schatzki's ring and dysphagia symptoms?**

Patients with Schatzki's ring and esophageal lumen less than 13 mm will almost always experience dysphagia, between 13 – 20 mm may or may not have dysphagia (about 50%) and greater than 20 mm will rarely have dysphagia.

❑❑ **With what lesion is the "steakhouse syndrome" commonly associated?**

Acute dysphagia due to food impaction is commonly associated with a Schatzki's ring.

❑❑ **What pathogenetic mechanisms have been implicated in the formation of Schatzki's ring?**

Pill-induced, gastroesophageal reflux disease and congenital.

❑❑ **What is the best diagnostic test to detect an esophageal ring?**

Barium esophagram. Use of a barium tablet or marshmallow may help even further to identify the ring and to estimate its luminal diameter.

❑❑ **How can a muscular ring be differentiated from Schatzki's ring radiographically?**

On barium swallow, the caliber of the muscular ring varies, and the stenosis may disappear with full distension. The Schatzki's ring does not vary in appearance.

❑❑ **What is the usual histology of a Schatzki's ring?**

As the rings are most often located at the gastroesophageal junction, the upper face usually has squamous epithelium, and the lower face is covered with columnar cells.

❑❑ **What are typical clinical signs of Schatzki's ring?**

Age greater than 40, intermittent and nonprogressive solid dysphagia, worse when eating is hurried.

❑❑ **What percent of patients with Schatzki's ring remain symptom-free after dilation at 1, 2 and 3-years follow-up?**

68%, 35% and 11%, respectively.

❑❑ **Where is the most common location of an esophageal web?**

Esophageal webs can appear anywhere in the esophagus but tend to occur most commonly in the proximal part.

❑❑ **What percentage of patients with dysphagia will be found to have an esophageal web?**

5% to 15%.

❑❑ **What is the Plummer-Vinson or Paterson-Kelly syndrome?**

Esophageal web that is associated with glossitis, iron deficiency anemia and koilonychia.

❑❑ **What types of cancers have been associated with Plummer-Vinson syndrome?**

Pharyngeal and cervical esophageal cancers.

❑❑ **What dermatological diseases have been associated with esophageal webs?**

Cicatricial pemphigoid and epidermolysis bullosa. Other associated skin diseases include Stevens-Johnson syndrome, psoriasis and idiopathic eosinophilic gastroenteritis.

❑❑ **After allogeneic bone marrow transplantation, what complication has been associated with the development of an esophageal web?**

Graft-versus-host disease.

❑❑ **T/F: Esophageal webs have a gender predilection.**

True. They are more common in women.

❑❑ **T/F: Esophageal webs that are associated with iron deficiency improve with iron supplements.**

False. The esophageal webs do not seem to consistently improve with iron therapy.

❑❑ **What esophageal disorders have been associated with webs?**

Inlet patch, Zenker's diverticulum and esophageal duplication cyst.

❑❑ **Which diverticulum is most commonly encountered in the esophagus?**

Zenker's diverticulum, that forms in the posterior midline between the inferior constrictor and the cricopharyngeus muscle (i.e., hypopharyngeal location).

❑❑ **What is the estimated prevalence of Zenker's diverticulum in the general population?**

0.01% to 0.11%.

❑❑ **At what age does a Zenker's diverticulum commonly present?**

Almost half of the cases will present during the seventh to eighth decade of life.

❑❑ **How commonly does squamous cell carcinoma occur in a Zenker's diverticulum?**

It is seen in approximately 0.4% of patients.

❑❑ **What surgical techniques are used to treat a Zenker's diverticulum?**

Diverticulopexy, diverticulectomy and cricopharyngeal myotomy. Endoscopic approaches have been described.

❑❑ **What is the most common cause of midesophageal diverticula?**

Esophageal motor dysfunction resulting in high intra-luminal pressure, outpouching and the formation of pulsion diverticula.

❑❑ **What is a traction diverticulum?**

Midesophageal diverticula were once considered to arise as a result of traction due to paraesophageal inflammation, most commonly from tuberculosis and fungal diseases.

❏❏ **What is the likely cause of an epiphrenic diverticula?**

As with midesophageal diverticula, esophageal motor disorders are believed to be the underlying mechanism for epiphrenic diverticula.

❏❏ **What is the clinical presentation of midesophageal diverticula?**

In most patients, the diverticula are asymptomatic and are incidentally discovered during barium esophagram. In a small number of patients, it can cause dysphagia and chest pain.

❏❏ **What percent of dysphagia cases are due to esophageal diverticula?**

Less than 5%.

❏❏ **What motility abnormalities have been documented in association with epiphrenic diverticula?**

Nutcracker esophagus, diffuse esophageal spasm, hypertensive lower esophageal sphincter, achalasia and non-specific motility disorders.

❏❏ **What is "feline esophagus?"**

Transient transverse folds of the esophagus that can be observed on both upper endoscopy and double contrast barium esophagram. These folds are termed "feline esophagus" due to the resemblance to the cats esophagus.

❏❏ **What are causes of "feline esophagus?"**

This appearance may be seen in asymptomatic patients as a normal variant and in patients with gastroesophageal reflux disease.

❏❏ **What are the clinical characteristics of "ringed esophagus?"**

This rare cause of dysphagia is commonly observed in males and is due to multiple esophageal rings. It has been associated with GERD and asthma.

❏❏ **What is esophageal intramural pseudodiverticulosis?**

Multiple, small (1mm - 3mm), flask shaped outpouching of the esophagus.

❏❏ **What is the pathogenesis of esophageal intramural pseudodiverticulosis?**

Cystic dilations of the esophageal gland ducts.

❏❏ **What infection can be detected in about one third of patients with esophageal intramural pseudodiverticulosis?**

Esophageal candidaiasis.

❏❏ **What esophageal lesion is almost always associated with esophageal intramural pseudodiverticulosis?**

Esophageal stricture located in the upper or mid-esophagus. The pseudodiverticula are often observed distal to the stricture.

❏❏ **What is the incidence of an inlet patch?**

It ranges between 4% to 10%.

❑❑ **What type of gastric mucosa can be found in an inlet patch?**

Gastric corpus or fundic mucosa that can include functional parietal and chief cells.

❑❑ **What complications have been described in association with an inlet patch?**

Uncommonly, proximal esophageal stricture, ulcer and esophageal adenocarcinoma.

❑❑ **What diagnosis should be considered in a newborn with nonbilious vomiting and an abdominal x-ray showing a distended stomach with an absence of air in the bowel?**

Gastric atresia. This condition most commonly affects the antrum and pylorus. The treatment is surgical.

❑❑ **T/F: Congenital hypertrophic pyloric stenosis may first become manifest as an adult.**

True. However, most cases of adult hypertrophic pyloric stenosis probably occur secondary to chronic pyloric ulcer disease, severe gastritis or cancer.

❑❑ **T/F: The therapy of adult and neonatal hypertrophic pyloric stenosis is the same.**

False. In neonates, the procedure of choice is a surgical pyloromyotomy. In adults, surgical resection of the pylorus is generally performed in order to rule out a small focus of cancer within the hypertrophied muscle.

❑❑ **T/F: Gastric duplication occurs more commonly in women.**

True. Most become symptomatic in infancy.

❑❑ **T/F: Gastric duplications are associated with gastric carcinoma.**

True. Surgical excision is the treatment of choice for gastric duplications.

❑❑ **Where are gastric diverticula most commonly located?**

Over 75% are located on the posterior wall within 2 cm of the gastroesophageal junction.

❑❑ **T/F: Most gastric diverticula are acquired and symptomatic.**

False. Most are thought to be congenital and are asymptomatic.

❑❑ **T/F: The histology of the remnant stomach in microgastria is normal.**

True. This condition is usually associated with congenital cardiac abnormalities and most patients die within weeks to months of birth.

❑❑ **What condition during pregnancy is associated with gastric atresia?**

Polyhydramnios.

❑❑ **What congenital gastric tumor contains all three embryonic germ layers?**

Gastric teratoma. These tumors are rarely found in the stomach, occur almost exclusively in males and are usually found extragastrically, near the greater curvature of the stomach.

❑❑ **T/F: Gastric teratomas are usually associated with other congenital abnomalities.**

False. The prognosis of these tumors is good. Surgical excision is the treatment of choice.

❑❑ **What is the difference between true and false diverticula?**

False diverticula do not include the muscularis propria in the sac wall.

❑❑ **T/F: Juxtapapillary diverticula have a strong association with gallstones.**

True. Also known as extraluminal duodenal diverticula or periampullary diverticula, they occur within 2 cm of the ampulla of Vater.

❑❑ **T/F: Intraluminal duodenal diverticula are lined by duodenal mucosa on the inside and outside of the structure.**

True. Also known as a windsock diverticula, this is a single saccular structure which originates in the second portion of the duodenum. They may be connected to the entire circumference or only part of the duodenal wall.

❑❑ **Jejunal diverticula are associated with what disorders?**

They are typically seen in disorders of small intestinal motility such as progressive systemic sclerosis and visceral myopathies and neuropathies.

❑❑ **A Meckel's diverticulum is the remnant of what embryological structure?**

The omphalomesenteric or vitelline duct.

❑❑ **T/F: A Meckel's diverticulum occurs on the mesenteric border of the gut.**

False. It occurs on the antimesenteric border.

❑❑ **T/F: The most common location for Meckel's diverticulum is 10 cm from the ileocecal valve.**

False. Most commonly they are 100 cm from the ileocecal valve.

❑❑ **T/F: The occurrence of and complications resulting from a Meckel's diverticulum is three times more likely in males than females.**

True.

❑❑ **T/F: Heterotopic tissue is present in one-half of all Meckel's diverticula.**

True. The most common types are gastric mucosa, pancreatic tissue or a combination of the two.

❑❑ **T/F: Detection of Meckel's diverticula by technetium-99m radionucleotide scanning is dependent on the presence of gastric mucosa within the diverticula.**

True. Tecnetium-99m is taken up by the ectopic gastric mucosa and may be enhanced by blocking anion secretion from the mucosa with histamine type 2 receptor antagonists.

❑❑ **What is the most common complication of a Meckel's diverticulum in children? In adults?**

In children, usually in infants and those younger than 5, gastrointestinal bleeding occurs most commonly. In adults, intestinal obstruction is more common.

❑❑ **What is the frequency of complications resulting from a Meckel's diverticulum in the adult population?**

Approximately 2%. They include obstruction, bleeding, diverticulitis, perforation and carcinoma.

❏❏ **T/F: Intestinal duplications are hypothesized to develop from aberrant recanalization of the gut during morphogenesis and share the same blood supply with the native intestine.**

True.

❏❏ **T/F: Duplications of the gastrointestinal tract are located on the mesenteric border of the gut.**

True.

❏❏ **T/F: The most common segment of the gut for intestinal duplication is the colon.**

False. The ileum is the most common segment followed by the jejunum.

❏❏ **T/F: Intestinal duplication may range from single cystic structures that do not communicate with the native bowel to tubular structures that share the lumen with the native bowel.**

True.

❏❏ **T/F: Gastric mucosa may line intestinal duplications.**

True.

❏❏ **T/F: Intestinal atresia and occlusion of the gut lumen is a common cause of intestinal obstruction in the neonate.**

True.

❏❏ **Duodenal atresia and stenosis are frequently associated with what congenital abnormalities?**

Esophageal atresia, midgut malrotation, imperforate anus, annular pancreas and Down's syndrome.

❏❏ **T/F: The distribution of gut atresia can range from the esophagus to the rectum.**

True.

❏❏ **What is the incidence of small bowel atresia?**

1 in 3000 to 5000 lives births.

❏❏ **Describe the several types of intestinal atresia.**

Type I	– diaphragm of mucosa and submucosa obstructs the lumen but the bowel wall and mesentery are intact.
Type II	– two blind bowel ends connected by a fibrous cord.
Type IIIA	– two blind bowel ends separated by a mesenteric gap.
Type IIIB	– "apple peel" atresia - proximal small bowel atresia and absence of the distal superior mesenteric artery.
Type IV	– "string of sausages" - multiple atretic regions throughout the small bowel.

❏❏ **Duodenal atresia is thought to develop at what gestational age?**

Recanalization of the intestinal lumen from the solid cord stage occurs at 4 to 8 weeks of gestation.

❏❏ **T/F: Polyhydraminos is frequently associated with gastrointestinal atresia of the distal gut.**

False. Proximal gut atresias are associated with polyhydraminos.

❑❑ **A double-bubble sign on abdominal radiograph or ultrasound in a neonate is classic for what type of intestinal atresia?**

Duodenal atresia.

❑❑ **Common presenting signs of a proximal (duodenal or proximal jejunum) atresia include:**

Jaundice and bilious vomiting. Distal atresias often present with abdominal distension.

❑❑ **What are the two major complications of gut malrotation?**

Volvulus around the vascular pedicle and duodenal obstruction secondary to Ladd bands.

❑❑ **T/F: Ladd bands are peritoneal bands that pass from the cecum across the duodenum to the right upper quadrant or to the duodenum and form after malrotation of the gut.**

True.

❑❑ **Describe the gut anatomy following nonrotation?**

The small intestine (jejunum and ileum) lies on the right side of the abdomen and the colon is entirely on the left. The cecum lies in the left iliac fossa. The small bowel mesentery remains suspended by a narrow pedicle, leaving a high risk for volvulus.

❑❑ **What is reversed rotation of the gut?**

The gut rotates clockwise, instead of the normal 270 degree counterclockwise rotation, resulting in the colon entering the abdominal cavity first. The colon then takes a position posterior to the superior mesenteric artery and the duodenum. The small bowel mesentery passes in front of the transverse colon.

❑❑ **T/F: Less than half of midgut malrotations present in infancy.**

False. Fifty percent to 80% present in infancy.

❑❑ **T/F: Biliary atresia and congenital heart disease are associated with gut malrotation.**

True.

❑❑ **T/F: Omphaloceles are sac-covered abdominal viscera herniating through the umbilical ring.**

True.

❑❑ **T/F: Gastroschisis is a small defect in the abdominal wall usually to the right of the closed umbilical ring through which there is massive evisceration of the intestines with direct exposure to amniotic fluid.**

True.

❑❑ **What is the gestational age when gastroschisis or omphaloceles develop?**

Between the fifth and tenth week of gestation.

❑❑ **What maternal serum level is associated with ventral fetal abdominal wall defects such as omphalocele and gastroschisis?**

An elevated alpha-fetoprotein level.

❏❏ **T/F: Volvulus of the small bowel in the absence of preexisting defects is more common in Africa, the Middle East and India because of the ingestion of bulky foods after periods of fasting.**

True. Volvulus of the small bowel is rare in the United States without preexisting defects.

❏❏ **T/F: Intussusception is one of the most common causes of bowel obstruction in children under the age of 2.**

True.

❏❏ **What is the cause and frequency of a pathologic lead point in pediatric intussusception?**

Most are idiopathic. Approximately 8% - 12% will have a structural abnormality such as a polyp, leiomyoma or lymphoma. Benign lymphoid tissue has also been suggested as a potential lead point.

❏❏ **T/F: Henoch-Schonlein purpura may lead to intususseption.**

True. The vasculitic bowel may result in an intramural hematoma that acts as a lead point for intussusception.

❏❏ **T/F: Small bowel intussusception is a major cause of intestinal obstruction in adults in the Western world.**

False. Approximately 5% of adult intestinal obstructions are caused by intussusception.

❏❏ **What is the frequency of a pathologic lead point in adult intussusception?**

Approximately 90% of adult intussusceptions will have an identifiable cause such as a polyp, tumor, Meckel's diverticulum and celiac disease with flaccid bowel.

❏❏ **T/F: Reduction of an intussusception in a pediatric patient is first attempted by barium enema.**

True. Barium enema is often successful in reducing an intussusception in a child.

❏❏ **T/F: Reduction of an intussusception in an adult is first attempted by barium enema.**

False. Since most adults will have a lead point, surgery in indicated.

❏❏ **What is the most common segment location for intussusception in pediatric populations?**

Ileocolic intussusception is the most common.

❏❏ **T/F: In adults with intussusception, the proper surgical management, in the absence of infarcted or gangrenous bowel, is manual reduction.**

False. Since many lead points in the adult population are malignant, manual reduction is not recommended. Instead, bowel resection of the affected segment is recommended.

❏❏ **What clinical findings may be found in intestinal lymphangiectasia?**

Steatosis, malabsorption, lymphocytopenia, hypogammaglobulinemia, protein-losing enteropathy, chylous ascites, chlyous pleural effusion and peripheral edema.

❏❏ **What medical conditions may lead to secondary lymphangiectasia?**

Abdominal/retroperitoneal carcinoma/lymphoma, retroperitoneal fibrosis, pancreatitis, tuberculosis, Crohn's disease, celiac disease, systemic lupus erythematosis and congestive heart failure.

❑❑ **Congenital lymphangiectasia is also referred to as what?**

Milroy's disease.

❑❑ **T/F: Gastroschisis is a small defect that occurs at the junction of the umbilicus and normal skin.**

True. It requires immediate operation because a membrane does not cover the bowel.

❑❑ **T/F: Long-term morbidity and mortality of gastroschisis are high because of necrotizing enterocolitis, bowel perforation or necrosis and prolonged total parenteral nutrition.**

True.

❑❑ **T/F: Omphaloceles are associated with extraintestinal birth defects whereas gastroschisis is rarely associated with other defects.**

True.

❑❑ **What percentage of Hirschsprung's disease involves the rectosigmoid colon?**

75% to 80%.

❑❑ **A child presents with chronic constipation, abdominal distension, volvulus and perforation. What is the most likely diagnosis?**

Hirschsprung's disease.

❑❑ **T/F: Anorectal manometry typically reveals a normal sphincter profile and an abnormal rectoanal inhibitory reflex in Hirschsprung's disease.**

True.

❑❑ **What cell type is absent in the submucosa and myenteric plexus of patients with Hirschsprung's disease?**

Ganglion cells that migrate from the neural crest region.

❑❑ **What pull-through operations have been used to surgically treat Hirschsprung's disease?**

Swenson technique, Duhamel procedure and Soave procedure.

❑❑ **The colon and the rectum account for what percentage of all gastrointestinal duplications.**

Five percent and 10%, respectively.

❑❑ **T/F: Asymptomatic rectal duplication should undergo surgical resection because of the risk of neoplasia.**

True.

❑❑ **T/F: Malrotation of the colon occurs if the midgut fails to complete the 180 degree counterclockwise rotation as it returns from herniation during the 10th to 12th week gestational period.**

False. It is a 270-degree counterclockwise rotation.

❑❑ **What associated anomalies have been reported in 30% to 60% of patients with malrotation?**

Small bowel atresia, intussusception, Hirschsprung's disease and abdominal wall defects.

❏❏ **An infant presents at one month of age with a proximal small bowel obstruction, volvulus or colonic ischemia. What is the most likely diagnosis?**

Malrotation.

❏❏ **T/F: Operative treatment of malrotation also includes an appendectomy because future diagnosis of appendicitis would be difficult.**

True.

❏❏ **T/F: The midgut volvulus formed by malrotation is reduced by untwisting it in a clockwise rotation.**

False. Reduction is performed in a counterclockwise rotation.

❏❏ **T/F: Imperforate anus occurs in 1:1,000,000 live births.**

False. It occurs in about 1:20,000 live births.

❏❏ **T/F: Congenital abnormalities, such as genitourinary, cardiac and gastrointestinal anomalies are rarely associated with imperforate anus.**

False. These anomalies occur in up to 50% percent of cases.

❏❏ **What are three common chromosomal abnormalities associated with imperforate anus?**

Down's syndrome, trisomy 8 mosaicism and fragile X syndrome.

❏❏ **T/F: Infants with imperforate anus cannot pass meconium at birth.**

True. However, some may have fistulae by which meconium can pass.

❏❏ **T/F: Imperforate anus is classified as either a high or low lesion according to the relation of the rectum to the levator ani muscle.**

True.

❏❏ **T/F: For the complete evaluation of the patient with imperforate anus, an intravenous pyelogram and voiding cystourethrogram are recommended.**

True.

❏❏ **Surgical treatment of high imperforate anus is successful what percentage of time?**

70% to 80%.

❏❏ **What are the prerequisites for volvulus formation?**

A dilated redundant colon and a narrow-based mesocolon.

❏❏ **Common symptoms of volvulus are abdominal pain, obstipation and abdominal distension.**

True.

❏❏ **What percentage of colonic obstructions in the United States are caused by a volvulus?**

Less than 10%.

❑❑ **T/F: A volvulus occurs when a stool-filled segment of bowel twists about its mesentery.**

False. A volvulus occurs when an air-filled segment forms a twist.

❑❑ **T/F: The sigmoid colon is involved in 90% of all the volvuli seen in the United States.**

False. The number is closer to 60%.

❑❑ **What segments of the population are at risk for a volvulus?**

The elderly, institutionalized and neuropsychiatric patients.

❑❑ **What maneuver should be performed to reduce a volvulus in a patient with peritoneal signs?**

Emergency exploratory laparotomy. Without peritonitis, sigmoidoscopy or a barium enema may reduce the volvulus.

❑❑ **What is the recurrence rate of a volvulus after non-operative reduction?**

Greater than 40%.

❑❑ **T/F: Cecal volvulus generally occurs in younger patients.**

True.

❑❑ **What percentage of volvuli involve the cecum?**

Less than 20%.

❑❑ **T/F: A cecal volvulus occurs because of an anomalous fixation of the right colon leading to a freely mobile cecum.**

True.

❑❑ **What are some precipitating factors for a cecal volvulus?**

Pregnancy, adhesions and an obstructing lesion of the left colon.

❑❑ **What percentage of a cecal volvulus involves a full axial twisting of the associated mesentery and its blood vessels?**

90%.

❑❑ **T/F: Colitis cystica profunda is characterized by the presence of submucosal mucus-filled cysts.**

True.

❑❑ **T/F: The rectum is rarely involved in colitis cystica profunda.**

False. Most lesions are found within 12 cm of the anal verge.

❑❑ **T/F: It is rare for patients with colitis cystica profunda to have rectal prolapse.**

False. Rectal prolapse occurs 54% of the time.

❑❑ **T/F: Pneumatosis cystoides intestinalis is characterized by multiple, thin-walled, non-communicating, gas-filled cysts with epithelial lining in the wall of the small or large intestines, or both.**

False. The gas-filled cysts have no epithelial lining.

❑❑ **T/F: Pneumatosis cystoides intestinalis is associated with chronic obstructive pulmonary disease, intestinal obstruction, collagen vascular disease (scleroderma) and iatrogenic conditions such as post-endoscopy or surgery.**

True.

❑❑ **T/F: Pneumatosis intestinalis is one cause of prolonged recurrent asymptomatic pneumoperitoneum.**

True.

❑❑ **A plain radiograph of the abdomen shows linear, curvilinear, or cystic lucencies in the bowel wall. What is the diagnosis?**

Pneumatosis intestinalis.

❑❑ **The amount of hydrogen in the cysts of pneumatosis intestinalis can approach 50% of the gas present.**

True.

❑❑ **What successful treatments have been reported for pneumatosis intestinalis?**

High-flow oxygen breathing, hyperbaric oxygen, antibiotics and surgical resection.

❑❑ **T/F: Surgical treatment has been shown to be curative in most cases of pneumatosis intestinalis.**

False. Surgery is not always successful and more extensive pneumatosis may occur; therefore, surgery is indicated in fulminant cases such as those with a likelihood of bowel necrosis, sepsis and death.

❑❑ **T/F: Malakoplakia is a rare chronic, granulomatous, inflammatory disorder that can affect the genitourinary and gastrointestinal tract.**

True. It can also affect the skin, lung, bone and brain.

❑❑ **What are the most common sites of the large bowel affected by malakoplakia?**

Rectum, descending and sigmoid colon.

❑❑ **What are the peak ages of incidence of malakoplakia?**

The age of incidence is bimodal with a small peak at 13 years of age and a late peak around the age of 57.

❑❑ **Histologic examination of a colonic lesion shows von Hansemann's cells and Michaelis-Gutmann's bodies. What is the diagnosis?**

Malakoplakia.

❑❑ **Name three predisposing conditions associated with malakoplakia.**

Chronic infection with *Escherichia coli*, sarcoidosis and tuberculosis.

❑❑ **T/F: A defect in macrophage phagocytic or digestive activity has been proposed as a mechanism for the pathogenesis of malakoplakia.**

True.

❏❏ **T/F: Congenital abnormalities of the gallbladder are frequently accompanied by congenital abnomalities of the extrahepatic biliary tree.**

True. In general, congenital abnormalities of the gallbladder are rare.

❏❏ **T/F: In common bile duct duplication, one duct usually drains the right lobe of the liver and the other duct drains the left lobe.**

True. These ducts open separately into the duodenum.

❏❏ **Define biliary atresia.**

Obliteration of the intra- or extrahepatic bile ducts. There is some evidence to suggest that the ducts originally were present but were destroyed by an unknown process.

❏❏ **What is the condition called when the liver parencyma contains just a few ducts?**

Intrahepatic biliary hypoplasia. Hypoplasia of the intra- and extrahepatic biliary system is thought to represent an interval stage in the evolution of biliary atresia.

❏❏ **T/F: The gallbladder is usually also involved in extrahepatic biliary atresia.**

True. Usually, only a fibrous remnant remains.

❏❏ **T/F: It is usually apparent at birth when biliary atresia is present.**

False. It usually does not become evident until several weeks after birth.

❏❏ **T/F: Choledochal cysts more commonly occur in men.**

False. These cysts are about four-times more common in women. There is also a higher incidence among Asians.

❏❏ **Describe the three types of choledochal cysts.**

Type 1 – fusiform dilation of the common bile duct.
Type 2 – diverticular outpouching of the common bile duct.
Type 3 – small saccular dilation of the distal common bile duct.

❏❏ **Which type of choledochal cyst is most common?**

Type 1.

❏❏ **What are two theories of pathogenesis of choledochal cysts?**

1) Pancreatic reflux and 2) Distal common bile duct obstruction (presumably, failure of recanalization of the distal bile duct during intrauterine development leads to narrowing of the distal bile duct with proximal dilation).

❏❏ **T/F: Type 1 choledochal cysts may be associated with intrahepatic bile duct dilatation (Caroli's disease).**

True.

❏❏ **What are potential risks of choledochal cysts if left unattended?**

Severe cholangitis and adenocarcinoma (about 10%). Surgical exision is the usual treatment of these cysts, which may become massive in size.

❑❑ **What is a Phrygian cap?**

A congenital deformity of the gallbladder of no clinical significance whereby the fundus of the gallbladder is kinked.

❑❑ **Air in the gallbladder in the setting of acute cholecystitis suggests the development of what clinical entity?**

Cholecystoenteric fistula due to necrosis of the gallbladder wall.

❑❑ **What syndrome produces pseudo-obstruction of the common bile duct?**

In Mirizzi's syndrome, a gallstone impacted in the cystic duct leads to compression and obstruction of the bile duct.

❑❑ **What are the cresent-shaped folds of the cystic duct mucosa that may block passage of stones into the common bile duct?**

Spiral valves of Heister.

❑❑ **Name three congenital defects associated with intrahepatic biliary atresia.**

Congenital rubella, trisomy 17 and 18 and alpha$_1$-antitrypsin deficiency.

❑❑ **What are the two main developmental abnormalities of morphology that account for most pancreatic congenital anomalies?**

Abnormalities of rotation and fusion.

❑❑ **At about what week of gestation does the embryological development of the pancreas first appear?**

About the fourth week of gestation, the pancreas first appears as two diverticula arising from the primitive foregut just distal to the stomach.

❑❑ **What are the names given to the pancreatic ducts that arise from the ventral and dorsal pancreatic buds?**

The ventral duct anastomoses with the dorsal duct to form the main pancreatic duct of Wirsung. The dorsal bud arises directly from the duodenal wall and undergoes varying degrees of atrophy to remain as the accessory duct of Santorini.

❑❑ **What percentage of the population have normal ductal anatomy?**

Approximately 60% to 70%.

❑❑ **What is the embryological cause of pancreas divisum?**

Pancreas divisum results from incomplete fusion of the dorsal and ventral pancreatic ductal systems.

❑❑ **What percentage of patients undergoing endoscopic retrograde cholangiopancreatography (ERCP) are found to have pancreas divisum?**

Pancreas divisum has been reported in up to 7% to 10% of patients undergoing ERCP. The prevalence may be even higher in patients undergoing ERCP for investigations of idiopathic pancreatitis.

❑❑ **What is the clinical presentation of patients with symptomatic pancreas divisum?**

Most patients with pancreas divisum are asymptomatic. Those patients that are symptomatic have symptoms suggestive of acute pancreatitis which is thought to occur secondary to a combination of the anomaly and stenosis of the minor duodenal papilla.

❑❑ At what age do patients with symptomatic pancreas divisum usually present?

The age of presentation varies widely but is most common between the third and forth decades of life.

❑❑ What is the best means of diagnosing pancreas divisum?

Endoscopic retrograde cholangiopancreatography with injection of the main and minor pancreatic ducts demonstrates incomplete fusion of the dorsal and ventral pancreatic ductal systems.

❑❑ What should be the initial therapeutic management of patients with symptomatic recurrent pancreatitis from pancreas divisum?

Therapeutic endoscopic sphincterotomy has been shown to decrease the frequency of recurrent attacks of pancreatitis in pancreas divisum.

❑❑ What is a heterotopic pancreas?

A heterotopic pancreas also known as ectopic or aberrant pancreas is defined as the presence of pancreatic tissue that lacks anatomic and vascular continuity with the main body of the pancreas.

❑❑ Where are the most common locations for ectopic pancreatic tissue?

Seventy percent of the ectopic pancreatic tissue is found in the upper gastrointestinal tract, including the stomach, duodenal and jejunum. However, it has been seen in many other abdominal locations.

❑❑ What is the most common presentation of patients with heterotopic pancreas?

Most cases of heterotopic pancreas are asymptomatic and the condition is generally discovered incidentally during the evaluation of other gastrointestinal disorders.

❑❑ What is the endoscopic appearance of heterotopic pancreatic tissue?

Ectopic pancreas appears as a well-defined dome-shaped defect with central umbilication.

❑❑ What are the histologic findings on endoscopic biopsy of the nodule seen in heterotopic pancreas?

Endoscopic biopsy of the nodule yields only normal gastric mucosa because the pancreatic tissue is submucosal or subserosal in origin.

❑❑ What should be the management of heterotopic pancreatic tissue when discovered?

Incidental lesions should be left alone since long term follow up has not established a relationship between ectopic tissue and symptoms in most patients.

❑❑ What is an annular pancreas?

An annular pancreas is a flat band of pancreatic tissue completely encircling the second portion of the duodenum.

❑❑ What is the clinical presentation of annular pancreas in the pediatric and adult populations?

In the newborn, the lesion is associated with polyhydramnios and typically presents with inability to tolerate feedings. In adults, obstructive symptoms such as nausea and vomiting occur, particularly postprandially.

❑❑ How is a diagnosis of annular pancreas established?

In neonates, a plain abdominal x-ray may reveal a classic "double-bubble" which is diagnostic of duodenal obstruction. In adults and older children, plain x-ray films are unhelpful and other studies such as endoscopic retrograde cholangiopancreatography are necessary to make the diagnosis.

❑❑ What is the management of an annular pancreas?

In newborns and adults, the management is surgical bypass of the obstructing lesion.

❑❑ What conditions are associated with multiple congenital cysts of the pancreas?

Multiple congenital cysts are associated with polycystic disease, cystic fibrosis and Von Hippel-Lindau syndrome.

❑❑ What is the management of a congenital cyst of the pancreas?

Surgical resection or drainage may be required for some patients with symptomatic solitary cysts; however, surgery is not usually necessary or advisable for patients with multiple cysts.

❑❑ What congenital anomalies are associated with annular pancreas?

Duodenal atresia and Down's Syndrome.

DISORDERS OF THE PELVIC FLOOR AND ANORECTUM

Yehuda Ringel, M.D. and William E. Whitehead, Ph.D.

☐☐ **T/F: Hemorrhoidal disease is more frequently associated with constipation than with diarrheal disorders.**

False. Studies suggest that diarrheal disorders are more frequently associated with hemorrhoidal disease.

☐☐ **Describe the classification of internal hemorrhoids according to their clinical severity.**

Internal hemorrhoids are classified according to their degree of protrusion and prolapse.
1) First degree internal hemorrhoids bulge into the anorectal lumen but do not protrude out of the anus.
2) Second degree hemorrhoids prolapse out of the anus with straining or defecation and spontaneously reduce back to their normal position.
3) Third degree hemorrhoids prolapse out of the anus with straining or defecation and require digital reduction.
4) Fourth degree hemorrhoids are irreducible.

☐☐ **Procidentia refers to complete prolapse of the rectum. What are other forms of rectal prolapse?**

Procidentia involves visible protrusion of all the rectal layers through the anus. Two other forms of rectal prolapse are mucosal prolapse in which only the distal rectal mucosa protrude through the anus and occult rectal prolapse which refers to internal intussusception of rectal tissue without visible protrusion through the anus.

☐☐ **A 62 year-old female patient complains of a mass that intermittently protrudes through her anus. What is the differential diagnosis?**

Prolapsing internal hemorrhoids, anorectal varices, mucosal prolapse, rectal prolapse, anal/rectal polyps, anal/rectal tumors and hypertrophic anal papillae.

☐☐ **T/F: Cirrhotic patients usually develop hemorrhoidal disease secondary to portal hypertension.**

False. Anorectal varices, not hemorrhoids, develop as a result of portal hypertension. They represent the communication between the portal circulation through the superior hemorrhoidal veins and the systemic circulation through the middle and inferior hemorrhoidal veins.

☐☐ **T/F: The classic endoscopic appearance of solitary rectal ulcer syndrome is a shallow, discrete 1 to 4 cm ulcer located at the posterior wall of the rectum 4 to 15 cm from the anal verge.**

False. Although the lesions in solitary rectal ulcer syndrome may be found on the posterior wall of the rectum, they are more commonly located on the anterior wall of the rectum.

☐☐ **What are functional and morphological abnormalities that can be associated with solitary rectal ulcer syndrome?**

Solitary rectal ulcer syndrome is associated with some form of rectal prolapse or mucosal prolapse and thicker muscularis propria in the rectal wall. The condition is commonly associated with high anal sphincter pressure, failure of the puborectalis to relax during defecation and delayed rectal evacuation.

☐☐ **What conditions predict a favorable response to biofeedback (pelvic floor retraining) therapy for fecal incontinence?**

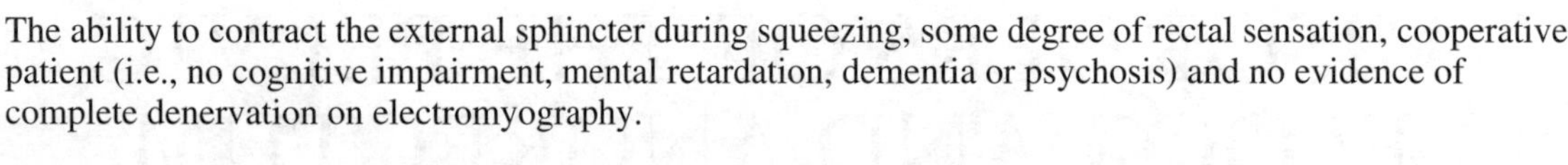

The ability to contract the external sphincter during squeezing, some degree of rectal sensation, cooperative patient (i.e., no cognitive impairment, mental retardation, dementia or psychosis) and no evidence of complete denervation on electromyography.

❑❑ T/F: Anal and rectal carcinomas are more common in men.

False. Rectal carcinoma is more common in men whereas anal canal tumors are nearly twice as common in women.

❑❑ T/F: Because of the anus' location at the very distal part of the gastrointestinal tract and its easy accessibility for digital examination, anal canal tumors produce symptoms early in the course of the disease and are usually diagnosed at an early stage.

False. In about 60% of the patients with anal canal tumors, the tumor is discovered late. Indeed, 15% to 30% are found to have metastatic spread at presentation. The symptoms are usually mild and nonspecific. Approximately 25% of patients with anal canal tumors are symptom free and the tumor is found incidentally during a routine examination.

❑❑ T/F: Adenocarcinoma is the most common malignant tumor of the anal canal.

False. The most common tumor of the anal canal is squamous cell (70-80%). Adenocarcinoma is a rare tumor in the anal canal.

❑❑ What are two medical therapies for chronic anal fissure and which one of them has been shown to be more effective?

Topical nitroglycerin and botulinum toxin injections. Both have been successfully used for the treatment of chronic anal fissure; however, the injection of botulinum toxin into the internal anal sphincter has been found to be more effective than topical application of 0.2% nitroglycerin ointment.

❑❑ What is the prevalence of fecal incontinence?

The prevalence of fecal incontinence in the Western Hemisphere is 2% to 7% and increases with age. Surveys have shown prevalence rates of 18% in the older female population and 45% to 47% in nursing home residents and hospitalized elderly patients.

❑❑ What information can be obtained from anorectal manometry?

Anorectal manometry is helpful in measuring anal and rectal function. This includes measures of anal sphincter tone (at rest, during squeezing and during increase in intra-abdominal pressure), rectal sensation thresholds, rectal compliance and the recto-anal inhibitory reflex.

❑❑ What information can be obtained from anal ultrasound?

Anal ultrasound is helpful in assessing the integrity of the anal sphincters. Anal ultrasound is not helpful in the assessment of anal function.

❑❑ What is the Pudendal Nerve Terminal Motor Latency (PNTML)?

PNTML is the time interval between stimulation of the pudendal nerve and the electromyographic response associated with contraction of the external anal sphincter muscle. A prolonged nerve latency may suggest pudendal neuropathy. The sensitivity and specificity of this test for diagnosing pudendal nerve injury as a cause of fecal incontinence are disputed.

❑❑ What are the differences between the internal and external anal sphincters and their role in maintaining continence?

The internal anal sphincter is composed of smooth muscle and is under the control of the enteric nervous system. Its main function is to maintain the resting tone of the anal sphincter. The external anal sphincter is composed of striated muscle innervated by the pudendal nerve (sacral branches S2 to S4) and is under voluntary control. The main role of the external anal sphincter is to contract voluntarily in response to a sudden increase in rectal or abdominal pressure so as to prevent inappropriate defecation.

❏❏ **What is the relative contribution of the internal and external anal sphincter muscles to the resting anal tone?**

About 70% of the anal canal resting tone is derived from the internal anal sphincter and the remainder by the external anal sphincter muscle.

❏❏ **A manometric evaluation in a patient with fecal incontinence reveals a failure to increase anal sphincter pressure when asked to squeeze but a normal increase in pressure in response to coughing. Besides poor motivation or comprehension, what is the most probable explanation?**

An increase in external anal sphincter pressure in response to an abrupt increase in intra-abdominal pressure is triggered by receptors in the pelvic floor and mediated through a spinal reflex arc. Lesions of the cauda equina or sacral plexus will result in loss of both the reflex response and the voluntary squeeze. Higher spinal cord lesions will result in the findings described in the question.

❏❏ **What are typical findings on physical examination and anorectal manometry in patients with proctalgia fugax?**

Proctalgia fugax is one functional disorder of the anorectum. The diagnosis is based on symptoms alone. There are no specific findings on physical examination or anorectal manometry testing.

❏❏ **A 40 year-old female complains of recurrent episodes of pain in the rectum that last for hours and are often brought on by sitting or lying down. Posterior traction of the puborectalis on rectal examination produces tenderness and pain. What is the diagnosis?**

The description is typical of levator ani syndrome. Levator ani syndrome is a functional disorder of the anorectum and its diagnosis is based on symptoms alone.

❏❏ **T/F: Levator ani syndrome and proctalgia fugax frequently coexist.**

True. Although the two disorders can be distinguished on the basis of duration, frequency and quality of pain, they coexist more often than expected by chance.

❏❏ **T/F: A multi-national working team (Rome Committee) recommends that the diagnosis of pelvic floor dyssynergia be based upon symptoms of difficult defecation in addition to manometric, electromyographic or radiologic evidence of failure of the pelvic floor to relax when attempting to defecate.**

True. Although these were the recommendations of a previous committee (Rome I), more recent recommendations (Rome II) also require evidence of adequate propulsive forces and incomplete evacuation.

❏❏ **T/F: A physical examination finding of a decrease in anal sphincter pressure while the patient is straining is usually sufficient to rule out the diagnosis of pelvic floor dyssynergia.**

True. However, the finding of an increase in anal sphincter pressure on digital rectal exam during straining is not reliable enough and further studies are indicated.

❏❏ **T/F: The majority of patients with pelvic floor dyssynergia will benefit from biofeedback (pelvic floor retraining) treatment.**

True. Approximately two-thirds of these patients can learn to relax the external anal sphincter and puborectalis muscles with biofeedback training and report associated decreases in both straining during defecation and the feeling of incomplete evacuation.

❑❑ **T/F: Rectocele and mucosal intussusception can frequently be seen in healthy normal subjects.**

True. Rectocele, mucosal prolapse and rectal intussusceptions have been reported in normal asymptomatic subjects. Therefore, these finding should be interpreted with caution since they may not necessarily suggest a causal relationship with defecation disorders.

❑❑ **T/F: Pelvic floor descent can be evaluated on physical examination.**

True. With the patient in the left lateral decubitus position, the level of the perineum relative to the ischial tuberosities is observed. The patient is asked to strain and the perineum should not descend beyond the outlet of the bony pelvis.

❑❑ **T/F: Fecal impaction can be definitely excluded by digital examination.**

False. Digital examination can miss 30% of fecal impactions in the elderly because a large amount of feces can accumulate above the reach of the examining finger.

❑❑ **What are indications for evacuation proctography (defecography) in the evaluation of anorectal and pelvic floor disorders?**

The American Gastroenterological Association Medical Position Statement on anorectal testing techniques suggests the use of evacuation proctography in patients with constipation in whom pelvic floor dyssynergia, enterocele or anterior rectocele are suspected as the cause of impaired defecation. There is no support for the use of this technique for other purposes.

❑❑ **What are the clinical findings of anorectal syphilis?**

Anal chancres in the skin around the anus, anal or rectal ulceration and rectal lesions resembling carcinoma have all been described. Enlarged and tender inguinal lymph nodes are often present. Serologic tests for syphilis should be performed prior to surgery for any atypical rectal lesion.

❑❑ **T/F: Vesicles on the perianal region and within the anal canal are commonly seen in anorectal herpes infections.**

False. Although perianal vesicles are a characteristic finding in anorectal herpes infection, they are uncommon within the anal canal. Ulcerations of the anal canal are more commonly seen in anorectal herpes infection.

❑❑ **T/F: The intersphincteric space is the most common anatomic location of anorectal abscesses.**

False. Perianal abscesses located just beneath the perianal skin are most common.

❑❑ **T/F: In at least one-half of ulcerative anal lesions in HIV-positive patients, no specific cause is found.**

True. Diagnostic considerations include syphilis, tuberculosis, *Mycobacterium avium-intracellulare*, herpes simplex, cytomegalovirus, fungi and neoplasm.

❑❑ **T/F: Anogenital condylomata acuminata caused by human papillomavirus (HPV) is associated with adenocarcinoma of the anus.**

False. HPV (types 16 and 18) is associated with squamous cell carcinoma of the anus as well as the cervix and vulva. Condylomata acuminata and anal cancer may coexist; thus, it is advisable to obtain biopsies from suspected lesions and examine the anal canal before beginning treatment.

❑❑ **What is anal sampling and how is it related to the continence mechanism?**

The anal canal is highly innervated and sensitive to pain, touch and temperature. This allows differentiation between gas, solids and liquids and allows for selective passage of rectal contents or voluntary contraction of the external anal sphincter to maintain continence. Loss of this anal sampling function may contribute to the development of fecal incontinence.

❑❑ **T/F: The most common cause of primary anorectal abscess and anorectal fistula is Crohn's disease.**

False. The most common case of primary anorectal abscess and anorectal fistula is primary anal cryptoglandular infection.

❑❑ **What is the most common type/location of anorectal fistula?**

Intersphincteric fistula.

❑❑ **T/F: Endoanal ultrasound is the most useful test to diagnose an anorectal fistula.**

False. Magnetic resonance imaging is the most accurate modality for diagnosing and localizing the position of an anorectal abscess or fistula.

❑❑ **T/F: A broad-spectrum antibiotic is the treatment of choice for an anorectal abscess.**

False. The primary treatment of an anorectal abscess is surgical. Except in patients with diabetes mellitus, leukemia and valvular heart disease, antibiotics are usually not required.

❑❑ **T/F: Up to 30% of women will have an anal sphincter defect on endoanal ultrasonography after their first vaginal delivery.**

True. In addition, about 10% will complain of urgency or incontinence.

FOREIGN BODIES AND CAUSTIC INJURY

Mohammed Mah'moud, M.D. and Rajeev Vasudeva, M.D.

❏❏ Where in the gastrointestinal tract is the most common site of foreign body impaction?

The esophagus is the most common site, especially at the level of the hypopharynx. Other common places are areas of physiologic narrowing and include the pylorus, retroperitoneal duodenum, ileocecal valve and the anus. The ileocecal region is the most frequent site of perforation beyond the esophagus.

❏❏ Where in the esophagus are objects likely to become lodged?

Objects may become lodged at any of the areas of physiologic narrowing (cricopharyngeus, aortic arch, the left main stem bronchus, immediately above the esophagogastric junction) or any other area of structural abnormality (stricture).

❏❏ Which adults are at an increased risk for swallowing foreign bodies?

Adults at increased risk include those who wear dentures, those who are mentally retarded, those with psychiatric illnesses and prisoners.

❏❏ What is the most common symptom in patients presenting with an esophageal foreign body?

Dysphagia is the most common symptom followed by odynophagia, choking and drooling.

❏❏ T/F: Most ingested foreign bodies that become lodged in the esophagus pass spontaneously.

True. Seventy percent of ingested foreign bodies pass spontaneously and fewer than 1% result in perforation.

❏❏ What is the most common physical finding in patients presenting with an ingested foreign body?

Usually the physical examination is normal; however, signs of crepitation should always be sought.

❏❏ A chest x-ray reveals an ingested foreign body aligning itself in the saggital plane. Is the object more likely to be located in the esophagus or trachea?

Trachea. Tracheal foreign bodies align themselves sagittally and are best seen on lateral projections.

❏❏ What is the best study for identifying a radiopaque foreign body in the esophagus?

Frontal view chest x-ray. Objects in the esophagus align themselves in the anteroposterior projections. Barium contrast studies are seldom helpful and should be avoided.

❏❏ What is the best imaging study to identify a toothpick in the abdomen?

Plain x-rays are usually not helpful. Ultrasonography may identify a toothpick as a hyperechoic straight line or a bright hyperechoic dot with sharp posterior shadowing when viewed on end. Alternatively, a CT scan may be helpful.

❏❏ How are pointed objects best removed?

Pointed objects should be removed with the pointed end trailing in order to avoid mucosal injury. Under these circumstances, you should consider utilizing an overtube or a hood attached to the tip of the endoscope.

❑❑ **T/F: Enzyme preparations such as papain should be tried prior to endoscopy in all cases of meat impaction.**

False. Besides being ineffective, it is important to avoid papain and other enzyme preparations because of the risk of perforation.

❑❑ **Prior to endoscopic removal of an ingested safety pin, what should be done by the endoscopist to increase the success rate?**

Rehearsal of the retrieval process (dry run) should always be performed in order to facilitate removal of the object.

❑❑ **T/F: Blindly pushing a foreign body into the stomach followed by endoscopic retrieval is routinely advocated.**

False. This technique should be avoided unless the lumen beyond the obstructing foreign body is adequately visualized and patent. In general, once the foreign body has passed into the stomach, it does not need to be retrieved as it will usually pass through the gastrointestinal tract without problem.

❑❑ **A 72 year-old woman is brought to the emergency room 72 hours after swallowing a pointed object. What is the best management at this point?**

Endoscopic removal should be attempted in this patient if it can be localized and is retrievable. Indications for prompt removal of ingested foreign bodies include the presence of complete esophageal obstruction and ingestion of sharp, pointed or toxic objects (disc batteries) lodged in the esophagus.

❑❑ **T/F: A 23 year-old man presents with fever, chills, neck pain and obvious subcutaneous emphysema two hours after accidentally swallowing a fish bone. Endoscopic removal by an experienced gastroenterologist is the most appropriate management for this patient.**

False. This patient has evidence of possible esophageal perforation. Therefore, surgery is the treatment of choice.

❑❑ **What is the most appropriate management for a patient who is found to have an ingested foreign body that is embedded in the esophageal wall?**

Surgery.

❑❑ **What are the most common symptoms of complete esophageal obstruction due to a foreign body?**

Sialorrhea, regurgitation and choking.

❑❑ **T/F: Immediate endoscopic removal is the best approach for management of ingested latex packets of cocaine.**

False. Endoscopic removal of such drug packets is unwise because of the potential for rupture upon manipulation.

❑❑ **What is the appropriate management of ingested elemental mercury in the intestine?**

Observation and possibly cathartics to hasten its elimination as long as there is no evidence of perforation or leakage outside the digestive tract.

❑❑ **What is the best approach to take when an esophageal stricture is found once the foreign body has been removed or pushed into the stomach?**

Dilatation of the stricture. If there is local mucosal trauma or bleeding or the patient is not cooperative or visualization of the field is suboptimal, the stricture is best dilated at a later time.

❑❑ **T/F: The location of the perceived discomfort is predictive of the most likely site of a foreign body lodged in the esophagus.**

False. As with dysphagia in general, the location of the perceived discomfort does not usually correlate with the anatomic location of the obstructing foreign body.

❑❑ **What size objects should be considered for endoscopic removal?**

Long objects greater than 6 cm in children and greater than 10 cm in adults should be removed. Rounded objects less than 2.5 cm usually pass through the pylorus in adults and can be managed conservatively.

❑❑ **When should endoscopy be utilized in the management of an ingested disc battery?**

Endoscopy should be performed promptly if the disc battery is lodged in the esophagus. If it has passed into the stomach, conservative measures may be employed and the patient observed. If the battery has remained in the stomach for more than 48 hours, is greater than 1.5 cm and has mercury, it should be promptly removed.

❑❑ **How long should you wait before contemplating endoscopic or surgical removal of a foreign body?**

Asymptomatic blunt objects that fail to leave the stomach after 2 weeks should be removed endoscopically. Surgical removal of blunt objects beyond the stomach that fail to advance after 7 to 10 days (sharp objects > 3 days) should be considered. Surgical intervention is otherwise indicated if fever, vomiting, overt bleeding or abdominal pain develop.

❑❑ **Which patients are more likely to ingest caustic substances?**

Children. It is estimated that 17,000 children, half of whom are under 4 years of age, accidentally ingest caustic substances each year. Although relatively uncommon in adults, it predominantly involves adults who are inebriated, mentally retarded, psychotic or suicidal.

❑❑ **What factors are implicated in the pathogenesis of caustic injury to the gut?**

The nature, concentration and physical state of the agent, the amount ingested, the time of exposure ("dwell time") and the amount of reexposure secondary to vomiting or reflux are important factors.

❑❑ **How do alkaline agents cause injury?**

Alkaline agents cause liquefaction (saponification) necrosis, which dissolves superficial mucosa, and rapidly diffuse into deeper tissues. Blood vessel thrombosis causes further cellular necrosis potentially resulting in full-thickness burns.

❑❑ **How do acidic agents cause injury?**

Acidic agents produce a coagulation necrosis of the surface epithelium which tends to limit deeper penetration.

❑❑ **What region of the gastrointestinal tract is more commonly affected by acidic agent ingestion?**

Acidic agents usually cause extensive damage to the stomach. The esophagus is relatively spared due to a combination of factors which include rapid transit through the esophagus, greater resistance of esophageal squamous epithelium to acid and the protection afforded by superficial coagulation necrosis preventing deeper injury. Nevertheless, 20% to 50% of patients may have significant esophageal burns from ingestion of highly concentrated sulfuric or hydrochloric acid.

❑❑ **T/F: There is good correlation between oral/pharyngeal burns and esophageal or gastric injury.**

False. The lack of oral or pharyngeal burns does not preclude the possibility of extensive esophageal or gastric injury.

❑❑ **T/F: Gastric lavage with water or administration of emetics play an important role in the management of caustic ingestions.**

False. However, if the patient is seen within the first hour of ingestion, gastric intubation, preferably under fluoroscopic guidance, with water lavage may be carried out. Emetics should always be avoided.

❑❑ **When should endoscopic examination be carried out in patients with suspected caustic ingestion?**

Although controversial, most experts now agree on the need to document extent of damage with early endoscopy within 12 to 24 hours.

❑❑ **T/F: Endoscopic findings accurately predict the depth of tissue injury.**

False. Grades of injury on endoscopy are not as precise as the pathologic degree of burn.

❑❑ **What are the 'Grades' of injury caustic by ingestion?**

The extent of injury can be divided into three degress of injury. First degree injury is characterized by mild friability, erythema and edama only. Second degree injury extends into the wall, occasionally to the muscularis propria. Ulceration, necrosis and exudate may be seen. Third degree injury involves the full thickness of the wall. A dark exudate with sloughing of the mucosa, hemorrhage, ulceration and necrosis are typically seen.

❑❑ **What is the role of antibiotics and corticosteroids in the management of caustic ingestions?**

The lack of controlled trials precludes definitive arguments in support of any therapeutic modality. The use of antibiotics and corticosteroids is fraught with controversy in the literature. However, corticosteroids may be considered if symptoms of laryngeal edema are present. Antibiotics are recommended in proven or suspected infection and in patients with second degree and third degree injury.

❑❑ **T/F: Administration of acid neutralizers is helpful immediately after caustic ingestion.**

False. The heat produced in the neutralization reaction may actually increase tissue injury. Additionally, since most alkali injuries occur very rapidly, acid neutralization is ineffective.

❑❑ **When do strictures usually develop following caustic ingestion?**

Most strictures (80%) present within the first 8 weeks after injury. However, they can occur insidiously over months to years after the initial event.

❑❑ **What are long-term complications of caustic ingestion?**

Long-term complications include recurrent or delayed strictures which occur in 15% to 38% of caustic exposures, especially in patients with more severe grades of injury, and the development of squamous cell carcinoma of the esophagus.

❑❑ **What is the usual latency period before squamous cell carcinoma develops?**

The latency period varies from 12 to 41 years and is shorter for injuries occurring after childhood. Specific surveillance protocols have not yet been defined.

❏❏ What are the usual sites of stricture development in the esophagus and stomach?

Strictures tend to develop at sites of pooling such as the cricopharyngeus, aortic arch, bifurcation of the trachea and lower esophageal sphincter in the esophagus and the antrum of fasting patients and the mid-body in patients who have food present at the time of caustic ingestion.

❏❏ What is the most sensitive imaging study to detect a suspected early perforation following caustic ingestion?

CT scan of the chest/abdomen with oral contrast.

GASTROESOPHAGEAL REFLUX DISEASE

Rajeev Vasudeva, M.D.

❏❏ T/F: Patients with gastroesophageal reflux disease (GERD) usually seek medical attention.

False. While an extremely common problem, the majority of patients with GERD do not seek medical attention. A recent survey of 2000 randomly selected subjects in Minnesota revealed the prevalence of GERD to be 58 per 100 individuals. In dramatic contrast, only 5% of individuals had sought medical attention.

❏❏ How often is endoscopic evidence of erosive esophagitis and Barrett's esophagus seen in patients with symptoms suggestive of GERD?

Up to one-half of patients with reflux symptoms will have erosive esophagitis, albeit usually mild, and 11% to 12% will have Barrett's esophagus.

❏❏ What are the major physiologic mechanisms that protect against esophageal acid injury?

Esophageal clearance mechanisms (peristalsis/saliva), esophageal mucosal/epithelial integrity, antireflux barrier (lower esophageal sphincter) competence and gastric emptying are the four major physiologic mechanisms.

❏❏ What are the three mechanisms of lower esophageal sphincter (LES) incompetence and how often is each primarily responsible for GERD?

Transient LES relaxation - 65%
Increased intraabdominal pressure - 17%
Spontaneous free reflux - 18%

❏❏ What factors are associated with severe esophagitis?

Low LES pressure, esophageal motor abnormalities and recumbent reflux are the most important determinants of severe endoscopic esophagitis. The presence of a hiatal hernia is also important.

❏❏ What esophageal histologic abnormalities are typical of GERD?

The basal zone occupying more than 15% of the total thickness of the epithelium and the papillae extending more than two-thirds of the distance to the surface. Eosinophils and neutrophils are also commonly present. Unfortunately, the sensitivity and specificity of these findings, either individually or in combination, is only fair at best.

❏❏ What role does the hiatal hernia play in the pathogenesis of GERD?

This has been a controversial issue for the past 2 decades. Initially thought to be the only mechanism by which reflux occurred, later it was considered to be unimportant. However, recently it has been shown that the right crus of the diaphragm contributes significantly to the anti-reflux barrier, thereby stressing the importance of a normally placed gastroesophageal junction. Some studies have shown that the hernia sac acts a reservoir for gastric contents (acid trap) and is associated with complicated forms of GERD such as severe esophagitis and peptic strictures, suggesting that it is a major contributory factor.

❏❏ T/F: There is a clear correlation between abnormal esophageal acid exposure on ambulatory pH monitoring, clinical symptoms and severity of esophagitis.

False. It appears that all three are independent although related aspects of GERD. No clear relationship exists between symptom severity, amount of reflux and presence of esophagitis.

❏❏ What is the cancer risk in Barrett's esophagus?

Barrett's esophagus is the major risk factor for esophageal adenocarcinoma whose incidence has been rising dramatically over the past two decades. A recent meta-analysis suggests that patients develop esophageal adenocarcinoma at a rate of approximately 1% per year (annual incidence rate). These patients have a 30 to 125 times increased risk of developing esophageal cancer compared to the general population.

❏❏ What are the recommended guidelines for endoscopic surveillance in Barrett's esophagus?

Although it is not clear that Barrett's esophagus influences survival adversely or that endoscopic surveillance can reliably detect early curable neoplasia, the American College of Gastroenterology recently published the following practice guidelines:

1) GERD should be treated aggressively prior to surveillance in order to minimize confusion due to inflammation.
2) Random, four-quadrant biopsies taken every 2 cm for standard histologic evaluation is recommended.
3) For patients with no dysplasia, surveillance endoscopy is recommended at 2 to 3 year intervals.
4) For patients with low grade dysplasia, surveillance endoscopy every 6 months for the 1st year and at yearly intervals thereafter if dysplasia has not progressed.
5) For patients with high grade dysplasia, the diagnosis should be confirmed by two expert pathologists. While esophageal resection is currently the standard of care, an intensive endoscopic surveillance (no specific interval recommended but may consider 3 months) may also be considered depending upon patient comorbidities and/or preference. Although not recommended in the practice guidelines, an experimental ablative therapy may also be considered as long as it is a part of an established research protocol.

❏❏ What is the natural history of high-grade dysplasia in Barrett's esophagus?

The natural history is poorly defined and therefore management of this condition is disputed. On one hand, some studies have shown that progression to cancer is frequent and rapid while other studies have shown no apparent progression to cancer and even regression. Therefore, management varies between esophageal resection, continued surveillance and experimental ablative therapies.

❏❏ T/F: There is a relationship between GERD and a multitude of pulmonary and otorhinolaryngologic symptoms.

True. A number of uncontrolled studies and anecdotal reports link GERD with several symptoms including laryngitis, hoarseness, globus, laryngeal cancer, chronic cough, asthma, aspiration, bronchitis, sinusitis and dental erosions; however, the association appears to be the strongest for chronic cough, hoarseness and asthma.

❏❏ In patients with noncardiac (unexplained) chest pain, what percentage is due to GERD and how effective is treatment?

Several studies show nearly 50% of patients may have underlying GERD. Uncontrolled studies reveal an improvement of 65% to 100% in symptomatology utilizing high-dose H_2 receptor antagonists and proton pump inhibitors.

❏❏ What are the mechanisms by which GERD is thought to produce respiratory symptoms?

Two mechanisms have been suggested: 1) Microaspiration of refluxed gastric contents into the airway (reflux theory) and 2) Reflux of gastric contents into the distal esophagus initiating a vagally-mediated reflex arc (reflex theory).

❏❏ In what way is the response to anti-reflux therapy in patients with extraesophageal symptoms different from classical GERD?

Despite the lack of adequate controlled data, the therapeutic response appears to be less. Therefore, high-dose proton pump inhibitors and a longer duration (several months) of treatment is required. Additionally, remission may be more difficult to maintain. The optimal management strategy remains to be defined.

❑❑ **What are the therapeutic recommendations in the management of confirmed or suspected reflux-related extraesophageal symptoms.**

A twice-daily proton pump inhibitor, with or without bedtime H_2 receptor antagonist to control nocturnal acid breakthrough, for at least three months should be attempted before considering a patient to have failed medical therapy or not to have GERD. Anti-reflux surgery may be considered as an alternative therapeutic modality in patients with documented GERD who have failed medical therapy. The efficacy of anti-reflux surgery in patients with extraesophageal GERD is unclear based upon the published literature.

❑❑ **In what situations should you consider diagnostic testing in patients with suspected GERD?**

1) Uncertain diagnosis.
2) Atypical symptoms (chest pain, ENT, pulmonary).
3) Symptoms associated with complications (dysphagia, odynophagia, unexplained weight loss, bleeding, anemia).
4) Inadequate response to therapy.
5) Recurrent symptoms.
6) Prior to anti-reflux surgery.

❑❑ **What are differences between the various diagnostic tests used in GERD?**

Diagnostic tests should be performed in individual patients to answer specific questions. While somewhat controversial, a barium swallow is the test of choice for evaluation of dysphagia given that its sensitivity is superior to endoscopy in identifying subtle mucosal rings. Endoscopy with biopsy is the best study for evaluating mucosal injury as well as identifying Barrett's esophagus. Ambulatory pH monitoring is the best study to confirm GERD, quantify reflux and allow symptom correlation. Esophageal manometry has a limited role but may be useful prior to anti-reflux surgery in order to identify severe esophageal peristaltic abnormalities.

❑❑ **What are the indications for ambulatory esophageal pH monitoring?**

1) Typical symptoms that do not respond to proton pump inhibitor therapy (on therapy).
2) Atypical symptoms (noncardiac chest pain, ENT/pulmonary manifestions).
3) Prior to anti-reflux surgery if confirmation of GERD is necessary (endoscopy-negative patients).
4) Recurrent symptoms following anti-reflux surgery.

❑❑ **T/F: Lifestyle modifications are extremely effective in the treatment of GERD.**

False. Lifestyle modifications are helpful in relieving symptoms in only about 20% of patients. No studies exist that demonstrate efficacy of lifestyle modifications in healing esophagitis, managing or preventing complications or maintenance of remission.

❑❑ **What is the role of prokinetic agents in GERD?**

Cisapride, the only practical prokinetic agent, is effective in relieving nocturnal heartburn and healing mild-to-moderate esophagitis and is comparable to H_2 receptor antagonists, in general. It seems to derive most of its benefit by enhancing gastric emptying. In combination with H_2 receptor antagonists, healing of esophagitis is superior to either agent alone, in short-term studies. However, the combination of cisapride and a proton pump inhibitor is not significantly better than a proton pump inhibitor alone and ends up being more expensive and cumbersome. Numerous drug interactions and the potential for cardiac toxicity further limit the use of cisapride.

❑❑ **How effective are H_2 receptor antagonists in GERD therapy?**

They eliminate symptoms in up to 50% with twice daily dosing. Healing of mild-to-moderate esophagitis requires at least twice daily dosing and usually more frequent and higher dosing is often required. Remission of esophagitis healing occurs in only about 15 to 25%.

❑❑ What is the recurrence rate of GERD on discontinuation of therapy?

GERD is a chronic relapsing condition and, in one study, 80% of patients were symptomatic at the end of 6 months after discontinuation of antisecretory therapy.

❑❑ What medical conditions predispose to the development of benign peptic strictures?

Progressive systemic sclerosis (Scleroderma), hypersecretory disorders (Zollinger Ellison syndrome), prolonged nasogastric intubation, and drugs such as nonsteroidal anti-inflammatory agents and quinidine.

❑❑ Where are peptic esophageal strictures usually located?

The distal esophagus involving the squamocolumnar junction. Other etiologies should be considered if strictures are located elsewhere.

❑❑ T/F: Medical therapy is effective in preventing the need for subsequent stricture dilatation.

True. While treatment with H_2 receptor antagonists and promotility agents does not decrease the need for subsequent dilatations, several recent studies have shown that proton pump inhibitors are effective in not only healing associated esophagitis but also decreasing the need for stricture dilatation.

❑❑ What are some of the reasons why proton pump inhibitors may fail to control gastric acidity?

1) There is significant intersubject variability in the bioavalability of proton pump inhibitors which may be decreased even further when taken with food.
2) The acid suppressive effect of proton pump inhibitors tends to be reduced in *Helicobacter pylori*-negative patients.
3) Although uncommon, hypersecretors may have a decreased effect.
4) The rate of proton pump inhibitor metabolism by the hepatic cytochrome P-450 2C enzymes. Rapid metabolizers show a decreased effect on acid control.
5) True proton pump inhibitor resistance (rare).

❑❑ What are some other reasons why PPI's may fail in controlling suspected GERD in the clinical setting?

1) Incorrect diagnosis.
2) Nonacid reflux.
3) Factors including significant gastric stasis, lower esophageal sphincter dysfunction or ineffective peristalsis may contribute to persisting symptoms. Also, many patients with GERD often have symptoms including bloating, distention, nausea which may be unmasked by proton pump inhibitors even though the classic reflux symptoms have improved.
4) Noncompliance.
5) Drugs such as aspirin, nonsteroidal anti-inflammatory agents and other drugs known to cause direct topical injury.
6) Hypersecretory states.

❑❑ What is the single most informative study in patients with medical refractory GERD?

24-hour simultaneous intraesophageal and intragastric pH-metry while on antisecretory medication. A similar study off medication may be considered if the diagnosis of GERD is in doubt.

❑❑ What are some similarities and differences in demographics between patients with long-segment Barrett's esophagus (LSBE) and short-segment Barrett's esophagus (SSBE)?

1) In general, the prevalence of LSBE is 3 to 5 times less than SSBE.

2)   The mean age of diagnosis is similar (55 to 65 years) with a strong propensity for males in LSBE (> 90%) and slightly less for SSBE (70%).
3)   Predominance of caucasians is noted for both although more striking in LSBE.
4)   Both smoking and alcohol ingestion are more prevalent in LSBE than is SSBE.

❑❑ **What are some of the similarities and differences in pathophysiology and clinical presentation between patients with long-segment Barrett's esophagus (LSBE) and short-segment Barrett's esophagus (SSBE)?**

1)   Symptoms of heartburn are similar but duration of heartburn greater than 5 years appears to be a distinguishing feature of LSBE.
2)   The pathophysiology and degree of acid reflux is different. Patients with LSBE typically are have a large hiatal hernia, very low lower esophageal sphincter pressure and decreased distal esophageal amplitude as compared to SSBE patients. Additionally, patients with LSBE have a combination of upright and supine reflux and more proximal esophageal acid reflux while SSBE have predominantly upright and distal esophageal reflux.

❑❑ **What are some of the differences in dysplasia risk between patients with long-segment Barrett's esophagus (LSBE) and short-segment Barrett's esophagus (SSBE)?**

The dysplasia prevalence is 15% to 24% in LSBE or 2 to 3 times higher than SSBE. The adenocarcinoma prevalence is 15% in LSBE or 7 to 15 times higher than the SSBE population.

❑❑ **What is the efficacy of antisecretory therapy in the healing and maintenance of remission of esophagitis based on severity?**

The rate of healing is inversely related to the severity of esophagitis. While H_2 receptor antagonists may heal milder grades of esophagitis, proton pump inhibitors are clearly superior in healing higher grades of esophagitis. In patients with severe esophagitis, the rate of healing is directly related to the dose of the agent. The degree of acid suppression required to maintain remission often is at least that required to heal acute esophagitis.

❑❑ **Which class of drugs provides the best long term remission rate in erosive esophagitis?**

Proton pump inhibitors. Of note, the maintenance dose requirement may increase with time according to one long-term Dutch study.

❑❑ **What are the indications for anti-reflux surgery?**

1)   Patient with severe GERD who are unwilling to accept life-long medical therapy.
2)   Patients with severe GERD who cannot tolerate proton pump inhibitors due to allergy or intolerable side effects.
3)   Patients who have GERD manifestations that require long-term high-dose proton pump inhibitor therapy.
4)   Patients who are young and require chronic proton pump inhibitor therapy or high-dose H_2 receptor antagonists for control of symptoms and complications of GERD.

❑❑ **T/F: Medical intractability remains a major indication for anti-reflux surgery in the era of proton pump inhibitors.**

False. Although once the most frequent reason for anti-reflux surgery, it is currently not a major indication for surgery. True intractability is uncommon in the era of proton pump inhibitors and the physician should reconsider the diagnosis of GERD in those who do not respond to these drugs. Anti-reflux surgery today is best reserved for patients who respond well to medical therapy.

GASTROINTESTINAL BLEEDING

James L. Achord, M.D., MACG, FACP and Maurice A. Cerulli, M.D.

❑❑ **What major clinical features help predict which patients who present with gastrointestinal bleeding can be managed without admission to the hospital?**

Absence of hypotension, melena or hematemesis and age less than 60 years.

❑❑ **Approximately what percentage of patients with esophageal varices that have never bled will experience a variceal hemorrhage in the 1 to 2 years following their diagnosis?**

Approximately one-third.

❑❑ **What endoscopic features of esophageal varices predict a high probability of hemorrhage?**

Large size and red wale markings.

❑❑ **What is the hepatic wedge pressure gradient below which bleeding from esophageal varices rarely occurs?**

12 mmHg.

❑❑ **T/F: An arteriovenous malformation (angiodysplasia) in a patient who has no evidence of gastrointestinal blood loss should be cauterized to prevent bleeding.**

False. The vast majority of angiodysplasia discovered at endoscopy are incidental findings and require no treatment.

❑❑ **If one considers all the diagnoses found in a large number of patients who present with upper gastrointestinal hemorrhage, what percentage have some form of acid-peptic disease?**

85%.

❑❑ **The national mortality rate from gastrointestinal bleeding has remained stable since 1945 and is approximately:**

10%.

❑❑ **T/F: Oral iron therapy produces a false positive fecal occult blood test.**

False. It may, however, cause visual interpretation errors.

❑❑ **What is the average amount of blood/day lost in the stool of healthy individuals on no medications as determined by the chromate-tagged red cell test?**

0.5 to 1.5 mL/day.

❑❑ **In experimental animals (and presumably in humans), at what rate must blood be lost into the gut lumen before arteriography is capable of demonstrating a bleeding site?**

0.5 to 1.5 mL/min. The corresponding rate for a nuclear medicine red blood cell scan is 0.1 to 0.4 mL/min.

❑❑ **Approximately what percentage of patients with a gastrointestinal hemorrhage will have no identifiable source despite careful evaluation including small bowel enteroscopy?**

10%.

❑❑ **T/F: Intense inhibition of acid secretion slows or stops acute upper gastrointestinal bleeding.**

False.

❑❑ **T/F: Intense inhibition of acid secretion prevents early rebleeding from peptic ulcer disease.**

True.

❑❑ **What percentage of acute hemorrhages due to Mallory-Weiss tears stop spontaneously?**

80% to 90%.

❑❑ **Considering all causes of upper gastrointestinal hemorrhage except variceal, what is the rebleeding rate (with or without endoscopy)?**

20%.

❑❑ **What is the advantage, if any, of esophageal variceal band ligation compared to sclerotherapy?**

Fewer complications with banding.

❑❑ **What is the presently accepted efficacy rate (of stopping hemorrhage) for sclerotherapy or banding of esophageal varices?**

85% to 90%.

❑❑ **What is the therapeutic efficacy (range) of a Sengstaken-Blakemore tube in controlling bleeding from esophageal varices?**

65% to 85%.

❑❑ **What are the two major complications of the Sengstaken-Blakemore tube for tamponade of bleeding esophageal varices?**

Aspiration pneumonia and perforation of the esophagus by erroneously inflating the gastric balloon in the esophagus.

❑❑ **What is the primary indication for angiographic infusion of vasopressors or embolization in the treatment of bleeding peptic ulcer disease?**

Failure of therapeutic endoscopy to control bleeding or rebleeding not controlled by a second therapeutic endoscopy in a patient who is of poor operative risk.

❑❑ **T/F: It is accepted as true that cure of *Helicobacter pylori* infection in a patient with a bleeding ulcer will prevent future bleeding episodes.**

True – although not in everyone. The nonsteroidal anti-inflammatory drug-status of the patient and location of the ulcer (i.e., gastric or duodenal) may play a role in those cases of recurrent ulcer bleeding.

❑❑ **T/F: It is the national standard of care that a repeat endoscopy be done in order to prove healing of a duodenal ulcer that has bled.**

False.

❏❏ **Given a patient with a third episode of bleeding from proven duodenal ulcer disease in the second portion of the duodenum, what diagnosis must be considered?**

Zollinger-Ellison Syndrome (gastrinoma).

❏❏ **What is the single most common risk factor for ulcer formation in patients who use nonsteroidal anti-inflammatory drugs regularly?**

Age greater than 65 or 70 years.

❏❏ **Upper gastrointestinal hemorrhage is a documented problem in truly stressful and prolonged illnesses and after extensive surgery, especially neurosurgery and cardiac procedures. What, if anything, can be done to reduce the frequency of such bleeding episodes?**

Intravenous or oral acid suppression. Sucralfate may also be useful in this setting.

❏❏ **A so-called "herald bleeding episode" in which significant bleeding that spontaneously ceases occurs, is characteristic of what post-surgical situation?**

An aorto-enteric fistula.

❏❏ **In a previously healthy, asymptomatic patient over the age of 40 years who presents with the sudden onset of severe lower abdominal cramping, an urge to defecate, passage of a fairly normal stool followed shortly by passage of gross blood, what should be your diagnosis of highest probability?**

Ischemic colitis.

❏❏ **What is the eventual outcome of ischemic colitis in the vast majority of patients?**

Spontaneous cessation of bleeding, usually without requiring blood transfusion and with no complications. Acute perforation (within 3 days) and late stricture formation are uncommon.

❏❏ **In a previously healthy, asymptomatic patient over the age of 60 years who presents with the sudden passage of gross blood with little or no abdominal discomfort, what should be your diagnosis of highest probability?**

Diverticular bleeding from the colon.

❏❏ **What is the most common cause of significant upper gastrointestinal bleeding in patients of child-bearing age?**

Duodenal ulcer disease.

❏❏ **If a patient with bleeding esophageal varices continues to bleed following two attempts at variceal banding or sclerotherapy, what is the recommended next therapeutic maneuver?**

Emergency portosystemic shunt, usually by surgery or by transjugular intrahepatic portosystemic shunt (TIPS), depending upon the cause of portal hypertension, severity of the liver disease and availability. A Sengstaken-Blakemore tube may be necessary in the interim.

❏❏ **In a patient with massive upper gastrointestinal bleeding who is found to have isolated gastric varices, what is your diagnosis of highest probability?**

Splenic vein thrombosis.

❏❏ **In a patient who is vigorously bleeding from esophageal varices despite pharmocotherapy and banding of varices and who is waiting for a surgical suite to become available for portosystemic shunt, what therapeutic maneuver is available that may control the hemorrhage?**

Sengstaken-Blakemore tube for tamponade.

❒❒ **What is the most common complication of upper gastrointestinal endoscopy in a patient with active upper gastrointestinal hemorrhage?**

Aspiration pneumonia.

❒❒ **In a patient over 50 years old who presents with intermittent hematochezia without iron deficiency anemia, persistently normal colored stools, and a clear history of blood on toilet tissue, what is the approximate frequency of significant lesions that will be discovered on colonoscopy compared to sigmoidoscopy?**

Less than 3%.

❒❒ **In an acutely bleeding patient, what is the first step in management?**

Support the intravascular volume (i.e., fluid resuscitation). Once hemodynamically stable, further evaluation can safely be performed.

❒❒ **T/F: Melena can only occur as a result of upper gastrointestinal hemorrhage.**

False. It may also occur due to a colonic lesion with slow transit resulting from partial obstruction.

❒❒ **A 26 year-old man presents with hematemesis, fever and severe pleuritic left chest pain a few hours after a severe vomiting episode. What is the most likely diagnosis?**

Boerhaave's syndrome.

❒❒ **A 56 year-old man with chronic heartburn for many years presents with dysphagia and iron deficiency anemia. What is the most likely diagnosis?**

Esophageal adenocarcinoma arising within Barrett's epithelium.

❒❒ **T/F: The incidence of recurrent ulcer hemorrhage is markedly reduced if *Helicobacter pylori* is eradicated.**

True.

❒❒ **T/F: A clean ulcer base has a very low incidence of rebleeding and requires no endoscopic therapy.**

True. The incidence of rebleeding is less than 5%.

❒❒ **What are some clinical predictors of ulcer rebleeding?**

Shock (hemodynamic instability), anemia, hematemesis and persistent bloody lavage.

❒❒ **What information can be gleaned from a bloody nasogastric aspirate associated with hematochezia?**

The patient is bleeding rapidly from the stomach or duodenum and has an increased risk of morbidity and mortality.

❒❒ **T/F: A negative nasogastric aspirate implies that a patient could not have bled from the stomach or duodenum.**

False. It is possible that a gastric or duodenal ulcer may not have bled for some time and there is no longer blood in the stomach.

❑❑ **T/F: Older patients have increased morbidity and mortality related to ulcer hemorrhage.**

True. This is due to the presence of comorbidities.

❑❑ **What effect do comorbid illnesses have on survival from ulcer hemorrhage and the risk of rebleeding after endoscopic therapy?**

Comorbid illnesses increase the risk of death from ulcer hemorrhage. They also increase the risk of rebleeding.

❑❑ **Which ulcer sites are at higher risk for rebleeding?**

Ulcers located high on the lesser curvature and posteriorly in the duodenal bulb are at higher risk due to their proximity to large arteries (left gastric, pancreatico-duodenal).

❑❑ **What is the range in size of a visible vessel?**

A visible vessel ranges in size from 0.3 mm to 1.8 mm.

❑❑ **What size vessel can be coagulated by monopolar electrocautery?**

Electrocautery can obliterate vessels up to 1 mm in diameter.

❑❑ **How is blood flow related to the size of the artery?**

The blood flow is related to the fourth power of the radius of the vessel.

❑❑ **Describe how arteries bleed in ulcer hemorrhage.**

There is fibrinoid necrosis of the vessel wall. The vessel bleeds from both sides and does not contract because it is not completely severed.

❑❑ **T/F: Endoscopic therapy should be utilized whenever a nonbleeding visible vessel is found.**

True. The high risk of rebleeding in this situation mandates endoscopic treatment.

❑❑ **What technique is needed for coagulation of vessels larger than 1 mm?**

Coaptive coagulation is needed for vessels larger than 1 mm and can be used for vessels up to 2 mm.

❑❑ **What is the mortality related to upper gastrointestinal hemorrhage?**

About 10%.

❑❑ **What specific causes of gastrointestinal bleeding are associated with increased mortality?**

Esophageal varices and gastric cancer.

❑❑ **What is the overall rate of rebleeding for ulcers?**

About 15% to 20%.

❑❑ **What is the rate of rebleeding after endoscopic treatment of an ulcer?**

About 10% to 30%.

❑❑ **What is a Dieulafoy lesion?**

A 'caliber-persistent' artery that protrudes from the mucosa with little or no surrounding ulceration. This lesion is usually treated with combination therapy using injection plus thermal therapy. Endoscopic band ligation may also be effective.

❑❑ **T/F: According to a consensus statement from the National Institutes of Health, heater probe, bipolar electrocautery, laser and injection therapy are about equal in the ability to control ulcer hemorrhage.**

True, in experienced hands.

❑❑ **T/F: Bleeding from gastric cancer is difficult to control.**

True. In general, bleeding from tumors of any type is difficult to manage nonsurgically.

❑❑ **A 70 year-old lady presents with hematemesis. At endoscopy, erythematous linear streaks are noted in the antrum giving a watermelon appearance. What is the most likely diagnosis and treatment of choice?**

Gastric antral vascular ectasia (GAVE) which may be treated by either laser or other thermal coagulation.

❑❑ **A 42 year-old man presents with melena. On examination, he is found to have pigmented spots on the buccal mucosa. What syndrome may he have?**

Peutz-Jegher's syndrome.

❑❑ **A 47 year-old woman presents with melena and is found to have increased lunulae (Terry's nails). What may be the cause of her bleeding?**

Variceal hemorrhage due to chronic liver disease.

❑❑ **What methods are available for the prevention of a first esophageal variceal hemorrhage?**

Therapy with non-selective beta blockers and long-acting nitrates has been shown to be effective. Prophylactic band ligation has also been shown to be effective, but only in a few small series; therefore, it currently is not recommended.

❑❑ **What endoscopic findings indicate increased risk for variceal hemorrhage?**

Size $\geq$ 5 mm, red wale signs, hematocystic spots.

❑❑ **Describe why varices bleed.**

As the varices become larger, the wall tension increases and the varix bursts. The red wale sign is due to the thinning of the vessel wall.

❑❑ **When a patient presents with melena and telangiectatic lesions in the lips, oral cavity , nailbeds or skin, what diagnosis should be entertained?**

Osler-Weber-Rendu syndrome.

❑❑ **Why does angiodysplasia occur mainly in the right colon?**

The increased wall tension of the right colon is due to the larger diameter. The veins become partially obstructed and over years become dilated and tortuous forming the angiodysplasia.

❑❑ **How common are angiodysplasia?**

More than 25% of asymptomatic individuals over age 60 have been found to have angiodysplasias.

❏❏ **T/F: Angiodysplasia can present as occult intestinal bleeding.**

True, in about 5%.

❏❏ **What is the most common site of diverticular hemorrhage?**

The proximal half of the colon accounts for most diverticular hemorrhage documented angiographically.

❏❏ **T/F: If a patient has one of six fecal occult blood test windows positive, this is a significant finding requiring colonoscopy.**

True.

❏❏ **T/F: Colonic biopsy can differentiate ischemic colitis from *Clostridium difficile* colitis.**

False.

❏❏ **A 31 year-old man presents with abdominal distention and hematemesis. Upper endoscopy reveals blood coming from beyond the 2nd portion of the duodenum. What is the most likely diagnosis?**

A jejunal volvulus with partial obstruction and ischemic necrosis.

❏❏ **A 51 year-old man presents with fever, right upper quadrant pain and hematemesis. Endoscopy reveals blood in the second part of the duodenum without any lesion noted. What is one possible cause of this scenario?**

Acute cholecystitis with a cystic artery aneurysm that has bled into the bile duct.

❏❏ **T/F: Varices may return after eradication.**

True. By 2 years, there appears to be a return of varices in 40% of patients.

❏❏ **What is the role of push enteroscopy in the evaluation and management of occult gastrointestinal intestinal bleeding?**

Enteroscopy may be useful after a negative colonoscopy and upper endosocopy. If a telangiectasia is found, it can be coagulated using thermal techniques.

❏❏ **A 23 year-old woman presents with right lower quadrant pain and hematochezia. Upper and lower gastrointestinal endoscopy are negative. Would a nuclear medicine scan be useful at this point?**

The patient could be bleeding from a Meckel's diverticulum which could be identified by such a scan.

❏❏ **T/F: Diverticular hemorrhage can be controlled by endoscopic means.**

True. If the bleeding site can be identified, injection around the orifice of the diverticulum or the endoscopic placement of clips may be helpful.

❏❏ **What size visible vessels should not be treated using endoscopically-delivered themal therapy?**

According to animal models, vessels larger than 2 mm are more difficult to coagulate by coaptive coagulation using a heater probe or bipolar probe. Combination therapy should be used for borderline vessels. Large vessels, particularly in dangerous places (high in the stomach, posteriorly in the duodenal bulb), should be referred for urgent surgical therapy.

GASTROINTESTINAL DERMATOSES

Michelle O. DiBaise, P.A.-C, MPAS

❑❑ **Perifollicular hyperkeratosis, also referred to as phrynoderma ("toad skin"), is seen in what nutritional deficiencies?**

Vitamin A, linoleic acid and B complex vitamins.

❑❑ **What are the three D's of pellagra?**

Dermatitis, diarrhea and dementia.

❑❑ **A deficiency in what two nutrients is responsible for pellagra?**

Niacin (most commonly) and tryptophan.

❑❑ **What, other than decreased nutritional intake of tryptophan or niacin, may cause pellagra?**

Alterations in tryptophan metabolism secondary to carcinoid, Hartnup's disease, use of isoniazid, 5-fluorouracil, 6-mercaptopurine or sulfapyridine.

❑❑ **Vitiligo has been associated with what two nutritional deficiencies?**

Vitamin B12 and folic acid.

❑❑ **What disease/nutritional deficiency leads to perifollicular purpura?**

Scurvy/vitamin C deficiency. Other findings include poor wound healing, corkscrew hairs and gingival bleeding.

❑❑ **Plummer-Vinson syndrome is associated with what findings?**

A post-cricoid web, koilonychia, angular stomatitis, sore tongue and iron deficiency.

❑❑ **What percent of patients with Plummer-Vinson Syndrome are at risk of developing a carcinoma?**

Between 5% and 10% will develop carcinoma at the site of the post-cricoid web. Patients with coexisting celiac disease may be at an even greater risk.

❑❑ **What is the classical dermatologic finding in patients with hemochromatosis?**

Bronze pigmentation of the skin.

❑❑ **What autosomal recessive condition leads to a perioral, acral and genital eczematous eruption, alopecia, glossitis and diarrhea?**

Acrodermatitis enteropathica.

❑❑ **What is the underlying cause of acrodermatitis enteropathica?**

Zinc deficiency.

❑❑ **What gastrointestinal conditions may lead to acquired zinc deficiency?**

Chronic inflammatory bowel disease with diarrhea and/or malabsorption, steatorrhea, pancreatic insufficiency, cirrhosis and surgically-induced conditions.

❑❑ **What percent of porphyria cutanea tarda (PCT) patients have associated chronic hepatitis C?**

71% to 91%.

❑❑ **What diagnoses should be considered when there are skin findings consistent with PCT in addition to acute episodes of abdominal pain, nausea, vomiting, paralysis and seizures?**

Variegate porphyria (VP) and hereditary coproporphyria (HCP).

❑❑ **What drugs can precipitate an attack of VP?**

Barbiturates, dapsone and estrogens.

❑❑ **What does CREST stand for?**

Calcinosis cutis, Raynaud's phenomenon, esophageal dysmotility, sclerodactyly and telangiectasias.

❑❑ **Patients with Ehlers-Danlos Syndrome (EDS) are at high risk for what gastrointestinal problems?**

Patients with Type IV (arterial subtype) EDS are at risk for rupture of the large intestine and/or rupture of the mesenchymal arteries in the abdomen.

❑❑ **Yellowish papules in flexural skin and rectal mucosa giving a "plucked chicken' appearance, ocular angioid streaks, hypertension and gastrointestinal hemorrhage are indicative of what disorder?**

Pseudoxanthoma elasticum. Other findings may include retinal hemorrhage and detachment, claudication, angina pectoris, abdominal angina and urinary tract bleeding.

❑❑ **What gastrointestinal symptoms are commonly seen in patients with cutis laxa?**

Hernias (inguinal, umbilical and obturator), diverticula of the gastrointestinal and genitourinary tracts and chronic diarrhea.

❑❑ **What gastrointestinal manifestations are seen in patients with Bloom Syndrome?**

This disorder is most frequently seen among Ashkenazi Jews. Approximately 20% of patients develop neoplasms (50% before age 20), most commonly lymphatic, nonlymphatic leukemia, lymphosarcoma, lymphoma and carcinoma of the oral cavity and digestive system. Patients are predisposed to multiple infections of the gastrointestinal and respiratory tracts. Other findings include sun sensitivity, facial telangiectasia, short stature and immunodeficiency.

❑❑ **What malignancies have been associated with Fanconi's anemia?**

Nonlymphatic leukemia and hepatoma.

❑❑ **Dyskeratosis congenita (Zinsser-Engman-Cole Syndrome) is an X-linked disease with multisystem abnormalities. What gastrointestinal findings may be seen?**

Mucosal leukoplakia, lingual hyperkeratosis, esophageal stenosis, squamous cell carcinoma of the mouth, anus and esophagus, and adenocarcinoma of the pancreas and stomach.

❑❑ What is the differential diagnosis of bullous lesions and/or ulcers of the oral mucosa?

Pemphigus vulgaris, bullous pemphigoid, epidermolysis bullosa, dermatitis herpetiformis, cicatricial pemphigoid, thermal burn, linear IgA dermatosis, herpes simplex, physical injury, syphilis, coxsackievirus, herpes zoster, deep mycoses, aphthous ulcers, Behçet's syndrome, Reiter's syndrome and erythema multiforme

❑❑ What conditions with dermatologic manifestations are associated with gastrointestinal bleeding?

Hereditary hemorrhagic telangiectasia, blue rubber bleb nevus syndrome, Ehlers-Danlos syndrome, pseudoxanthoma elasticum, Kaposi's sarcoma (Human Herpes Virus 8), vasculitides (Henoch-Schoenlein disease and polyarteritis nodosa) and Dego's disease (malignant atrophic papulosis).

❑❑ What conditions are associated with both gastrointestinal polyps and dermatologic manifestations?

Gardner's syndrome presents with multiple epidermal inclusion cysts, lipomas, osteomas of the face. Peutz-Jegher's syndrome presents with freckling around the mouth and on the lips. Cronkhite-Canada syndrome presents with patchy alopecia and nail changes. Neurofibromatosis or Von Recklinghausen's Syndrome, Type I presents with axillary and inguinal freckling, café au lait spots and neurofibromas. Cowden's disease is an autosomal disorder associated with multiple tricholemmomas (resembling warts) around the mouth, nose and ears.

❑❑ What skin signs may aid in the diagnosis of acute pancreatitis?

Cullen's sign (periumbilical bruising) and/or Grey Turner's sign (flank bruising).

❑❑ What cutaneous signs may herald gastrointestinal malignancy?

1)   Dermatomyositis in adults (controversial) - gastric and colonic carcinomas.
2)   Acanthosis nigricans - adenocarcinoma of the stomach and bowel, but is predominantly associated with obesity, medications and endocrinopathies.
3)   Sister Mary Joseph nodules (umbilical metastases) - carcinoma of the stomach, colon and ovary.
4)   Muir-Torre syndrome - autosomal dominant disorder presenting with multiple sebaceous tumors is associated with colon cancer.
5)   The sign of Leser-Trélat (controversial) - sudden onset of multiple, pruritic seborrheic keratoses has been reported to occur with malignancy of the stomach, breast, prostate, lung and colon.
6)   Acrokeratosis of Bazex - symmetrical psoriasisiform eruption affecting the hands, feet, ears, nose is seen predominantly in males and is associated with tumors of the pharynx, esophagus, tongue and lungs.
7)   Erythema gyratum repens - raised, erythematous, concentric eruption that moves on the skin and is likened to a "wood grain" pattern has been associated with tumors of the breast, lung, bladder, prostate, cervix, stomach, esophagus and multiple myeloma.
8)   Ataxia telangiectasia - oculocutaneous telangiectasia, xerosis, gray hair, atrophic or sclerotic skin, recurrent impetigo with progressive cerebellar ataxia and an increased incidence of tumors of the oral cavity, breast, stomach and pancreas.
9)   Sweet's syndrome (acute febrile neutrophilic dermatosis) - presents as erythematous to bluish papules or nodules that coalesce to form well-demarcated plaques, likened to a "relief of a mountain range." Twenty percent of cases are associated with malignancy. Most commonly seen with acute myelocytic leukemia, it has also been reported to occur with gastric carcinoma and adenocarcinoma of the rectum.
10) Acquired ichthyosis - excessively dry skin with tessellated or tile-like scale predominantly on the lower extremities can be seen in many underlying gut tumors, but most commonly is associated with lymphoma.

❑❑ From what cells do carcinoid tumors arise?

Enterochromaffin or Kulchitsky cells.

❏❏ In what sites do carcinoid tumors reside?

While the appendix is the most common site, the ileum, the second most common site, is more likely to be the origin of the classic carcinoid syndrome and is the most frequent site of the origin of metastases. Other sites for carcinoid tumors are the rectum, duodenum, stomach, colon, biliary tract and pancreas.

❏❏ What differences occur in the carcinoid syndrome depending on where the tumor originates in relation to the embryologic foregut, midgut and hindgut?

The foregut tumors (bronchus, stomach, pancreas), in addition to serotonin, also produce histamine leading to peptic ulcer disease, brighter and more persistent flushing reactions, lacrimation, sweating, vomiting and asthma. Midgut tumors (small intestine to midcolon) are associated with a bluish flushing with mixed erythema and pallor, hypotension and bronchoconstriction. Hindgut tumors (descending colon and rectum) are not associated with flushing or other manifestations of carcinoid syndrome.

❏❏ What conditions should be considered in a patient with a painful, erythematous nodule of the lower extremity and known inflammatory bowel disease?

1) Pyoderma gangrenosum begins as a painful nodule or pustules then develops into an ulcer with a serpiginous, erythematous to violaceous border and boggy, necrotic base and may not resolve once the bowel disease is under control.
2) Erythema nodosum lesions are erythematous, painful nodules predominantly on the extensor surfaces of the lower extremities and may precede the onset of inflammatory bowel disease.

Both disorders are more common in patients with ulcerative colitis than Crohn's disease. Pyoderma gangrenosum has also been found in patients with chronic active hepatitis, diverticulitis, primary biliary cirrhosis, gastric and duodenal ulcers, rheumatoid arthritis, myeloma, and collagen-vascular diseases. Erythema nodosum has also been found in patients with sarcoidosis, bacterial, viral, AFB and fungal infections, Behçet's, oral contraceptive use, and lymphoma.

❏❏ What haplotypes are most commonly associated with dermatitis herptiformis?

HLA-B8, -DR3, -DQw2.

❏❏ What gastrointestinal condition is associated with dermatitis herpetiformis?

Gluten-sensitive enteropathy.

❏❏ What treatment options are available for dermatitis herpetiformis?

Dapsone, sulfapyridine (in dapsone intolerant patients) and a gluten-free diet have all been offered as treatment options. A gluten-free diet will resolve the intestinal and skin lesions; however, the skin lesions respond more rapidly to medication. It can take five months to a year for the diet to eliminate the need for medication in most, but not all, patients with this condition.

❏❏ What diagnosis should be considered in a patient with periorofacial, intertriginous and perigenital circinate lesions with vesicles, crusting and postinflammatory pigmentation in association with glossitis, weight loss, diarrhea and diabetes?

Glucagonoma. Arising in the islet cells of the pancreas, glucagonoma is associated with a distinctive dermatitis referred to as necrolytic migratory erythema (NME). It is histologically similar to the lesions seen in acrodermatitis enteropathica and since the rash of NME may be an early sign in slow-growing tumors, this differential should be kept in mind.

❏❏ What gastrointestinal manifestations may be seen in patients with urticaria pigmentosa?

Gastric hypersecretion due to elevated plasma histamine leading to gastritis and peptic ulcer disease, diarrhea, abdominal pain, malabsorption in 30%, and abnormal liver tests, in particular alkaline phosphatase.

❏❏ What skin changes may be seen in patients with Hepatitis C?

Leukocytoclastic vasculitis, cryoglobulinemia, pruritis, porphyria cutanea tarda, erythema nodosum, urticaria, erythema multiforme, polyarteritis nodosa, lichen planus, jaundice and excoriations from itching.

❏❏ What skin changes may be seen in patients with Primary Biliary Cirrhosis?

Melanosis, predominantly in exposed areas, clubbing, scleroderma-associated features, lichen planus, jaundice, excoriations from itching, xanthomas on the hands feet and trunk, xanthelasma and occasionally tuberous xanthomas.

❏❏ What skin changes may be seen in patients with Wilson's disease?

Azure lunulae or bluish color of the lunular area of the nails and Kayser-Fleischer rings of the cornea.

GASTROINTESTINAL PATHOLOGY

Cory A. Roberts, M.D.

❏❏ Where in the esophagus are you most likely to find heterotopic gastric mucosa?

The cervical region is the most common location. This is also referred to as an inlet patch.

❏❏ What is the pathology of achalasia?

It is characterized, in part, by nearly complete absence of the myenteric plexus within the esophagus.

❏❏ What infectious agent and disease present a nearly identical clinical and pathologic scenario as idiopathic achalasia?

Infection with *Trypanosoma cruzi* causes Chagas' disease which results in findings similar to achalasia.

❏❏ In a patient with achalasia, what type of esophageal tumor occurs at an increased rate compared to control populations?

Squamous cell carcinoma.

❏❏ What is the most common type of esophagitis in biopsy specimens and what are the histologic features?

Reflux esophagitis is the most common type and is characterized by epithelial hyperplasia, elongation of the papillae, basal hyperplasia, spongiosis, vascular ectasia within the papillae and epithelial infiltration by neutrophils and eosinophils.

❏❏ In a biopsy of Barrett's esophagus, at what pH should one use an alcian blue stain to demonstrate the specific mucin seen in the specialized intestinal metaplastic cells?

The alcian blue stain should be at an acidic pH of 2.5.

❏❏ How frequently would you expect to see specialized columnar epithelial metaplasia in a biopsy of reflux esophagitis?

In about 10% of cases.

❏❏ List some risk factors for development of squamous cell carcinoma of the esophagus.

Smoking, alcohol, history of lye stricture, achalasia, previous radiation, Plummer-Vinson's syndrome, diverticula and tylosis.

❏❏ T/F: In progressive systemic sclerosis (scleroderma), the esophagus is commonly involved.

True. About 80% of patients have some esophageal abnormality.

❏❏ What is the typical age, race and gender of patients who develop squamous cell carcinoma of the esophagus?

Greater than 50 years old, African-American and male. It is interesting that whites have a higher incidence compared to blacks of adenocarcinoma arising in Barrett's esophagus.

❏❏ **What are the typical histological findings in the esophagus of a patient with progressive systemic sclerosis?**

Smooth muscle atrophy, fibrosis and hyaline thickening with luminal narrowing of small arterioles.

❏❏ **What is the most common type of tissue heterotopia in the stomach?**

Pancreatic tissue is most common and is usually present in the submucosa of the distal stomach, antrum or pylorus.

❏❏ **What organism is associated with development of lymphoma of gastric mucosa-associated lymphoid tissue (MALT)?**

Helicobacter pylori.

❏❏ **What stain(s) would you use to highlight *Helicobacter pylori* in a gastric biopsy tissue section?**

A number of stains can be used. Silver-based stains work very well but are more expensive. Inexpensive and easily performed stains commonly used are Giemsa and Diff-Quik.

❏❏ **What three forms of hypertrophic gastropathy are characterized by enlarged rugal folds?**

Menetrier's disease, hypertrophic-hypersecretory gastropathy and gastric gland hyperplasia in Zollinger-Ellison syndrome.

❏❏ **Describe the usual histologic appearance of Menetrier's disease?**

Gastric glandular atrophy with pronounced hyperplasia of the overlying superficial mucus producing cells.

❏❏ **What are the usual demographic characteristics and clinical presentation of the typical patient with Menetrier's disease?**

It is three times as common in men as women; typically ranges in age from the fourth to sixth decade of life; and, presents with weight loss, abdominal pain and occasionally peripheral edema.

❏❏ **Where in the stomach would you be most likely to find an adenomatous gastric polyp?**

The antrum.

❏❏ **T/F: Gastric polyps are frequently a component of familial adenomatous polyposis and Gardener's syndrome.**

True. Gastric polyps of some type (adenomatous, fundic gland, or hyperplastic/regenerative) are present in more than half of the patients. Most commonly, the polyps are of the fundic gland type.

❏❏ **According to Lauren, what are the two general categories of gastric carcinomas?**

Intestinal type (50%) and diffuse type (33%) with combinations making up the remainder. The classic linitis plastica is the most characteristic type of diffuse gastric carcinoma and is characterized by an infiltrating signet ring cell carcinoma.

❏❏ **Where are gastrinomas typically found in patients with Zollinger-Ellison syndrome?**

The majority are in the pancreas or duodenum.

❏❏ **What are the typical microscopic findings in the antrum in a patient with Menetrier's disease?**

Sorry, this is a trick question. The antrum is typically spared and the transition to the other involved areas is abrupt.

❑❑ **Describe the typical histologic features of so-called chemical gastritis?**

The foveolae are hyperplastic with increased luminal serrations, the antral glands are atrophic, the lamina propria is fibrotic with splayed smooth muscle fibers and there are increased number of congested and somewhat ectatic superficial capillaries.

❑❑ **How is autoimmune gastritis associated with pernicious anemia inherited?**

It is autosomal dominant with incomplete penetrance. It has a particularly high incidence in people of northern European descent.

❑❑ **What tumor of the stomach is seen at an increased rate in patients with autoimmune gastritis?**

Carcinoid.

❑❑ **What is the characteristic ultrastructural finding in carcinoid tumor cells?**

Dense core neurosecretory granules.

❑❑ **What is the most common site of origin of primary lymphoma in the gastrointestinal tract?**

The stomach in about 50% of the cases.

❑❑ **What is the most common site of origin of gastrointestinal stromal tumors (GIST)?**

The stomach accounts for about half of all cases.

❑❑ **A spindle cell tumor in the wall of the stomach is found to be CD117 positive via immunohistochemistry. What is the most likely diagnosis?**

Gastrointestinal stromal tumor (GIST).

❑❑ **What structure, if it persists, is the origin of persistent fibrous cord (from umbilicus to the bowel wall), enteroumbilical fistula and Meckel's diverticulum?**

The vitelline or omphalomesenteric duct.

❑❑ **What is the typical histology of a Meckel's diverticulum?**

This is a congenital anomaly which results from persistence of the proximal vitelline duct; is found within 90 cm of the ileocecal valve on the antimesenteric border; and, is usually lined by small intestinal mucosa. However, gastric, duodenal, colonic or pancreatic mucosa may also be found.

❑❑ **What is the "rule of two's" as it refers to Meckel's diverticulum?**

Meckel's diverticulum is found within two feet of the ileocecal valve, is two inches long, causes symptoms in 2% of cases, and is found in 2% of the population.

❑❑ **T/F: Hirschsprung's disease is more common in males than females.**

True. Hirschsprung's disease is characterized by a loss of both the submucosal (Meissner's) and myenteric (Auerbach's) plexuses with resultant nerve trunk hyperplasia. The gender incidence varies - males are four times more likely to have a short segment of affected colon while patients with long segments are more frequently female. In addition, 10% of Hirschsprung's disease is found in patients with trisomy 21 (Down's syndrome).

❑❑ **What is the main histologic finding in patients with gluten-sensitive enteropathy?**

Markedly blunted villi with an increased number of intraepithelial lymphocytes and plasma cells within the lamina propria.

❑❑ **What antibodies may be present in patients with celiac sprue?**

Anti-gliadin, anti-endomysial and anti-reticulin. There may also be antibodies to tissue transglutaminase.

❑❑ **What HLA type is found in 80% of patients with celiac sprue?**

HLA B8.

❑❑ **What would you expect to see histologically in the small bowel from a patient with disaccharidase deficiency?**

Normal small bowel mucosa.

❑❑ **Where would you look in a small bowel biopsy for the causative agent of Whipple's disease?**

The *Tropheryma whippelii* organisms reside in macrophages which are "stuffed" with organisms amidst an expanded lamina propria. These organisms can be confused with mycobacterial organisms. An acid fast stain is useful to differentiate between the two.

❑❑ **A 67 year-old man on chronic hemodialysis presents for further evaluation of chronic diarrhea. A small bowel biopsy contains glassy eosinophilic material which stains positively with a Congo red stain. What is the diagnosis?**

Gastrointestinal amyloidosis. Thioflavin T or S would also stain the amyloid.

❑❑ **What diagnostic methodology is necessary to diagnose microvillous inclusion disease on a biopsy?**

Electron microscopy. This autosomal recessive condition is characterized by absence of surface villi and, ultrastructurally, microvillous inclusions are found within the cytoplasm of the enterocytes. Unfortunately, death prior to the age of two is common unless small bowel transplantation occurs.

❑❑ **What is the inheritance pattern of abetalipoproteinemia?**

Autosomal recessive.

❑❑ **What condition of the large intestine typically occurs in premature infants, can be associated with umbilical artery catheterization and results in abdominal distention, loss of bowel sounds, bloody stools and the presence of pneumatosis intestinalis?**

Neonatal necrotizing enterocolitis.

❑❑ **If you suspect a patient has an adenocarcinoma of the small bowel, where would you most commonly expect to find it?**

The duodenum is the most common site of primary adenocarcinoma of the small bowel.

❑❑ **What specific race and disease might you expect to find in a patient with an endocrine tumor of the duodenum which is of the delta-cell type?**

African-American patients with von Recklinghausen's disease have an increased incidence of delta-cell type endocrine tumors of the duodenum. Delta cells produce somatostatin.

❑❑ **A tumor is resected from the ileum and your friendly pathologist tells you that grossly the tumor is well circumscribed, nodular and has a distinctly yellow cut surface. What type of tumor do you suspect this is?**

This is the classic appearance of a carcinoid tumor.

❑❑ **What autosomal dominant condition is found in people of Mennonite descent in Canada, is associated with diarrhea and dehydration in young childhood and can be deadly?**

Torkelson syndrome. These patients sometimes show evidence of common variable immunodeficiency. Histologically, the changes are nonspecific and include blunting of the villi, edema and focal acute inflammation.

❑❑ **What is acrodermatitis enteropathica?**

This is an autosomal recessive condition that is found in children, usually responds to administration of zinc sulfate and shows ultrastructural rod-like fibrillar inclusions within Paneth cells.

❑❑ **What pinworm would you expect to find either as an incidental finding in the appendix or, less commonly, associated with acute appendicitis?**

Enterobius vermicularis. This organism is found in about 3% of appendectomy specimens in the United States.

❑❑ **A patient has an appendectomy for acute appendicitis. Histologic sections of the appendix show multinucleated giant cells which are called Warthin-Finkeldey cells. What viral illness do you suspect?**

Warthin-Finkeldey cells occur in the prodromal stage of measles infection in the appendix. The patient will likely develop a typical measles rash in the near future.

❑❑ **What is a mucocele of the appendix?**

This is an etiologically nonspecific term that, unfortunately, engenders a great deal of confusion. It is probably best thought of simply as a descriptive term describing a dilated appendix filled with thick mucin. The causes include retention cysts, mucinous cystadenomas and mucinous cystadenocarcinoma.

❑❑ **A patient has a peritoneum which is filled with mucinous material. Histologically, sections demonstrate bland-appearing glandular epithelium floating in the middle of large pools of mucin. What is your diagnosis?**

Pseudomyxoma peritonei.

❑❑ **What is the difference between acquired and congenital diverticula?**

Acquired diverticula either lack a muscularis propria or it is greatly attenuated while congenital diverticula, such as a Meckel's diverticulum, contain all three layers of the intestinal wall.

❑❑ **What is the term given to describe the presence of numerous submucosal gas filled cysts which create polypoid projections in the mucosa of the bowel?**

Pneumatosis intestinalis. In children, it is associated with necrotizing enterocolitis and in adults there is usually an associated gastrointestinal disorder or chronic obstructive pulmonary disease.

❑❑ **How frequently is the ileum involved in Crohn's disease?**

About three-fourths of patients will have ileal involvement.

❑❑ **What is the term given to describe the type of colitis that is characterized by thickening of the subepithelial collagen band?**

Collagenous colitis.

❑❑ **What is the term given to describe the colitis characterized by increased numbers of intraepithelial lymphocytes that is characteristically seen in middle-aged women with watery diarrhea?**

Lymphocytic or microscopic colitis.

❑❑ **What is the normal, allowable number of lymphocytes per 100 epithelial cells in the surface epithelium of the colon?**

Five.

❑❑ **Discuss some of the microscopic features you would expect to see in a biopsy of solitary rectal ulcer syndrome (mucosal prolapse syndrome)?**

In spite of the name of "solitary", about one out of ten cases are not solitary at all but rather are multiple. The crypts are dilated with irregular branching which can impart a villiform appearance. The goblet cells are often mucin depleted and the lamina propria exhibits fibrosis and vascular congestion.

❑❑ **Behcet's syndrome in the colon is characterized by what histologic/endoscopic findings?**

It is characterized by ulcers occurring in various parts of the large intestine with an associated "lymphocytic vasculitis" of the submucosal veins. This can result in a colitis which may mimic Crohn's disease.

❑❑ **What is the most common polyp in children?**

Juvenile or retention polyp; however, again in spite of the name "juvenile", more than 30% of cases are diagnosed in adults. The most common site of occurrence is in the rectum.

❑❑ **T/F: Arteriovenous malformations in the large intestine are most commonly found in the rectum.**

False. The vast majority are in the cecum and ascending colon.

❑❑ **What are some of the basic histologic features of an adenomatous polyp?**

Decreased mucin production, nuclear pseudostratification and hyperchromasia, basal nuclear debris and either a tubular, villous or tubulovillous architecture.

❑❑ **Name three histologic features that help determine the presence of so-called pseudoinvasion of the stalk in an adenomatous polyp as opposed to true malignant invasion?**

1) The glands are surrounded by a loose lamina propria stroma not a desmoplastic tissue response.
2) There are associated hemosiderin-laden macrophages.
3) The glands in the stalk are identical to those that are more superficially located.

❑❑ **In what fashion is Peutz-Jeghers syndrome inherited?**

Autosomal dominant. It is characterized by multiple hamartomatous polyps of the gastrointestinal tract and abnormal pigmentation of mucosa and skin.

❑❑ **What is the malignant potential of the hamartomatous gastrointestinal polyps seen in Peutz-Jeghers syndrome?**

While these patients face a higher risk for development of a carcinoma, it is not related to the polyps. Rather, these unfortunate patients incur an increased rate of malignancy in other organs such as the breast or pancreas.

❑❑ **On what chromosome is the gene for familial adenomatous polyposis located?**

Chromosome 5q21.

❑❑ **What is the name of the syndrome characterized by the combination of adenomatous polyposis of the colon and associated tumors of the central nervous system, typically gliomas?**

Turcot's syndrome.

❑❑ **Where is the allele called DCC (deleted in colon cancer) located?**

On chromosome 18q where it encodes for a molecule in the cell adhesion molecule family. The expression of this protein is absent or markedly reduced in almost 75% of colon cancers.

❑❑ **In some patients with a genetic predisposition to development of adenocarcinoma of the colon, there is an abnormality of the DNA on chromosome 2. What is the abnormality?**

Microsatellite instability.

❑❑ **In a patient with an Astler-Coller stage B2 carcinoma of the colon, what would you expect the approximate five-year survival to be?**

Remember the Astler-Coller staging system:
Stage A - limited to the mucosa
Stage B1 - tumor extension into the muscularis propria without penetration or involved nodes
Stage B2 - tumor penetrates through the muscularis propria without involvement of regional lymph nodes
Stage C1 - penetration into the muscularis propria but not through it with positive lymph nodes
Stage C2 - penetration by tumor through the muscularis propria with associated involved lymph nodes
Stage D - distant metastatic spread.

A B2 tumor is associated with an approximate 50% five-year survival.

❑❑ **What is another name for hereditary non-polyposis colorectal cancer syndrome?**

Lynch syndrome.

❑❑ **Where in the colon do most carcinomas in the Lynch syndrome occur?**

They are typically right-sided.

❑❑ **What is the name of the syndrome composed of colorectal carcinoma with multiple sebaceous tumors and keratoacanthomas?**

The Muir-Torre syndrome.

❑❑ **What are the components and inheritance of Cowden's syndrome?**

It is characterized by the presence of oral mucosal papillomas, trichilemmomas of the face and acral hyperkeratosis. Approximately one-third of the patients have intestinal polyposis. Inheritance is autosomal dominant.

❑❑ **What is the Cronkhite-Canada syndrome?**

This syndrome is characterized by the presence of numerous gastrointestinal polyps and abnormalities of the nails termed onychodystrophy.

INFECTIOUS DISORDERS

John K. DiBaise, M.D., Eric B. Goosenberg, M.D., David S. Hodges, M.D.,
Elizabeth A. Lien, M.D., David McFadden, M.D.,
A. Steven McIntosh, M.D. and Bola Olusola, M.D.

❑❑ **Which infectious forms of esophagitis are most common in AIDS patients?**

Candida albicans, herpes simplex virus and cytomegalovirus.

❑❑ **What are the most common risk factors for *Candida albicans* esophagitis?**

Immunosuppression, most commonly due to AIDS or cancer chemotherapy, or suppression of normal oropharyngeal flora by antibiotic use.

❑❑ **Comparing *Candida albicans* esophagitis in AIDS patients to cancer patients receiving immunosuppressive chemotherapy, which group is more likely to have disseminated infection?**

Patients receiving chemotherapy. Isolated lymphopenia, seen in AIDS patients, limits *Candida* infection to the superficial layers of the esophagus, while chemotherapy-induced granulocytopenia is far more likely to allow dissemination of infection.

❑❑ **What underlying medical conditions increase the risk of developing *Candida albicans* esophagitis?**

Gastric hypochlorhydria, diabetes mellitus, adrenal dysfunction, alcoholism and conditions associated with impaired esophageal peristalsis such as achalasia, esophageal cancer and scleroderma.

❑❑ **How should an immunocompetent patient who recently received a course of antibiotic therapy and now has *Candida* esophagitis be treated?**

A non-absorbable oral agent such as nystatin is usually adequate.

❑❑ **How should an AIDS patient with oral thrush, dysphagia and *Candida* esophagitis be treated?**

A systemically absorbable anti-fungal agent such as fluconazole or ketoconazole should be given. Gastric achlorhydria may impair the absorption of ketoconazole, but this can be overcome with concurrent ingestion of a phosphoric acid-containing cola beverage.

❑❑ **How should a cancer patient with granulocytopenia and clear evidence of *Candida* esophagitis be treated?**

Intravenous amphotericin B can prevent and treat disseminated infection and it also is effective for systemic aspergillosis. Flucytosine may need to be added to amphotericin in life-threatening disease. Parenteral fluconazole is adequate for the treatment of candidiasis but does not cover aspergillosis.

❑❑ **T/F: Non-candida fungal infections (e.g., *Aspergillus, Blastomyces, Cryptococcus* and *Histoplasma*) of the esophagus occur only in severely immunocompromised individuals.**

True.

❑❑ **T/F: Biopsies of esophageal ulcers looking for Herpies simplex infection should be targeted toward the center of the ulcer, as the heaped-up margins are typically composed of normal epithelial cells.**

False. The opposite strategy is true. Herpes simplex preferentially infects the epithelial cells, which are present at the ulcer margins.

❑❑ **T/F: In the absence of immunosuppression, an individual with nasolabial herpetic lesions and concurrent esophageal symptoms should have endoscopic biopsies and cultures done before a diagnosis of *Herpes* esophagitis can be made.**

False. In this situation, a clinical diagnosis of Herpes esophagitis is likely enough to treat empirically.

❑❑ **How should Herpes simplex esophagitis be treated?**

Intravenous or high-dose oral acyclovir for 7 to 10 days is generally effective. The development of resistant strains of Herpes simplex may necessitate the use of intravenous foscarnet. Oral famciclovir or valacyclovir have excellent bioavailablilty and may replace acyclovir in the future.

❑❑ **T/F: Biopsies and culture specimens of esophageal ulcers, looking for cytomegaloviral (CMV) infection, should be targeted toward the center of the ulcer, as the heaped-up edges are typically normal epithelial cells.**

True.

❑❑ **T/F: A patient with known CMV infection who presents with new symptoms of dysphagia and odynophagia should be treated empirically for a diagnosis of CMV esophagitis without further diagnostic evaluation.**

False. Nausea, vomiting, fever, epigastric pain, fever and weight loss are usually the more prominent symptoms than are classic symptoms of esophageal infection. Endoscopy should be done to rule out a separate explanation for esophageal symptoms.

❑❑ **T/F: Patients with reactivation of herpes zoster infection on the chest wall who also have esophageal symptoms should be suspected of having zoster-associated esophagitis.**

True. Zoster-associated esophageal ulcers that endoscopically resemble those of Herpes simplex infection have been reported in this setting. These ulcers generally resolve with resolution of the skin eruptions.

❑❑ **What is the most common pathophysiology of esophageal involvement in tuberculosis?**

Esophageal tuberculosis is most often the result of spread from an infected mediastinal lymph node. Infection reaches the esophagus by way of a fistula or due to lymphatic obstruction. This infection has become much more common as a complication of AIDS.

❑❑ **What viral infections are associated with gastric ulcers?**

Cytomegalovirus and Herpes simplex type 1.

❑❑ **A biopsy from a gastric ulcer reveals granulomas. What is the differential diagnosis?**

Infection (tuberculosis, histoplasmosis), Crohn's disease, sarcoidosis and foreign body reaction.

❑❑ **Menetrier's disease is associated with what viral infection?**

Menetrier's disease in childhood is usually associated with gastric cytomegalovirus infection.

❑❑ **An acutely ill patient is found to have purulent gastric inflammation on endoscopy. What is the diagnosis?**

Phlegmonous gastritis. This has been associated with alpha-hemolytic streptococcus in about 50% of the cases. A variant, emphysematous gastritis, results from infection with gas-producing organisms.

❏❏ **What part of the gastrointestinal tract is most commonly involved in mucormycosis?**

The stomach. The typical lesion is a deep bleeding ulcer with black indurated edges.

❏❏ **A 23 year-old woman develops severe abdominal pain after eating sushi. Upper endoscopy reveals a small worm protruding from the mucosa. What is the diagnosis?**

Anisakidosis. This is acquired by eating sushi or other types of raw fish.

❏❏ **T/F: Histoplasmosis of the gastrointestinal system mainly affects the stomach.**

False. The colon and the ileum are the most common sites. The stomach is rarely involved.

❏❏ **What food is usually implicated in the vomiting syndrome caused by *Bacillus cereus*?**

Fried rice.

❏❏ **Improperly canned products may contain what potentially lethal infection?**

Clostridium botulinum. Its spores are resistant to heat and its neurotoxin can block acetylcholine at the neuromuscular junction, resulting in fatal respiratory muscle paralysis.

❏❏ **What potentally lethal infection is usually transmitted by drinking unpasteurized or poorly pasteurized milk/milk products?**

Listeria monocytogenes. Populations at risk include pregnant women and immunosuppressed persons. Meningitis can be a fatal occurrence with this infection.

❏❏ **What is the primary etiologic agent for large food-borne outbreaks of bacterial gastroenteritis in the United States?**

Salmonella.

❏❏ **Name three clinical syndromes associated with neurologic abnormalities (parathesias, ataxia, hypotension, seizures, muscle paralysis) that occur following ingestion of toxin-containing fish.**

Puffer fish poisoning (tetrodotoxin), paralytic shellfish poisoning (saxitoxin) and ciguatera poisoning (ciguatoxin)

❏❏ **What is the most common fish poisoning in the United States?**

Ciguatera. This is commonly seen in Florida, Hawaii and the Caribbean.

❏❏ **Which contaminated fish poisoning may cause flushing, vertigo and burning sensation and is effectively treated with antihistamines?**

Scromboid. Histamine-like substances cause the symptoms and histamine levels can be assayed in the implicated fish. Spoiled tuna, mackerel and skipjacks are often implicated. If any of these fish has an unpleasant odor or clouded eyes, it should be avoided.

❏❏ **Which strain of *E. coli* may cause hemorrhagic colitis and hemolytic uremic syndrome and has a high fatality rate?**

E. coli 0157:H7, also called enterohemorrhagic *E. coli*. It does not invade epithelial cells but produces at least two cytotoxins. It is usually asociated with consumption of inadequately cooked ground beef or raw milk.

❏❏ **What are differences between the enterotoxins produced by *Vibrio cholera* and *Clostridium perfringens*?**

Clostridial enterotoxin has maximal activity in the ileum and minimal activity in the duodenum, just the opposite of cholera toxin.

❐❐ What is the most common vehicle for *Clostridium perfringens* gastroenteritis?

Meat or poultry that is cooked, stored and then reheated. Heat-resistant spores that survive the cooking process germinate within the food during the cooling period. On reheating, sporulation of the cells occurs with subsequent enterotoxin production.

❐❐ If an individual travels to an underdeveloped country and develops fever and bloody stools, what is the most likely infection?

Shigellosis. While enterotoxigenic *E. coli* accounts for most cases of traveler's diarrhea worldwide, it produces a non-bloody diarrhea.

❐❐ T/F: A causative agent is found in most patients with traveler's diarrhea suffering from prolonged diarrhea.

False.

❐❐ Which newly described protozoan parasite is responsible for traveler's diarrhea in visitors to a number of underdeveloped countries?

Cylclospora cayetanensis.

❐❐ What parasitic infections are hazards in travelers to St. Petersburg, Russia (formerly Leningrad)?

Giardia lamblia and Cryptosporidium.

❐❐ What is the approach to patients with persistent traveler's diarrhea in whom a specific pathogen cannot be identified?

1) Treatment with an antibiotic directed at common bacterial pathogens.
2) Empiric course of antiprotozoal therapy if the above approach does not alleviate symptoms.
3) Endoscopic evaluation if the above fails.

❐❐ What is the current recommendation for the treatment of traveler's diarrhea?

For mild to moderate diarrhea (fewer than 4 bowel movements per day without blood or fever), either loperamide or bismuth subsalicylate can be used effectively. For more severe diarrhea, an antimicrobial drug should be used, usually a fluoroquinolone or trimethoprim-sulfamethoxazole. Antimotility agents should not be used when bloody stools or high fever are present.

❐❐ What is the risk of using antibiotics in patients with uncomplicated, nontyphoidal *Salmonella* gastroenteritis?

It increases the incidence and duration of intestinal carriage of the organism.

❐❐ With what clinical disorders should antibiotics definitely be used when *Salmonella* gastroenteritis is diagnosed?

1) Lymphoproliferative disorders.
2) Malignant disease.
3) Immunosuppressed hosts (AIDS, congenital or acquired forms).
4) Transplant patients.
5) Abnormalities of the cardiovascular system - prosthetic heart valves, vascular grafts, aneurysms, rheumatic or congenital valvular heart disease.
6) Foreign bodies implanted in the skeletal system.

7)   Hemolytic anemias.
8)   Extreme ages of life.
9)   Severe sepsis.

❑❏ **What condition predisposes to *Yersinia enterocolitica* septicemia?**

Iron overload states, such as in hemochromatosis, cirrhosis and hemolytic processes.

❑❏ **What intestinal infection can mimic acute appendicitis?**

Yersinia enterocolitica. This infection is most common in children. Abdominal pain frequently localizes to the right lower quadrant with peritoneal signs, mimicking acute appendicitis.

❑❏ **What infection is associated with raw or improperly stored seafood or food contaminated with seawater?**

Vibrio parahemolyticus.

❑❏ **What is the cause of tropical sprue?**

Current evidence suggests that tropical sprue results from an infectious disease of the small intestine caused by several offending agents, all of which are toxigenic strains of coliform bacteria, including *Klebsiella pneumoniae, Enterobacter cloacae* and *E. coli.* Travelers who acquire tropical sprue persist with bacterial contamination after return to a temperate climate until antibiotic treatment is given.

❑❏ **What is the treatment of tropical sprue?**

Tetracycline or non-absorbable sulfonamides given for several months. Additionally, daily oral folic acid and weekly parenteral B12 should be given when megalobastic anemia is present.

❑❏ **What symptoms may precede gastrointestinal complaints in Whipple's disease?**

Arthralgias and fever. Migratory arthralgias of the large joints may precede the onset of diarrhea by several years.

❑❏ **What is the diagnostic procedure of choice for Whipple's disease?**

Upper endoscopy with multiple biopsies of duodenum or proximal jejunum. Biopsies show infiltration of the lamina propria with PAS-positive macrophages containing Gram-positive, acid-fast negative bacilli.

❑❏ **In the absence of histologic evidence of Whipple's disease on small bowel biopsy, what further testing can be used to detect *Tropheryma whippelii*?**

Polymerase chain reaction of biopsied tissue.

❑❏ **Why should rectal biopsy not be used to diagnose Whipple's disease?**

PAS-positive macrophages resembling those seen in Whipple's disease may be found in the rectal lamina propria of normal people and in patients with benign conditions such as melanosis coli and colonic histiocytosis.

❑❏ **What condition resembles Whipple's disease histologically?**

Intestinal infection with *Mycobacterium avium intracellulare* in patients with AIDS. The histologic lesions in these two conditions are similar; however, *T. whippelii* will not take up acid-fast stain.

❑❏ **What is the most serious sequela in a patient treated for Whipple's disease?**

Neurologic sequelae, including irreversible dementia, may occur several months or years after successful treatment. This suggests that, unless an antibiotic that readily penetrates the blood-brain barrier is used, the central nervous system may provide a safe haven for residual Whipple's bacilli.

□□ What is the treatment of Whipple's disease?

Double-strength trimethoprim-sulfamethoxazole twice daily for a year. This antibiotic readily crosses the blood-brain barrier and should effecively eradicate central nervous system involvement. For patients intolerant of this drug, a third-generation cephalosporin such as ceftriaxone can be used.

□□ What is the treatment of a central nervous system relapse in Whipple's disease?

Repeat initial therapy with double-strength trimethoprim-sulfamethoxazole. If unsuccessful, chloramphenicol, which also results in high central nervous system concentrations, is given at a dose of 250 mg four times a day.

□□ What is the appearance of cryptosporidia on mucosal biopsy specimens?

On light microscopy, the trophozoites appear as multiple, round, tiny basophilic bodies lying on the brush border of enterocytes.

□□ After successful treatment of intestinal cryptosporidiosis in immunocompromised patients, what causes recurrence?

Seeding from the biliary tract, where cryptosporidia can also reside.

□□ How is *Isospora belli* detected in the stool?

Oocysts in the stool fluoresce bright yellow with auramine-rhodamine stain and appear pink with red-purple sporocysts on a modified acid-fast stain.

□□ What area of the intestinal tract is most commonly involved in histoplasmosis?

Terminal ileum.

□□ T/F: Histoplamosis can occur in an immunocompetent host.

True. Histoplasmosis is a very common infection in the midwestern and south-central United States, where 80% of inhabitants are infected. However, gastrointestinal disease is seen only in immunocompromised individuals.

□□ When should infection with microsporidiosis be considered?

When no other pathogens are identified in an immunocompromised patient with severe diarrhea, malabsorption and weight loss.

□□ What is the most specific diagnostic tool for detecting microsporidia in intestinal biopsy specimens?

Electron microscopy. Under light microscopy, the organism is difficult to identify.

□□ What type of surgery increases susceptibility to infection with salmonella?

Gastric surgery resulting in achlorhydria.

□□ Why should patients with underlying liver disease be warned about eating raw seafood, especially raw oysters?

Vibrio vulnificus infection can be acquired through direct consumption of seafood, usually raw oysters. Subsequent septicemia has a 50% mortality rate. This infection can be lethal in patients with underlying liver disease.

❏❏ **What severe intestinal complications may occur in typhoid fever?**

Perforation (3% of cases) and hemorrhage (20% in pre-antibiotic era). These events are not related to the severity of the disease and tend to occur in the same patient, with bleeding serving as a harbinger of a possible perforation.

❏❏ **What infectious agent causes most cases of sporadic bacterial gastroenteritis in the United States?**

Campylobacter jejuni. This accounts for 4% to 11% of all diarrhea cases in the United States.

❏❏ **The most common sites for intestinal involvement of tuberculosis are:**

Distal ileum and cecum.

❏❏ **What small intestinal parasite, once ingested, has part of its life cycle in the lungs?**

Ascaris lumbricoides. Duodenal larvae migrate through the epithelium into portal venous blood and eventually reach the lungs causing a pnuemonitis. Larvae then migrate up the bronchioles to the pharynx, are swallowed and develop into adults in the small intestine.

❏❏ **What tapeworm may cause vitamin B12 deficiency?**

Diphyllobothrium latum. The worm ingests vitamin B12 and thus competes with the host for available vitamin B12 .

❏❏ **What parasitic infestation may result in variceal bleeding?**

Shistosomiasis. Granulomatous fibrosis occurs around entrapped ova in pre-hepatic portal venules with relative sparing of hepatic parenchyma. This results in presinusoidal portal hypertension.

❏❏ **What are the types of diarrheagenic *E. coli*?**

Enterotoxigenic (ETEC), Enteropathogenic (EPEC), Enteroinvasive (EIEC), Enterohemorrhagic (EHEC), Enteroaggregative (EAEC) and Diffusely adherent *E. coli*.

❏❏ **What regions of the gastrointestinal tract do they tend to involve?**

Enterotoxigenic - small intestine.
Enteropathogenic - small intestine.
Enteroinvasive   - large intestine.
Enterohemorrhagic - large intestine.
Enteroaggregative - unkown.

❏❏ **What clinical syndromes are associated with ETEC?**

Diarrhea in small children in the developing world and traveler's diarrhea.

❏❏ **How does enteropathogenic *E. coli* (EPEC) cause disease?**

It causes adherence and effacement of enterocytes.

❏❏ **T/F: Stools from patients with enterotoxigenic *E. coli* are bloody.**

False. They are watery without blood or pus.

❑❑ **What is the site of infection with enteroinvasive *E. coli*?**

The colonic mucosa. Ulceration may occur as a result of this infection.

❑❑ **What other member of the Enterobacteriaceae is enteroinvasive *E. coli* like?**

Shigella. In fact, it may be misidentified as a *Shigella.*

❑❑ **Which *E. coli* strain is associated with hemolytic-uremic syndrome?**

Enterohemorrhagic *E. coli* (*E. coli* 0157:H7).

❑❑ **What are the components of hemolytic-uremic syndrome?**

The classic triad includes: 1) acute renal failure, 2) thrombocytopenia and 3) microangiopathic hemolytic anemia.

❑❑ **What is the classic histopathology characteristic of EHEC?**

Hemorrhage and edema in the lamina propria of the colon. On barium enema, a thumbprinting pattern in the ascending and transverse colon may be seen as a result of edema and mucosal hemorrhage.

❑❑ **What might a colonic biopsy from a patient with EHEC show?**

Biopsies from many patients have shown focal necrosis and infiltration of neutrophils. Pseudomembranes may also be seen.

❑❑ **What is the major virulence factor of EHEC?**

Shiga toxin.

❑❑ **How is *E. coli* 0157:H7 transmitted?**

It is usually transmitted via contaminated beef but may also be transmitted through contaminated juice, water and vegetables. Person-to-person transmission is also possible. The main reservoir is cattle.

❑❑ **T/F: There a seasonality associated with EHEC infection.**

True. In the developed countries of the northern hemisphere, it is more common in the summer.

❑❑ **What is the infectious dose of *E. coli* 0157:H7?**

One hundred to 200 organisms are sufficient to cause infection.

❑❑ **How long is the organism shed in the stool?**

One study showed that 66% were culture-negative after 7 days, even in the absence of antibiotic therapy.

❑❑ **What are the frequencies of the various syndromes for diagnosed cases of *E. coli* 0157:H7?**

10% nonbloody diarrhea; 90% hemorrhagic colitis.

❑❑ **What percentage of patients infected with *E. coli* 0157:H7 develop hemolytic-uremic syndrome (HUS)?**

In patients < 10 years old, approximately 10% develop HUS. It appears to be less common in adults.

❑❑ **T/F: All individuals with *E. coli* 0157:H7 should be treated with antibiotics.**

False. There is evidence that this may increase the incidence of HUS in children. Anti-diarrheal agents may also increase the risk of HUS.

❑❑ How does infection with *E. coli* 0157:H7 present?

The initial complaint is that of nonbloody diarrhea and vomiting in about half of these patients. In some individuals, this may be preceded by crampy abdominal pain and fever. After 1 to 2 days, the diarrhea becomes bloody and the abdominal pain may increase. The bloody diarrhea lasts about 4 to 10 days.

❑❑ What is the clinical outcome in patients infected with *E. coli* 0157:H7?

Most patients recover without apparent sequelae. In those < 10 years old, approximately 10% develop HUS. Three to five percent of affected children will die and 12% to 30% experience renal insufficiency, hypertension or central nervous system manifestations.

❑❑ How is *E. coli* 0157:H7 detected in the clinical lab?

The Center for Disease Control and Prevention recommends that bloody diarrheal stools and stools from patients with HUS be screened for *E. coli* 0157:H7 on sorbitol maconkey agar. This organism does not ferment sorbitol and thus is colorless on this medium.

❑❑ What are the species and groups of *Shigella*?

S. sysenteriae (group A)
S. flexneri (group B)
S. boydii (group C)
S. sonnei (group D)

❑❑ Which species of *Shigella* is the most common isolate in the United States?

S. sonnei (60% to 80%).

❑❑ How does *Shigella* produce disease?

Virulent *Shigella* invade the intestinal mucosa. This is the primary virulence factor. *Shigella* spp. can also produce an exotoxin, the shiga toxin.

❑❑ T/F: Blood cultures are usually positive with *Shigella* infection.

False. The organism rarely invades beyond the mucosa.

❑❑ Where in the intestinal tract does *Shigella* infection occur?

Within 12 hours, the bacteria transiently multiply within the small bowel. During this time, fever and abdominal pain may occur. After a few days, the bacteria are found diffusely in the colon producing microabscesses which coalesce and mucosal ulcerations. When the bacteria are in the colonic stage, urgency, tenesmus and bloody mucoid stools occur.

❑❑ T/F: There is a seasonality to *Shigella* infection.

True. It is more common in the summer.

❑❑ What is the typical clinical course of *Shigella* infection?

Early, fever and abdominal cramping occur and are followed by voluminous watery diarrhea (while bacteria are in the small bowel). Later, there is a decrease in fever but increase in stools of smaller volume. After a few days, bloody mucoid stools may occur with fecal urgency and tenesmus (when bacteria are in the colon stage).

❏❏ **How often do patients with *Shigella* develop fever or bloody stools?**

Nearly all patients with *Shigella* experience abdominal pain and diarrhea. Fever occurs in about 50%, mucus in stools in about 50% and grossly bloody stools in about 40%.

❏❏ **What are the laboratory findings in patients with *Shigella*?**

Sometimes the peripheral white blood cell count is elevated. Microscopic evaluation of feces show may polymorphonuclear leukocytes. On stool culture, since *Shigella* does not ferment lactose, colonies appear colorless on lactose-containing media. Serologic studies are not helpful in establishing the diagnosis but may be an epidemiologic tool for defining the extent of an epidemic.

❏❏ **T/F: Patients with *Shigella* infections should receive antibiotic treatment.**

True. All patients should be treated in order to shorten the duration of illness and to decrease spread of the infection.

❏❏ **What antibiotics are used to treat *Shigella*?**

Trimethoprim-sulfamethoxazole if acquired in the United States (160/800 b.i.d for 3 to 5 days). If acquired outside of the United States or if resistant to trimethoprim-sulfamethoxazole, a fluoroquinolone can be used.

❏❏ **Untreated, how long do patients with *Shigella* excrete the microorganism?**

About 1 to 4 weeks. The organism is carried in the colon. Long-term carriers are uncommon. Carriers usually respond to antibiotic treatment.

❏❏ **What host factor lowers the infectious dose in *Salmonella* infections?**

Lack of gastric acid. Acid is the first line of defense in *Salmonella* infections.

❏❏ **Describe the histology of nontyphoidal *Salmonella* infection.**

Massive neutrophil infiltration in both large and small bowel mucosa. Degranulation of neutrophils contributes to inflammation.

❏❏ **Who is at increased risk for infections due to *Salmonella*?**

AIDS patients, patients following organ transplantation or with a lymphoproliferative disease or chronic granulomatous disease, those with phagocytic overload (bartonellosis, malaria and schistosomiasis), sickle cell disease and neonates. In addition, those with decreased stomach acid, those receiving antibiotics and those with inflammatory bowel disease are at an increased risk.

❏❏ **Describe the clinical features of *Salmonella* gastroenteritis?**

Symptoms (nausea, vomiting and diarrhea) begin within 48 hours of ingestion of contaminated food or water. The diarrhea varies in volume but most are without blood or mucus. Fever and abdominal cramping occur in about 90% of cases. Fever resolves in 2 to 3 days and the diarrhea is usually self-limiting.

❏❏ **What is seen in the laboratory evaluation of a patient with *Salmonella*?**

Fecal leukocytes are seen on microscopic evaluation of stools. *Salmonella* sp. are nonlactose fermenters; therefore, the colonies appear colorless on lactose-containing media. Less than 5% of immunocompetent individuals will have positive blood cultures with nontyphoidal *Salmonella* infections.

❏❏ **How long will a patient carry *Salmonella* after resolution of *Salmonella* gastroenteritis?**

Nontyphoidal strains may be carried about 4 or 5 weeks. Less than 10% will still carry the organism by 10 to 12 weeks.

❑❑ What are the recommendations for treatment of *Salmonella* gastroenteritis?

Otherwise healthy persons with mild symptoms should not be treated with antibiotics because antibiotics may lead to longer carriage of the microorganism. Those with infection severe enough to be hospitalized or with the previously mentioned underlying conditions should be treated with fluoroquinolones or trimethoprim-sulfamethoxazole.

❑❑ What is the reservoir of *Campylobacter jejuni*?

Campylobacter is a zoonosis. It is most commonly acquired from poultry but also may be transmitted through raw milk, other dairy products and undercooked meat.

❑❑ T/F: There is a seasonality to *Campylobacter jejuni* infections.

True. Infections occur year round, but increase in summer and early fall.

❑❑ What are the sites of tissue injury in *Campylobacter* infections?

Jejunum, ileum and colon. Inspection shows diffuse, bloody edematous and exudative enteritis.

❑❑ What is seen on laboratory evaluation of a patient with *Campylobacter jejuni* infection?

Gram stain of stool shows Gram-negative (gull wing) bacteria. The sensitivity of diagnosis with Gram stain is 50% to 75%. Stool culture must be done using special media under microaerophilic conditions. Blood cultures are positive in less than 1%.

❑❑ What are some of the sequelae of *Campylobacter jejuni* infection?

There have been rare reports of septic abortion, cholecystitis, pancreatitis and cystitis. Those with immunoglobulin deficiencies may develop recurrent infection. A reactive arthritis may occur several weeks after infection in persons with HLA-B27. Guillian-Barré syndrome is uncommon. Of those with Guillian-Barré syndrome, 10% to 40% occur following C. *jejuni* infection.

❑❑ Describe the pathology of lesions seen with *Entamoeba histolytica* infection.

Colonic lesions range from nonspecific thickening of the mucosa to the classic flask-shaped ulcer. Twenty to fifty percent of patients have classic ulcers extending through the mucosa and muscularis mucosa and into the submucosa.

❑❑ Describe the extraintestinal pathology of *Entamoeba histolytica*.

Liver abscesses containing proteinaceous debris surrounded by a rim of trophozoites. Pleuropulmonary amebiasis can occur as a complication of amebic liver abscess. Intraperitoneal rupture of liver abscesses can also occur. Rarely pericardial, genitourinary and cerebral amebiasis occurs.

❑❑ How is infection with *E. histolytica* treated?

Ten day course of metronidazole followed by an intraluminal agent such as diloxanide furoate or paromomycin.

❑❑ What pathologic lesions are seen with *Cryptosporidium* infection?

In immunocompromised patients, cryptosporidium can be found on biopsies taken throughout the intestinal tract, hepatobiliary system and respiratory tract. In otherwise healthy individuals, it is mostly confined to the intestine. Villous atrophy, blunting, fusion or loss of villi, crypt hyperplasia and lengthening have all been observed. There may also be infiltration of the lamina propria with lymphocytes, neutrophils, plasma cells and macrophages.

❑❑ How is *Cryptosporidium* diagnosed in the laboratory?

Stools should be examined by modified acid fast stain. Intestinal biopsy can also be performed.

❑❑ How is infection with *Cyrptosporidium* prevented?

Water filtration. The organism is resistant to chlorination.

❑❑ What organism is associated with most cases of antibiotic-associated pseudomembraneous colitis?

Clostridium difficile.

❑❑ How is *C. difficile* colitis treated?

A seven to ten day course of oral metronidazole or oral vancomycin. For cases of suspected relapse, after reconfirmation of the diagnosis, retreatment with the standard course of oral metronidazole or vancomycin is recommended.

❑❑ What organism is most commonly associated with recurrent pyogenic cholangitis?

Clonorchis sinensis.

❑❑ Name four causes of multiple liver abscesses.

Gallstones, obstructing carcinoma of the bile duct, primary sclerosing cholangitis and congenital biliary anomalies such as Caroli's disease.

❑❑ Which lobe of the liver are liver abscesses most commonly found?

Right.

❑❑ How do amoeba cause focal infection of liver cells?

Amoeba multiply and block intrahepatic portal nodules.

❑❑ In the setting of an amoebic liver abscess, a sudden rise in bilirubin suggests what two clinical entities?

Superinfection or abscess rupture into the pertitoneum.

❑❑ In addition to intravenous antibiotics, what adjuvant therapy is necessary to ensure amoebic eradication?

A 20-day course of an intraluminal antibiotic such as iodoquinol. This is given in order to eradicate amoeba persisting in the gut.

❑❑ Alkaline phoshatase elevation disproportionate to bilirubin elevation is indicative of what clinical entity?

Space occupying lesion of the liver.

❑❑ A histologic finding of a liver abscess showing sulfur granules is suggestive of what organism?

Actinomyces israeli.

❏❏ **What are the intermediate hosts in hydatid disease?**

Man, sheep and cattle.

❏❏ **What parasite can predispose to intrahepatic gallstones?**

Ascaris lumbricoides.

❏❏ **What is the intermediate host for *Fasciola hepatica*?**

Lymnaeca trunculata - snail. Patients are infected by eating watercress infected with ingested forms of the fluke.

❏❏ **When is surgical treatment indicated for patients with infestation of the biliary tract by *Clonorchis sinensis* (Chinese liver fluke)?**

Surgical treatment is reserved for complications, such as biliary obstruction, due not only to the parasites themselves but also to secondary formation of stones and acute cholangitis. Some patients present with pancreatitis, presumably caused by passage of the stones or the worms. In addition to cholecystecomy and clearing the bile ducts of stones and flukes, improved biliary drainage by choledochoduodenostomy or transduodenal sphincteroplasty is thought to reduce the rate of recurrent biliary obstruction, which otherwise exceeds 40%.

❏❏ **What is one antibiotic that has been shown to have high concentration in bile and is useful in treating cholangitis?**

Ciprofloxacin.

❏❏ **What antibiotic can lead to the development of biliary sludge?**

Ceftriaxone precipitates a calcium salt that has the ultrasonic appearance of biliary sludge.

❏❏ **What factors are associated with the development of black pigment stones?**

Chronic hemolysis, as can occur in hereditary spherocytosis, thalassemia and the presence of mechanical heart valves; cirrhosis; total parenteral nutrition; and, advanced age.

❏❏ **What bacterial infection and anatomical deformity play a role in the formation of brown pigment stones?**

Escherichia coli and a juxtapapillary duodenal diverticulum.

❏❏ **What bacterial enzyme is responsible for hydrolysis of conjugated bilirubin and may play a role in the development of pigmented stones?**

Beta-glucuronidase.

❏❏ **What bacteria can cause acute cholecystitis and also be non-pathogenic in a carrier state?**

Salmonella.

❏❏ **Name two viruses that predispose to acute cholecystitis in an immunocompromised host.**

Cytomegalovirus and *cryptosporidium.*

❏❏ **What are the three most common organisms isolated from blood cultures in patients with cholangitis?**

Escherichia coli, *Klebsiella* and *Pseudomonas*. Anaerobes are isolated in approximately 15%.

❑❑ **What is the mechanism of biliary obstruction in tuberculosis?**

Obstructive jaundice is a rare complication of tuberculosis. The obstruction is caused by tuberculous infection in lymph nodes in the porta hepatis or the retroduodenal area that compresses the bile duct.

❑❑ **Eosinophilia, elevated alkaline phosphatase and cholangiography findings of filamentous filling defects with blunted tips in the bile duct suggest what infection?**

Clonorchis sinensis or *Fasciola hepatica.*

❑❑ **Which of the following primary duct stones has the highest culture rate of bacteria - black, brown, or cholesterol?**

Brown.

❑❑ **Charcot's triad plus what other two clinical features defines Reynold's pentad?**

Hypotension and altered mental status.

❑❑ **In Oriental cholangitis, which side of the hepatic ductal system most commonly develops strictures and intrahepatic stones?**

The left hepatic duct due to its more acute angle at the bifurcation.

❑❑ **Bacillary angiomatosis with peliosis is caused by what organism?**

Bartonella henselae or *Bartonella quintana.*

❑❑ **What is the treatment of Bacillary angiomatosis with peliosis in a patient with fever, abdominal pain and elevated liver tests?**

Antibiotic therapy with erythromycin or doxycycline.

❑❑ **What species of *Microsporidia* is responsible for causing AIDS cholangiopathy?**

Enterocytozoon bieneusi.

❑❑ **What are the most common viral infections of the pancreas?**

Mumps, Coxsackie B, Enterovirus, Epstein-Barr Virus, and Cytomegalovirus. In addition, the Hepatitis viruses A, B and C have also been reported to infect the pancreas.

❑❑ **What fungal infections can involve the pancreas and/or cause pancreatitis?**

Aspergillosis and Actinomycosis.

❑❑ **What parasitic infestations may involve the pancreas?**

Ascaris lumbricoides, Echinococcus granulosis, Giardia lamblia and *Plasmodium falciparum.*

❑❑ **T/F: The most common bacteria that cause pancreatic infections are Gram-negative enteric organisms.**

True. *Escherichia coli,* enterobacter and enterococcal species occur most commonly; however, *Staphylococcus aureus* is also frequently isolated.

❑❑ **A visiting shepherd from South America is transferred to your service with fevers, weight loss and diarrhea. A CT scan of the abdomen reveals a large calcified cyst with fenestrations in the pancreas and several smaller cysts nearby. What is your diagnosis?**

Hydatid cysts of the pancreas.

❏❏ What organism is responsible for hydatid cyst disease?

Echinococcus granulosus, or occasionally *E. multilocularis*, a parasitic worm that normally resides in the intestine of dogs.

❏❏ How is the diagnosis of hydatid disease made?

Diagnosis is based on history of exposure from endemic areas and characteristic radiographic findings. A negative serologic test does not necessarily exclude the diagnosis.

❏❏ What is the treatment of hydatid cysts of the pancreas?

Surgical excision, if technically possible, or high dose mebendazole or albendazole are the mainstays of treatment.

❏❏ T/F: The signs and symptoms of an acute pancreatic infection differ from those that occur with acute pancreatitis.

False. Epigastric pain, fever, nausea and/or vomiting are frequent symptoms. Signs include leukocytosis and elevations in serum amylase and lipase.

❏❏ How does the human immunodeficiency virus affect the pancreas?

Indirectly through secondary infections (*Mycobacterial* spp, fungi), infiltrative processes (lymphoma, Kaposi's sarcoma) or drugs used in its treatment (2',3' dideoxyinosine).

INFLAMMATORY BOWEL DISEASE

Renee L. Young, M.D.

□□ **T/F: Oral aphthous ulcerations may be seen in patients with Crohn's disease or ulcerative colitis.**

True. Oral aphthae occur in at least 10% of patients with active ulcerative colitis and typically resolve when this disease goes into remission. Aphthous ulcerations occur more commonly in Crohn's disease.

□□ **Kidney stones develop with increased frequency in Crohn's disease. What types of stones may be seen?**

Oxalate kidney stones are seen in 5% to 10% of Crohn's disease patients. Steatorrhea promotes excess colonic absorption of oxalate which leads to the development of oxalate kidney stones. Urate stones are seen less frequently and are often associated with the presence of an ileostomy and/or dehydration.

□□ **T/F: Crohn's disease patients are predisposed to gallstone formation.**

True. Fifteen percent to 30% of patients with small bowel Crohn's develop gallstones. Ileal dysfunction or resection leads to alterations in the bile salt pool.

□□ **Which patients with Crohn's disease are most at risk for the development of amyloidosis?**

Those with longstanding suppurative or fistulous complications.

□□ **Amyloidosis is an unusual but life threatening complication of inflammatory bowel disease. What is the most common presentation of this rare complication?**

Nephrotic syndrome. Amyloid may also be diffusely deposited in bowel, spleen, liver, heart and thyroid.

□□ **T/F: Primary sclerosing cholangitis is associated with both ulcerative colitis and Crohn's disease.**

True. Primary sclerosing cholangitis is seen less frequently in Crohn's disease. With either disease, it can be complicated by the development of cholangiocarcinoma.

□□ **In what trimester of pregnancy are relapses most frequently seen in women with Crohn's disease?**

First trimester. Approximately 75% of women in remission remain in remission throughout pregnancy, while only one-third of women with active Crohn's disease at the time of conception will achieve remission during pregnancy.

□□ **T/F: Crohn's disease almost always flares after delivery in recently pregnant women.**

False. The activity of the disease in the puerperium reflects disease activity at term.

□□ **On the basis of radiology and endoscopic findings, most patients with Crohn's disease can be subdivided into three anatomic groups. Name those groups and the approximate percentage of each.**

Colon alone - 15% to 25%
Small intestine and colon - 40% to 55%

Small intestine alone - 30% to 40%.

❑❑ What percentage of Crohn's colitis involves the entire colon, exclusive of small bowel disease?

Twenty-five percent. Crohn's disease involving the colon alone has more frequent involvement of the distal colon than those patients with ileocolitis. Only one-fourth of patients with Crohn's colitis exhibit skip lesions.

❑❑ T/F: "Skip" areas are characteristic of Crohn's disease. These areas appear normal grossly, radiologically, endoscopically and histologically.

False. "Skip" areas of the intestine may have normal or abnormal histology.

❑❑ T/F: Involvement of the rectum in a patient with colitis rules out Crohn's disease.

False. Although rectal sparing is characteristic of Crohn's disease and helps distinguish it from ulcerative colitis, the rectum can be involved.

❑❑ T/F: The siblings of a Crohn's disease patient are more likely to develop Crohn's.

True. They are about 17 to 35 times more likely to develop Crohn's disease than the general population.

❑❑ T/F: The incidence of Crohn's disease is declining.

False. Most recent studies throughout the world show a rising incidence of Crohn's disease and a declining incidence of ulcerative colitis.

❑❑ T/F: Smoking cessation has been associated with an increased relative risk for the occurrence of Crohn's disease.

False. Smoking is associated with an increased relative-risk for the occurrence of Crohn's disease by a factor of 2 to 5.

❑❑ Granulomas are a pathognomonic feature of Crohn's disease. Do these granulomas most resemble those seen in tuberculosis or sarcoidosis?

Sarcoidosis. The granulomas found in sarcoid and Crohn's disease lack central caseation.

❑❑ Describe the earliest endoscopic features of inflammation in Crohn's disease.

Mild mucosal hyperemia and edema are the earliest findings followed by aphthae or discrete ulcerations in more advanced cases.

❑❑ Describe how the mucosal surface acquires the "cobblestone" appearance frequently seen in Crohn's disease.

Longitudinal and transverse serpiginous ulcerations form and the intervening edematous mucosa swells.

❑❑ Crohn's disease consists of transmural involvement of the intestinal tract. The bowel wall becomes thickened and the lumen narrows. Surgeons describe "creeping fat" in Crohn's disease. What is "creeping fat"?

In Crohn's disease, the mesentery becomes thickened, edematous, hypervascular and fatty. Finger-like projections of this inflamed mucosa "creep" along the serosal surface of the intestine and encase the involved segment of the intestine.

❑❑ T/F: Sulfasalazine has been proven to maintain remission in Crohn's disease.

False. Most clinicians realize a benefit, especially in Crohn's colitis; however, sulfasalazine has been shown to be a remission-maintaining drug in ulcerative colitis only.

❑❑ **The gastrointestinal presentation of Crohn's disease in children and adolescents is similar to adults. Children, however, have prominent systemic complaints that often precede their gastrointestinal complaints by months to years. Name some systemic manifestations of Crohn's disease in children and adolescents.**

Arthralgias and arthritis are seen in approximately 15%. Weight loss, failure to thrive, growth failure, fever and anemia are all manifestations of Crohn's disease in children, particularly when the small bowel is involved.

❑❑ **Small bowel barium x-ray in Crohn's disease may demonstrate separation of barium-filled loops of small bowel. Why does this occur?**

Edema of the bowel wall, especially the deeper layers of the bowel, produces this separation.

❑❑ **When differentiating gastrointestinal tuberculosis from Crohn's disease, which of the following can be seen in both: fistulae, granulomas and/or normal chest x-ray?**

All may be seen in both conditions. Fistulization occurs less frequently in tuberculosis. Granulomas can be seen in mesenteric lymph nodes in tuberculosis when there are no granulomas of the bowel. Crohn's disease, however, only produces granulomas of the lymph nodes when they are also present in the bowel wall.

❑❑ **T/F: 6-mercaptopurine and azathioprine are efficacious in treating active Crohn's disease and maintaining remission; however, acute pancreatitits develops in about 3%. Patients who develop pancreatitis while on one of these drugs should be challenged with the other drug.**

False. Pancreatitis is reversible on withdrawing the drug but recurs upon rechallege with 6-MP or azathioprine. Pancreatitis secondary to one drug is an absolute contraindication to either drug.

❑❑ **What is the phenomenon called when a child develops inflammatory bowel disease at an earlier age than his/her parent?**

Genetic anticipation - a child develops the disease at an earlier age than did the affected parent.

❑❑ **T/F: Ulcerative colitis is more common in nonsmokers than smokers.**

True. The relative risk of developing ulcerative colitis in nonsmokers compared with smokers is 2.6. The risk is particularly high in former smokers and especially former heavy smokers.

❑❑ **T/F: There an association between ulcerative colitis and autoimmune disorders.**

True. There is an increased incidence of thyroid disease, pernicious anemia and diabetes.

❑❑ **What percentage of ulcerative colitis patients are p-ANCA positive?**

Perinuclear antineutrophilic cytoplasmic antibody occurs in 60% to 80% of ulcerative colitis patients and 20% to 30% of patients with Crohn's disease. This antibody is of the IgG type and its titer does not change with disease activity. However, the titers have been reported to decline after colectomy for greater than 10 years or after very long-standing disease remission. The significance of this antibody remains to be defined. Anti-saccharomyces cereviseae antibody (ASCA), an antibody associated with Crohn's disease, is currently undergoing evaluation for specificity and sensitivity in the diagnosis of inflammatory bowel disease.

❑❑ **Which is more common in patients with ulcerative colitis - pancolitis or distal colitis?**

Distal colitis. The disease is limited to rectosigmoid in 40% to 50%, is pancolonic in 20% and is left-sided in 30% to 40%.

❑❑ T/F: The rectum is always involved in ulcerative colitis.

False. There are rare exceptions when, in severe acute disease, the proximal colon is more severely involved than the rectum. Another etiology of apparent rectal sparing is in patients being treated with topical agents.

❑❑ T/F: The shortening and narrowing of the colon in patients with history of recurrent attacks of ulcerative colitis is due to fibrosis.

False. Fibrosis is uncommon in ulcerative colitis unlike Crohn's disease. The foreshortened colon is a result of abnormalities in the muscle layer.

❑❑ Inflammation is predominantly confined to the mucosa in ulcerative colitis. What specific area of the epithelium do the neutrophils attack?

The crypts, giving rise to cryptitis.

❑❑ T/F: Pseudopolyps spare the rectum.

True. The reason for this is unknown.

❑❑ T/F: Active ulcerative colitis with diarrhea is almost always associated with macroscopic blood.

True. If blood is not present, the diagnosis should be questioned.

❑❑ Why will patients with proctitis or proctosigmoiditis sometimes complain of constipation instead of bloody diarrhea?

Colonic motility is altered by inflammation. In distal proctitis, there is slowing of proximal colon transit and prolonged transit in the small bowel. Distal transit remains rapid.

❑❑ A 62 year-old woman presents with diarrhea and, during her evaluation, a flexible sigmoidoscopy is performed. The mucosa in the sigmoid is granular and slightly friable. Biopsies show a thick subepithelial collagen band. What is the diagnosis?

Collagenous colitis usually reveals a normal appearing mucosa on endoscopic exam; however, it can cause friable and granular mucosa. It can be differentiated from ulcerative colitis and infectious colitis by the thickened subepithelial collagen band. A normal collagen layer is 3 µm to 6.9 µm thick. In collagenous colitis, the layer is 7 to 93 µm thick. The diagnosis of collagenous colitis is usually not made unless the collagen layer is at least 10 µm thick. Of note, the disease can be patchy and more prominent in the colon than the rectum.

❑❑ A 20 year-old woman presents with rectal pain and pus coming from her rectum. Proctoscopic exam reveals granular rectal mucosa and a biopsy shows an intense neutrophil infiltration and Gram positive cocci. What is the diagnosis?

Gonococcal proctitis, included in the differential of ulcerative colitis, rarely presents with diarrhea but instead with rectal pain. Biopsy confirms the diagnosis.

❑❑ A patient with active ulcerative colitis and erythema nodosum was hospitalized and treated with intravenous steroids. All symptoms subsided and the patient was discharged on sulfasalazine and oral steroids. The patient returned with erythema nodosum over her lower extremities but no symptoms of active colitis. What is the etiology of the erythema nodosum?

Erythema nodosum is usually associated with active colitis and presents as multiple tender and inflamed nodules usually over the shins. It occurs in 2% to 4% of cases of active colitis. Erythema nodosum can also occur as a reaction to sulfasalazine. Mesalamine is another rare cause of erythema nodosum.

❏❏ **What haplotype is most often associated with primary sclerosing cholangitis?**

HLA-DR3 B8.

❏❏ **Which of the following inflammatory bowel disease patient-types is most often associated with primary sclerosing cholangitis: fulminant colitis requiring colectomy, proctitis, mild pancolitis?**

Mild pancolitis. In fact, the inflammatory bowel disease may remain undiagnosed until after the diagnosis of their liver disease in some patients. Colectomy is not protective against future development of primary sclerosing cholangitis.

❏❏ **T/F: Pseudopolyps or inflammatory polyps are a premalignant condition.**

False.

❏❏ **What type of ulcerative colitis patient is at greatest risk of developing colorectal cancer?**

Pancolitis with frequent exacerbations > Pancolitis with infrequent exacerbations > Left-sided colitis > Proctocolitis.

❏❏ **When should colonoscopic surveillance for dysplasia begin for patients with chronic inflammatory bowel disease?**

In patients with pancolitis, after 8 years of disease. In those patients with disease confined to the left colon, surveillance should begin after about 15 years of disease. Repeat surveillance, if no dysplasia is found, should be undertaken every 1 to 3 years.

❏❏ **T/F: The incidence of pyoderma gangrenosa is higher in ulcerative colitis compared to Crohn's disease.**

True. The incidence, while higher in ulcerative colitis, is only 1% to 5%. It is most often associated with extensive disease of long-standing duration. One-half to one-third of patients with pyoderma have inflammatory bowel disease.

❏❏ **T/F: Pericholangitis is the most common hepatic complication of inflammatory bowel disease.**

True, with a prevalence as high as 50% to 80%. These patients usually present with asymptomatic elevations of alkaline phosphatase.

❏❏ **T/F: The development of calcium oxalate stones in Crohn's disease occurs most often in patients with ileostomies.**

False. The presence of an ileostomy in a Crohn's patient predisposes to the development of urate stones resulting from decreased urine volumes related to high ostomy outputs. Calcium oxalate stones require an intact colon. With an absent or diseased ileum, fat malabsorption leads to unabsorbed fatty acids in the gut lumen. Calcium binds to the fatty acids instead of oxalate. Oxalate then binds to sodium (instead of calcium) and forms sodium oxalate, which is absorbed in the colon.

❏❏ **Granulomas in Crohn's disease occur more commonly in the mucosa or submucosa?**

The submucosa. This explains why granulomas are found more commonly in surgical specimens rather than endoscopic specimens.

❏❏ **T/F: Perforation of the colon occurs most often during the first acute attack of ulcerative colitis.**

True. Free perforation can occur without toxic megacolon and occurs more frequently in the left colon.

❑❑ A dermatologist refers you a patient with pyoderma gangrenosum. The patient has no gastrointestinal symptoms. What should you do?

Evaluate for the presence of inflammatory bowel disease. At least one-third of patients with pyoderma have inflammatory bowel disease.

❑❑ T/F: Infliximab, a mouse-human chimeric tumor necrosis factor antibody, is currently approved for treating ulcerative colitis unresponsive to other agents.

False. The approved use of infliximab is currently for the treatment of fistulizing Crohn's disease or Crohn's disease unresponsive to other treatments.

❑❑ T/F: Sacroileitis is symptomatic only when patients have active inflammatory bowel disease.

False. Of the extraintestinal manifestations of IBD, sacroileitis is not one that follows the course of the bowel disease activity.

❑❑ T/F: Patients with ulcerative colitis and are p-ANCA positive often have a more aggressive course.

True. These p-ANCA positive patients may have a more treatment-resistant (5-ASA products) disease and are more likely to develop chronic pouchitis after ileal pouch anastamosis.

❑❑ What effect does sulfasalazine have on fertility in males?

Sulfasalazine reduces the total sperm count and sperm motility. These effects are reversible with discontinuation of the drug.

❑❑ T/F: Fertility problems occur commonly in women with Crohn's disease.

True. Fertility is normal in ulcerative colitis but impaired in Crohn's disease. The exact explanation is yet unknown but contributing factors include impaired ovulation, fallopian tube blockage, dyspareunia and avoidance of pregnancy on medical advice.   Nevertheless, many women with inflammatory bowel disease become pregnant without difficulty and deliver healthy babies.

❑❑ Describe the clinical presentation of gastroduodenal Crohn's disease.

Nearly all cases of gastroduodenal Crohn's present with symptoms of peptic ulcer disease. Most cases are associated with more distal small bowel involvement.

❑❑ T/F: All inflammatory bowel disease medications should be stopped if a woman with the disease becomes pregnant or desires to become pregnant.

False.   A flare of inflammatory bowel disease during pregnancy is associated with higher infant mortality; thus, it is desirable to continue the medications. Patients with quiescent disease before pregnancy tend to have well-controlled disease during pregnancy. Many of the drugs used to treat inflammatory bowel disease have not been extensively studied in pregnancy. The 5-ASA preparations are considered safe to use during pregnancy. There is data on azathioprine in pregnant renal transplant patients that suggests this drug is safe in pregnancy. Methotrexate, ciprofoxacin and metronidazole are contraindicated during pregnancy. Extensive counseling should take place with each patient concerning the risks, benefits and alternatives of medication use during and after pregnancy.

❑❑ T/F: Olsalazine frequently causes watery diarrhea.

True. Sixteen percent of patients on olsalazine develop watery diarrhea. Gradual titration of the dose and the administration of olsalazine with meals may reduce the incidence of diarrhea.

❏❏ **In patients with ulcerative colitis requiring colectomy, which patients should not be considered for ileoanal pouch construction?**

Women with multiple pregnancies, women with difficult deliveries, older patients and patients with diminished anal sphincter tone. The most important contraindication to the ileoanal pouch anastomosis is poor anal sphincter function. The patient groups listed are all at risk for anal sphincter dysfunction.

❏❏ **Crohn's disease patients that develop short fibrotic symptomatic strictures should be sent for surgical intervention and stricturoplasty. List contraindications of stricturoplasty.**

Sepsis, perforation, phlegmon, fistula (enteroenteric or enterocutaneous - in the area of the stricturoplasty), multiple strictures in a short segment that might lend itself better to a single resection, gross ulceration and fragile mucosa at the site, colonic stricture and carcinoma.

❏❏ **A 41 year-old man with a 15 year history of pancolonic ulcerative colitis that is currently in remission undergoes surveillance colonoscopy. A single biopsy shows definite high-grade dysplasia (confirmed by a second expert pathologist). What should you recommend to the patient?**

Colectomy should be performed when high-grade dysplasia is found either in flat mucosa or a mass lesion (DALM).

❏❏ **A 30 year-old woman with long-standing, well-controlled ulcerative colitis undergoes surveillance colonoscopy. The colonoscopy is essentially normal but biopsies reveal low-grade dysplasia (confirmed by a second expert pathologist). What should you recommend to the patient?**

When low-grade dysplasia occurs in flat mucosa or a mass lesion (DALM), the high risk of progression to high-grade dysplasia or cancer warrant a policy of early colectomy. Some have recommended more rigorous surveillance colonoscopy in this situation, but this is controversial.

❏❏ **T/F: Adenomatous polyps occur in patients with and without inflammatory bowel disease. The management of adenomas in patients with ulcerative colitis differs from that in patients without the colitis.**

True. Colitis-associated cancer typically arises from flat mucosa or a dysplasia-associated lesion or mass (DALM). A polyp should be presumed to represent a DALM if it occurs in involved mucosa. Pedunculated or sessile polyps that occur in uninvolved mucosa in patients who do not have pancolitis should be managed as they would in a patient without colitis. If a sessile adenoma is found within involved bowel, a colectomy may be the most prudent clinical action. When a pedunculated adenoma arises in involved bowel, the bowel around the polyp should be sampled after performing a polypectomy. If there is no evidence of dysplasia in the surrounding mucosa or elsewhere, a colectomy is not necessary.

❏❏ **T/F: Prophylactic use of mesalamine or metronidazole has been proven to prevent postoperative recurrence of Crohn's disease.**

False.

MALDIGESTION AND MALABSORPTION

Themistodes Dasopoulos, M.D. and Eli D. Ehrenpreis, M.D.

❏❏ **What are common signs and symptoms of malabsorptive disorders?**

Patients usually describe diarrhea (typically large volume) and associated weight loss. Associated symptoms include fatigue due to anemia, bloating and flatulence, bruising from vitamin K deficiency, skin rashes, muscle wasting and paresthesias.

❏❏ **What clinical features suggest a functional cause in chronic diarrhea?**

Duration of symptoms greater than one year, straining with defecation, lack of significant weight loss and absence of nocturnal diarrhea.

❏❏ **How is the fecal osmotic gap calculated and how is it used?**

The following formula is used: $290 - 2([Na^+] + [K^+])$. The normal osmolality of stool within the distal intestine (estimated as 290 mOsm/kg) should be used rather than the measured stool osmolality, because, in the collected specimen, bacterial fermentation of unabsorbed carbohydrates into osmotically active organic acids raises the measured osmolality. An osmotic gap > 125 mOsm/kg occurs in pure osmotic diarrhea whereas an osmotic gap < 50 occurs in pure secretory diarrhea.

❏❏ **How is steatorrhea defined?**

Steatorrhea is defined as a daily fecal fat output > 7 grams/day (9% of dietary fat intake). A fecal fat > 14 grams/day is indicative of markedly impaired fat digestion or absorption.

❏❏ **Describe a bedside test for laxative use/abuse.**

Alkalinization of 3 ml of stool supernatant or urine with one drop of concentrated (1 N) sodium hydroxide will result in a pink or red color if phenolphthalein is present. More sophisticated stool and urine tests are available for the detection of other laxatives. Stool sulfate, phophate and magnesium analysis detects those factitious diarrheas caused by osmotic cathartics.

❏❏ **What is pancreatic cholera?**

Pancreatic cholera is a rare type of secretory diarrhea caused by the release of vasoactive intestinal peptide into the circulation by a neuroendocrine tumor. It should be suspected in diarrhea lasting longer than 4 weeks with the clinical features of secretory diarrhea, a volume always greater than 1 liter/day, marked hypokalemia, hypochlorhydria and severe dehydration.

❏❏ **What serologic tests are available for the diagnosis of celiac sprue?**

The antiendomysial IgA antibody, detected by indirect immunofluorescence, is the most sensitive and specific serologic test for celiac sprue. ELISA antigliadin IgA and IgG antibodies are inexpensive but less sensitive and specific. The antigliadin IgG antibody should be checked in patients with known or suspected IgA deficiency. The prevalence of IgA deficiency is increased approximately 10-fold among patients with celiac sprue.

❏❏ **Describe the classic endoscopic appearance of the small intestine in celiac sprue.**

Scalloping, nodularity and/or absence of the small intestinal plicae (circular folds).

❑❑ **Name five causes of chronic diarrhea in which an endoscopically normal colonic mucosa is present.**

Microscopic colitis (lymphocytic and collagenous), amyloidosis, Whipple's disease, granulomatous infections, and helminthic infections.

❑❑ **Name some diseases associated with chronic diarrhea that may be diagnosed by small intestinal biopsy.**

Crohn's disease, giardiasis, celiac sprue, intestinal lymphoma, eosinophilic gastroenteritis, hypogammaglobulinemic sprue, Whipple's disease, lymphangiectasia, abetalipoproteinemia, amyloidosis, mastocytosis, and various mycobacterial, fungal, protozoal and parasitic infections.

❑❑ **Describe some clinical manifestations of celiac sprue.**

In addition to the signs and symptoms common to all malabsorptive disorders, the following may be seen in patients with celiac sprue: occult blood in the stool, thrombocytosis (hyposplenism), demyelinating central nervous system lesions, seizures and liver enzyme abnormalities.

❑❑ **What is the relationship between celiac sprue and dermatitis herpetiformis (DH)?**

More than 90% of patients with DH and the granular pattern of IgA deposition at the derma-epidermal junction, and at least 10% of patients with a linear pattern have coexisting celiac sprue. Many lack significant symptoms of the disease because the lesion is often mild and limited to the proximal intestine. Conversely, fewer than 10% of patients with celiac sprue have DH.

❑❑ **Name some diseases associated with celiac sprue.**

Dermatitis herpetiformis, type I diabetes mellitus, Down's syndrome, selective IgA deficiency, autoimmune thyroid disease and microscopic colitis. Less convincing but possible associations have been reported between celiac sprue and juvenile rheumatoid arthritis, epilepsy with cerebral calcification, primary biliary cirrhosis, primary sclerosing cholangitis and IgA nephropathy.

❑❑ **Which D-xylose test is preferable, the 1-hour serum test, or the 5-hour urine test?**

The 1-hour serum D-xylose test is preferable. The 5-hour urine test can be falsely abnormal in patients with renal insufficiency, incomplete urine specimen collection and a variety of other conditions.

❑❑ **What is the auto-antigen recognized by the antiendomysial antibody?**

The antigen is tissue transglutaminase (TTG), a calcium-dependent enzyme that catalyzes cross-links between glutamine and lysine residues in substrate proteins. TTG is believed to cross-link gliadin, rendering it immunogenic.

❑❑ **T/F: The mucosal lesion seen in celiac sprue is specific for that disorder.**

False. Identical or very similar mucosal lesions (villous atrophy and infiltration of the lamina propria with chronic inflammatory cells) can be seen with other inflammatory disorders including tropical sprue, giardiasis, diffuse lymphoma, autoimmune enteritis, Crohn's disease, bacterial overgrowth, viral gastroenteritis, and the marked gastric acid hypersecretion associated with gastrinoma. However, a completely flat mucosa is most suggestive of celiac sprue.

❑❑ **Name clinical conditions associated with bacterial overgrowth of the small intestine.**

1) Small intestinal stagnation due to anatomical derangements (Billroth II gastrectomy, duodenal or jejunal diverticulosis, surgical blind loop, obstruction).
2) Motor disorders (scleroderma, intestinal pseudo-obstruction, diabetic gastroenteropathy).
3) Intestinal fistulae or resected ileocecal valve.
4) Other conditions such as achlorhydria, immunodeficiency states and chronic pancreatitis.

❑❑ **What is the suggested pathophysiology of "diabetic diarrhea"?**

Since most patients with diabetic diarrhea also have autonomic neuropathy, this condition was classically thought to be due to disordered motility. More recently, sympathetic denervation with decreased enterocyte α-2 adrenergic receptors has been described and this is thought to result in decreased intestinal absorptive function. Steatorrhea and bile salt malabsorption may also occur in these patients. Other causes of diarrhea in diabetic patients include bacterial overgrowth, celiac sprue, microscopic colitis, pancreatic dysfunction and, rarely, islet cell tumors (glucagonoma, vipoma, somatostatinoma).

❑❑ **How does eosinophilic gastroenteritis present?**

Eosinophilic gastroenteritis may involve any layer of the gut wall, from the mucosa to the serosa. Manifestations of eosinophilic gastroenteritis include nausea, vomiting, diarrhea, weight loss, iron deficiency, malabsorption, protein-losing enteropathy, pyloric outlet or intestinal obstruction, and eosinophilic ascites.

❑❑ **A 72 year-old woman presents with memory loss and a borderline low vitamin B12 level (< 250 pg/mL) is found. How can a definitive diagnosis of vitamin B12 deficiency be made?**

Elevated serum methylmalonic acid and homocysteine levels establish the presence of vitamin B12 deficiency at the tissue level.

❑❑ **What are the most common causes of chronic diarrhea?**

Irritable bowel syndrome, inflammatory bowel disease, microscopic colitis, malabsorption due to small intestinal or pancreatic diseases, enteric infection, medications and post gastrectomy/ vagotomy state.

❑❑ **What is the most consistent laboratory abnormality that may occur in small bowel bacterial overgrowth?**

Vitamin B12 malabsorption is the most consistent abnormality and can be documented with a Schilling test. Normalization of the Schilling test after treatment with antibiotics (also called the stage IV Schilling test) confirms that bacterial overgrowth is the source of vitamin B12 malabsorption. Interestingly, serum folate levels are frequently elevated because of bacterial production of folate.

❑❑ **What tests are available to diagnose small bowel bacterial overgrowth syndrome?**

The gold standard for the diagnosis of bacterial overgrowth is quantitative small bowel culture. Bacterial concentrations greater than 10^5 colony forming units/ml indicate bacterial overgrowth. Several different breath tests (C^{14}-D-xylose, glucose-H^2 and lactulose-H^2) are also available; however, there is controversy regarding the sensitivity and specificity of these tests. A therapeutic trial of antibiotics is often also used as a 'diagnostic' tool.

❑❑ **Explain the mechanism of calcium oxalate stone formation in Crohn's disease.**

This condition is termed enteric hyperoxaluria. Bile salt malabsorption due to ileal disease or resection may result in fat malabsorption. Intraluminal fatty acids bind calcium cations, which would otherwise bind to intestinal oxalate. Free oxalate thus enters the colon where it is absorbed and then renally excreted, causing calcium oxalate stones. Prevention of calcium oxalate stones in patients with Crohn's disease involves limitation of fat and oxalate intake, as well as calcium supplementation. A patient who has undergone a colectomy cannot develop enteric hyperoxaluria.

❑❑ **How does ileal resection lead to diarrhea?**

1) Resection of less than 100 cm leads to bile salt wasting. Bile salts are deconjugated in the colon where they cause a secretory diarrhea. Bile salt wasting is compensated by increased bile salt synthesis in the liver leading to normal fat absorption.
2) Resection of greater than 100 cm of ileum leads to depletion of the bile salt pool, steatorrhea and a secretory diarrhea related to the laxative effect of hydroxylated fatty acids.

❑❑ **What disorders can be diagnosed on the basis of an endoscopic small bowel biopsy?**

Whipple's disease, common variable immunodeficiency, abetalipoproteinemia and *Mycobacterium avium* complex infection causes characteristic lesions that involve the small bowel mucosa diffusely. Characteristic, but patchy lesions, may also be seen with lymphoma, lymphangiectasia, eosinophilic enteritis, mastocytosis, amyloidosis, Crohn's disease, collagenous sprue, giardiasis and cryptosporidiosis. These diseases may therefore be missed on endoscopic small bowel biopsy.

❑❑ **Name some complications specific to celiac sprue?**

Development of malignancy (small bowel lymphoma, extra-intestinal lymphoma, small bowel adenocarcinoma, esophageal squamous cell carcinoma), refractory sprue, collagenous sprue and ulcerative jejunoileitis.

❑❑ **What is collagenous sprue?**

Collagenous sprue is a rare disorder that presents with symptoms identical to celiac sprue. However, small intestinal biopsies show excess collagen deposition in the lamina propria beneath the epithelial layer. Patients with this condition have a poor prognosis as they do not respond to a gluten-free diet.

❑❑ **What mechanisms may be responsible for diarrhea in Crohn's disease?**

Small bowel inflammation, small bowel bacterial overgrowth, surgical resection, fistulae, cholerrhetic diarrhea and steatorrhea.

❑❑ **What are some components of prescription and non-prescription medications that may cause malabsorption in certain individuals?**

Gluten, lactose and polyols (sorbitol, mannitol, and xylitol).

❑❑ **A 15 year-old boy presents with chronic diarrhea. You elicit a history of recurrent upper respiratory infections. What is your next test?**

A sweat test to rule out cystic fibrosis.

❑❑ **What are the sites of protein digestion?**

Lumen of the stomach and small intestine (pepsin, pancreatic proteases), brush border of the enterocyte (peptidases), and cytoplasm of the enterocyte (peptidases).

❑❑ **What are the sites of carbohydrate digestion?**

Intestinal lumen (salivary and pancreatic amylase), brush border of the enterocyte (sucrase, lactase, glucoamylase).

❑❑ **What are the enzymes involved in fat digestion?**

Acid lipases (lingual lipase, gastric lipase) and the pancreatic lipases. Pancreatic carboxyl ester lipase hydrolyzes triglycerides, cholesterol, vitamin esters and other substrates. Pancreatic phospholipase A2 hydrolyzes phosphatidylcholine, phosphatidylethanolamine, phosphatidylserine and cardiolipin.

❑❑ **What medications may result in malabsorption of vitamins and other nutrients?**

Antacids, mineral oil, cholestyramine, methotrexate, chemotherapeutic agents, phenytoin, orlistat, sulfasalzine and sucralfate.

❑❑ **Name some medications that can cause secretory diarrhea.**

Laxatives, cholinergic agents, quinidine and quinine, colchicine, metoclopramide, misoprostol, olsalazine, theophylline and thyroid preparations.

❑❑ What enteric infections may cause a protracted diarrhea?

Enteropathogenic *E. coli*, Giardia, Amoeba, Cryptosporidium, Microsporidia and Isospora. Aeromonas and *Yersinia enterocolitica* can both present with an acute or chronic watery diarrhea syndrome, or colitis. *Clostridium difficile* infection frequently relapses.

❑❑ What are the mechanisms causing diarrhea in Zollinger-Ellison (ZE) syndrome?

High volumes of secreted hydrochloric acid, fat maldigestion due to inactivation of pancreatic lipase, and bile acid precipitation due to the low duodenal pH. Diarrhea occurs in up to one-third of patients with the ZE syndrome, may precede the other symptoms and may be the major clinical manifestation of the disease.

❑❑ What is the Cronkhite-Canada syndrome?

The Cronkhite-Canada syndrome is a non-inherited polyposis syndrome characterized by hamartomatous polyps found throughout the gastrointestinal tract and by a severe protein-losing enteropathy due to a diffuse mucosal injury of obscure etiology. Clinical features also include cutaneous hyperpigmentation, alopecia and nail atrophy.

❑❑ A 44 year-old man with chronic diarrhea has a fecal osmotic gap < 50 and fecal sodium > 90. The diarrhea ceases with fasting. What is the diagnosis?

The fecal osmotic gap and sodium concentration are consistent with a secretory diarrhea. However, the cessation of diarrhea with fasting argues against secretory diarrhea. Ingestion of sodium sulphate or sodium phosphate would cause an osmotic diarrhea that mimics a secretory diarrhea because of the high sodium content.

❑❑ How is the Schilling test performed?

An intramuscular dose of nonlabeled vitamin B12 (usually 1000 micrograms) is administered in order to saturate liver binding sites. Oral radiolabeled vitamin B12 is then administered and urine radioactivity is measured over 24 hours. Appearance of less than 10% of the radiolabeled vitamin B12 in the urine is considered diagnostic of vitamin B12 malabsorption. If vitamin B12 malabsorption is corrected by administration of intrinsic factor, this establishes intrinsic factor deficiency (Stage II Schilling test). If vitamin B12 malabsorption is corrected with pancreatic enzymes (Stage III) or with antibiotics (Stage IV), then the test establishes pancreatic insufficiency or bacterial overgrowth, respectively. If the test does not correct with any of these maneuvers, then the cause of malabsorption is ileal disease or resection.

❑❑ What tests are useful for determining enteric protein loss?

Twenty-four hour stool collection for determination of chromium[51]-albumin clearance and α_1-antitrypsin clearance.

❑❑ What tests are available to test pancreatic function?

The pancreatic stimulation tests (secretin test, cholecystokinin test and Lundh test meal) require intestinal intubation and collection of pancreatic secretions, and are time consuming. The so-called "tubeless" tests include the bentiromide test, the pancreolauryl test and the dual-label Schilling test.

❑❑ Name some causes of lactase deficiency.

Acquired deficiency in adulthood, small intestinal disease or resection, and autosomal recessive congenital deficiency.

❑❑ Describe the clinical features and genetic defect of abetalipoproteinemia.

Abetalipoproteinemia is a rare autosomal recessive disorder of lipoprotein metabolism characterized by extremely low levels of serum cholesterol and triglycerides and the absence of apoB-containing lipoproteins. Clinical manifestations include malabsorption, neurological symptoms such as spinocerebellar dysfunction, retinopathy that causes impairment of night and color vision, and acanthotic erythrocytes. Mutations of the microsomal triglyceride transfer protein have been shown to cause abetalipoproteinemia.

❑❑ **What are the clinical features of intestinal lymphatic obstruction?**

Hypoalbuminemia, hypoglobulinemia, lymphopenia, peripheral edema, ascites, and even anasarca. The differential diagnosis of intestinal lymphatic obstruction includes congenital intestinal lymphangiectasia, cardiac disease, Whipple's disease, Crohn's disease, mesenteric tuberculosis, mesenteric sarcoidosis, lymphoma and lymphenteric fistula.

❑❑ **What are causes of iron deficiency occurring after gastric surgery?**

Gastric acid dissociates iron salts from food and dissolves them. The achlorhydric stomach cannot release food-bound iron. In addition, patients who have undergone antrectomy have defective meat digestion so that heme proteins (myoglobin, hemoglobin) cannot be digested properly by pancreatic proteases to liberate the heme-iron complexes. Finally, iron deficiency may result from decreased food intake and blood loss from gastritis.

❑❑ **Name some systemic diseases associated with malabsorption.**

Thyrotoxicosis, hypothyroidism, Addison's disease, hypoparathyroidism, diabetes mellitus, scleroderma and AIDS.

❑❑ **What is the ^{14}C-glycocholic acid breath test?**

This test is used in the diagnosis of bacterial overgrowth. ^{14}C-glycocholic acid undergoes peptide hydrolysis by bacteria, releasing ^{14}C-glycine. ^{14}C-glycine is then absorbed and metabolized to ^{14}CO$_2$ which is then excreted in expired air. Increased ^{14}CO$_2$ excretion occurs with bacterial overgrowth but also can be seen with bile acid malabsorption. Measurement of fecal radioactivity helps distinguish between these two possibilities.

❑❑ **How is tropical sprue treated?**

Initial treatment includes correction of fluids, electrolytes and deficient nutrients. Tetracycline and folic acid are given as pharmacotherapy. The beneficial effect of treatment with folic acid suggests that folate deficiency plays a role in perpetuating the intestinal lesion of tropical sprue. It is recommended that treatment be continued for several months.

❑❑ **What are clinical features of Whipple's disease?**

Diarrhea with steatorrhea, fever, arthritis, lymphadenopathy, pericarditis, endocarditis, myocarditis, dementia, depression, choreoathetosis and ophthalmoplegia. This condition is caused by a Gram positive bacillus called *Tropheryma whippelii*. Treatment ususally consists of double-strength trimethoprim-sulfamethoxazole twice daily for one year.

❑❑ **What are causes of PAS-positive macrophages present in the lamina propria seen on intestinal biopsy?**

In the past, the finding of lamina propria PAS-positive macrophages was diagnostic of Whipple's disease. More recently, it has been recognized that PAS-positive macrophages are also seen with atypical mycobacterial infections. The acid-fast stain distinguishes between the two.

❑❑ **What are the most common causes of short bowel syndrome in children?**

Congenital short bowel (2/3) and necrotizing enterocolitis (1/3).

❑❑ **What is the most common cause of short bowel syndrome in adults?**

Crohn's disease requiring multiple bowel resections (60%-80%). The next most common cause is small intestinal resection secondary to thrombosis of the mesenteric arteries and veins.

❑❑ **What is the pathophysiology and clinical features of D-lactic acidosis?**

D-lactic acidosis is a rare complication of short bowel syndrome that occurs as a result of carbohydrate overfeeding and, possibly, antibiotic use. Malabsorbed carbohydrate is metabolized by colonic bacteria to short-chain fatty acids and lactate which, in turn, lower colonic pH. A lower colonic pH favors the growth of D-lactate-producing enteric flora. D-lactate is absorbed but is poorly metabolized due to a lack, in humans, of D-lactic acid dehydrogenase. Patients present with acidosis with a normal L-lactate level, nystagmus, ophthalmoplegia, ataxia, confusion and inappropriate behavior. The mediator of the neurologic symptoms is unknown. Treatment consists of bicarbonate administration and fasting. Prevention may be attempted with a low carbohydrate diet and, possibly, probiotics.

❑❑ **What pancreatic enzyme formulations are used for the treatment of the pain of chronic pancreatitis?**

Non-enteric-coated formulations are potentially beneficial in the treatment of chronic pain in some patients with chronic pancreatitis. Enteric-coated formulations are used to treat pancreatic maldigestion. To prevent steatorrhea, the recommended dose is 30,000 IU of lipase with each meal.

❑❑ **What are the mechanisms of malabsorption in patients with scleroderma?**

Villous atrophy, enterocyte dyfunction and submucosal collagen deposition. Bacterial overgrowth often occurs secondary to small intestinal stasis, loss of the migrating motor complex and the presence of small intestinal diverticula. Pancreatic insufficiency may also be present.

❑❑ **What are the mechanisms of diarrhea in patients with radiation enteritis?**

Altered absorption of fluids and electrolytes, bile-salt malabsorption, bacterial overgrowth due to stasis, entero-enteric fistuale and short bowel syndrome secondary to resection.

❑❑ **What is the rationale for using medium-chain triglycerides (MCT) as nutritional supplements in patients with malabsorption syndromes?**

Normal fat digestion and absorption requires a multi-step process including emulsification in the stomach, release of free fatty acids by gastric acids, breakdown of triglycerides by pancreatic lipases, formation of micelles with bile salts in the duodenum, and enterocyte absorption. MCT are rapidly hydrolyzed and absorbed directly without requiring pancreatic lipase, bile salts or micelle formation.

❑❑ **What conditions are associated with vitamin B12 malabsorption?**

Pernicious anemia, bacterial overgrowth, old age (incomplete release of food-bound vitamin B12), gastric surgery (achlorhydria, decreased intrinsic factor), therapy with proton pump inhibitors and H_2 receptor antagonists (incomplete release of food-bound vitamin B12; rare), HIV infection (ileal disease, achlorhydria), Crohn's disease (ileal disease or resection) and other diseases of the small intestine, multiple sclerosis (idiopathic), and chronic pancreatitis (incomplete cleavage of the R protein-intrinsic factor complex).

MISCELLANEOUS INFLAMMATORY CONDITIONS OF THE GUT

John K. Marshall, M.D., FRCPC, David McFadden, M.D.,
Isaac Raijman, M.D. and Rajeev Vasudeva, M.D.

How common is pill-induced esophageal injury?

The prevalence is very difficult to determine; however, the incidence is believed to be 3.9 per 100,000 population per year based upon one prospective Swedish study.

Which patients are more likely to develop drug-induced esophageal injury?

Most reports reveal a predominance of elderly and female patients. The elderly are more prone due to a higher prevalence of esophageal motility disorders and obstructing lesions of the esophagus. In addition, the elderly ingest more drugs in general, produce less saliva and are more likely to forget proper dosing instruction and spend more time in the recumbent position. Drug-induced injury is about twice as common in females due to greater use of potassium supplements and alendronate.

What are the major pathogenic factors contributing to drug-induced esophageal damage?

The chemical content, formulation of the drug and the manner in which the drug was taken by the patient are the major factors. Most patients with drug-induced esophageal injury have no detectable esophageal dysmotility or structural abnormality.

What are the common locations in the esophagus for drug-induced esophageal injury?

The level of the aortic-arch (more prevalent in older patients) and the distal esophagus.

What are the most common clinical manifestations of drug-induced esophageal injury?

Retrosternal chest pain is the most common manifestation (61% - 72%) followed by odynophagia (50% - 74%) and dysphagia (20% - 40%). Symptoms can develop within hours to days after starting the medication. In almost all cases, the diagnosis can be determined on the basis of the history.

What medications are commonly implicated in drug-induced esophageal injury?

The most common is tetracycline or one of its derivatives. Other medications include nonsteroidal anti-inflammatory drugs, potassium chloride, iron sulfate, quinidine, corticosteroids, pancreatic enzymes, cloxacillin, dicloxacillin, oral contraceptives and alendronate.

What is the best diagnostic modality in drug-induced esophageal injury?

Although not necessary in every patient, endoscopy is clearly the best diagnostic modality with considerable superiority in sensitivity over a barium contrast esophagogram.

T/F: In chemotherapy-related esophagitis, esophageal involvement correlates with involvement of oropharyngeal mucosa.

True. It is very unusual to have esophageal damage in the absence of oral changes.

❑❑ How does radiation dosage correlate with esophageal symptoms and signs?

30 Gy- retrosternal burning and odynophagia
40 Gy- mucosal erythema and edema
50 Gy- incidence and severity of esophagitis increases
60-70 Gy- strictures, perforations and fistulae

❑❑ What other factors potentiate radiation-induced eophageal damage?

The manner of delivery with an accelerated fractionation schedule may result in more injury. Concomitant chemotherapy may also potentiate radiation injury and is particularly common with doxorubicin.

❑❑ What are late effects of esophageal radiation?

Motor dysfunction of the esophagus, strictures, fistulae and squamous cell carcinomas may appear months to years after radiation.

❑❑ A 35 year-old man with acute lymphocytic leukemia underwent bone marrow transplantation 120 days ago and now presents with dysphagia and retrosternal pain. Barium swallow reveals a mid-esophageal stricture. What is the most likely etiology?

Chronic graft versus host disease is the most likely etiology and is manifested by webs, rings and strictures of the upper and mid esophagus. The clinical presentation resembles that of progressive systemic sclerosis. Immunosuppressive drugs are commonly employed in this situation and endoscopy with dilatation in selected cases may be helpful.

❑❑ T/F: Lymphocytic and collagenous colitis are distinct clinical entities.

This question continues to be debated. Although they differ slightly in the histologic criteria for diagnosis, growing evidence suggests that lymphocytic and collagenous colitis are two manifestations of the same disorder, with similar presentation, response to treatment and prognosis.

❑❑ How does lymphocytic/collagenous colitis typically present?

Patients with lymphocytic/collagenous colitis are typically middle-aged or elderly females with large-volume watery diarrhea. A prior history of nonsteroidal anti-inflammatory drug ingestion is common and was suggested to be a risk factor in a published case-control study.

❑❑ What is the sensitivity of rectal biopsy for detecting collagenous/lymphocytic colitis?

Only 27% of cases of collagenous colitis are detected on rectal biopsy. To exclude the diagnosis, full colonoscopy is usually required. Histologic changes are seen in the cecum in 82% of patients and the transverse colon in 83%.

❑❑ What proportion of patients with celiac disease have features of lymphocytic colitis on colonic biopsies?

20% to 30%.

❑❑ T/F: Lymphocytic colitis usually responds to a gluten-free diet.

False.

❑❑ What treatments may be prescribed for lymphocytic/collagenous colitis?

Patients should avoid secretagogues such as caffeine and lactose. Medical treatment options include sulfasalazine and other 5-aminosalicylate derivatives, cholestyramine, bismuth subsalicylate and systemic corticosteroids. Anti-diarrheal agents such as diphenoxylate and loperamide are often ineffective. Refractory cases have required surgical diversion of the fecal stream.

❑❑ Which of the above treatment options is/are supported by evidence from controlled clinical trials?

None.

❑❑ Characterize the natural history of lymphocytic/collagenous colitis.

Lymphocytic and collagenous colitis usually enter remission spontaneously in the short-term but may ultimately follow a chronic relapsing course. Between one-quarter and two-thirds of patients will require long-term medication for chronic intermittent diarrhea.

❑❑ T/F: Collagenous/lymphocytic colitis is associated with an increased risk of inflammatory bowel disease.

False.

❑❑ T/F: Collagenous/lymphocytic colitis increases the risk of developing colorectal carcinoma.

False.

❑❑ Following proximal diversion of the fecal stream, how common is diversion colitis?

Approximately one-third of patients will develop diversion colitis in the excluded segment.

❑❑ T/F: Diversion colitis occurs more commonly after colectomy for inflammatory bowel disease than for cancer.

True. Diversion colitis develops more frequently among patients who undergo surgery for inflammatory bowel disease (89%) than for cancer (23%).

❑❑ How does the endoscopic appearance of diversion colitis differ from that of ulcerative proctitis?

Diversion colitis cannot be differentiated endoscopically from ulcerative proctitis. Endoscopy typically reveals an erythematous and friable rectal mucosa with superficial ulceration.

❑❑ What histologic feature is the hallmark of diversion colitis?

Lymphoid follicular hyperplasia with germinal centers is found in almost all cases. Cryptitis and neutrophil infiltration develop in at least 60% after 3 months.

❑❑ What causes diversion colitis?

Diversion colitis occurs when a segment of bowel is excluded from the fecal stream. Current evidence implicates deficiency of luminal short-chain fatty acids such as acetate, propionate and butyrate. Butyrate normally provides 70% of the oxidative energy for colonocytes.

❑❑ How is diversion colitis treated?

The best treatment for diversion colitis is to restore the fecal stream. Short-chain fatty acid enemas induce remission in many patients but are not commercially available. A suggested formulation contains 60mmol/L acetate, 30mmol/L propionate and 40mmol/L butyrate. Hydrocortisone enemas are ineffective and there is little evidence exists to support the use of aminosalicylate preparations.

❑❑ How does acute radiation proctosigmoiditis present?

Acute injury presents with diarrhea and tenesmus during radiation treatment or within six weeks of exposure. The endoscopic appearance of the rectum is normal.

❏❏ What are the clinical manifestations of chronic radiation proctitis?

The typical symptoms of chronic injury are rectal bleeding, diarrhea and tenesmus. Rectal strictures may develop as can fistulae to the vagina, bladder or uterus.

❏❏ Describe the typical endoscopic appearance of chronic radiation proctitis.

Mucosal pallor with friability and telangiectasia.

❏❏ How long after radiation exposure does chronic radiation proctitis develop?

On average, symptoms develop after one year, fistulae after 18 months and strictures after 3 years.

❏❏ What treatments are effective in controlling hemorrhage from radiation proctitis?

Oral 5-aminosalicylic acid and corticosteroid enemas do not appear to control bleeding or tenesmus. Local instillation of 4% formalin, sucralfate and 5-ASA may be effective. Nd:YAG or argon laser ablation or electrocoagulation of the rectal mucosa are useful endoscopic approaches. Hyperbaric oxygen therapy may also be beneficial by attenuating tissue hypoxia from obliterative endarteritis. Proctectomy may be considered for refractory cases but the colo-anal anastomosis is prone to leakage.

❏❏ At what age is the incidence of milk protein allergy highest?

The peak incidence is at 6 weeks. Symptoms may include vomiting, colic, diarrhea and rectal bleeding from colonic ulcers. Since the allergy is usually IgE-mediated, eczema, urticaria and angioneurotic edema may also be seen.

❏❏ How is the diagnosis of milk protein allergy made?

Resolution of symptoms with milk withdrawal and recurrence within 48 hours of rechallenge makes the diagnosis. Rechallenge is often omitted since it may result in anaphylaxis. If performed, rechallenge should be conducted in a hospital setting.

❏❏ At what age can children with milk protein allergy resume drinking cow's milk?

Allergy to milk protein usually resolves by between 9 months and 3 years.

❏❏ Which laxatives are associated with melanosis coli?

Anthraquinones, including cascara sagrada, aloe, rhubarb, senna and frangula.

❏❏ How soon does melanosis appear and how quickly does it resolve?

Melanosis coli can develop within 4 months of starting a laxative and usually resolves within approximately 9 months after they are discontinued.

❏❏ Name the pigment that is deposited in the mucosa in melanosis coli?

The identity of the pigment is unknown. It has been found to bear some biochemical similarity to lipofuscin, melanin and the hepatic pigment of Dubin-Johnson syndrome.

❏❏ Describe the location and endoscopic appearance of the solitary rectal ulcer syndrome (SRUS).

Endoscopy reveals a lesion on the anterior rectal wall between 6 and 10 cm from the anal verge. The lesion itself is variable and may appear as a single ulcer, a cluster of ulcers, a polypoid lesion or an area of erythema.

❏❏ What are the typical histologic findings in the SRUS?

The appearance on biopsy is described as fibromuscular obliteration of the lamina propria. As this term suggests, the lamina propria is replaced with fibroblasts, smooth muscle and collagen with hypertrophy and disorganization of the muscularis mucosa.

□□ Describe hypotheses regarding the pathogenesis of SRUS.

Self-digitation has been suggested as the cause of SRUS and is documented in up to 50% of patients. An alternate hypothesis suggests that SRUS results from prolapse and ischemia of the rectal mucosa in the setting of a high fecal voiding pressure. The latter may result from inadequate relaxation of the puborectalis during defecation.

□□ How is SRUS treated?

Initial conservative therapy with bulk laxatives, avoidance of straining and reassurance is recommended. Topical anti-inflammatory medication is generally ineffective. For refractory cases, the surgical procedure of choice is an abdominal rectopexy.

□□ What complications of nonsteroidal anti-inflammatory drugs (NSAIDs) have been described in the colon?

Acute colitis, ischemic colitis, perforation of colonic diverticula and diaphragm-like stricture formation have been reported after NSAID ingestion. NSAIDs may also exacerbate or trigger relapse of Crohn's disease and ulcerative colitis.

□□ Which disease-modifying anti-rheumatic drug has been associated with an acute colitis?

Gold salts may induce an acute colitis characterized by ulceration and friability of the rectosigomoid mucosa. Symptoms typically resolve within 2 weeks of drug withdrawal.

□□ Name five classes of drugs which have been associated with ischemic injury of the colon.

Nonsteroidal anti-inflammatory drugs, oral contraceptives, vasopressin, ergotamine, cocaine, dextroamphetamine, neuroleptics and digitalis.

□□ What is typhlitis?

The Greek word *typhlos* refers to a blind sac. Typhlitis is an acute necrotic inflammation of the cecum. It has also been called neutropenic enterocolitis, necrotizing enterocolitis and ileocecal syndrome.

□□ In what clinical setting does typhlitis occur?

Typhlitis classically affects leukemic patients with severe neutropenia but has been described in a number of other immunosuppressed states.

□□ How does typhlitis present?

Typical symptoms include fever, abdominal pain, distension, vomiting and bloody diarrhea. An associated mucositis may involve the oropharynx. Plain films may reveal cecal thumbprinting or pneumatosis. Computed tomography and ultrasound demonstrate bowel wall thickening.

□□ How is typhlitis treated?

The primary management is medical, with hydration, broad-spectrum antibiotics and nasogastric decompression. Refractory cases may require a right hemicolectomy with mucous fistula.

□□ What is the mortality rate from acute typhlitis?

40% to 50%.

❑❑ **What event often precedes the development of acute cholecystitis?**

Cystic duct obstruction often precedes the development of acute calculous cholecystitis.

❑❑ **What other factors are associated with acute calculous cholecystitis?**

Supersaturated bile, decreased lecithin and increased lysolecithin in the gallbladder, increased production of prostaglandins (E2), increased fluid secretion within the gallbladder and circulating platelet-activating factor. Ischemia may play a significant role in some patients as a result of decreased blood supply caused by obstruction of the cystic artery as the gallbladder enlarges from inflammatory changes. Underlying atherosclerosis of the cystic artery may also contribute.

❑❑ **T/F: Bacterial involvement of the gallbladder is a primary event in the development of acute calculous cholecystitis.**

False. Bacterial inflammation is considered a secondary event and is found in as many as 80% of patients with acute calculous cholecystitis undergoing cholecystectomy.

❑❑ **What is the most common location of a gallbladder perforation?**

The fundus of the gallbladder due to its larger diameter and thus greater tension.

❑❑ **What percentage of cholecystectomies are performed for acute calculous cholecystitis?**

Approximately 20%. There are about 500,000 cholecystectomies performed annually in the United States.

❑❑ **T/F: In the elderly, biliary symptoms usually precede the development of acute cholecystitis.**

False.

❑❑ **T/F: Gallstones are more common in diabetics.**

False. However, diabetics have an higher incidence of related complications compared to the non-diabetic population.

❑❑ **What percentage of patients with acute calculous cholecystitis have associated choledocholithiasis?**

Approximately 10%.

❑❑ **T/F: Jaundice occurs commonly in adults with acute calculous cholecystitis.**

False. Approximately 20% of adults with acute calculous cholecystitis develop jaundice. This increases to approximately 50% in children.

❑❑ **How specific is laboratory data in patients with acute calculous cholecystitis?**

Laboratory data is nonspecific and may, in fact, be normal. Remember that in patients with a rapidly rising bilirubin and no evidence of biliary obstruction, gallbladder perforation with secondary increased absorption of bilirubin through the peritoneal cavity should be considered.

❑❑ **T/F: An elevated amylase is always indicative of acute pancreatitis in the setting of acute calculous cholecystitis.**

False. Hyperamylasemia may reflect a gangrenous gallbladder.

❑❑ **What percentage of gallstones may be visualized on a routine scout film of the abdomen?**

Only 10% to 20% of patients will have radiolucent gallstones.

❑❑ What is the diagnostic test of choice for acute calculous cholecystitis?

Ultrasound remains the test of choice for diagnosing acute calculous cholecystitis. Suggestive findings include pericholecystic fluid, thickened gallbladder wall, stones or sludge and enlargement of the organ. Murphy's sign is also useful but it may be absent in the presence of gangrenous cholecystitis

❑❑ T/F: Hepatobiliary scanning of the gallbladder is useful in diagnosing acute acalculous cholecystitis.

True. A positive test occurs when there is no filling of the gallbladder, usually within 1 hour. However, in some normal patients it may take up to 4 hours for the gallbladder to fill. Causes of false positives include parenteral nutrition, prolonged (> 24 hrs) or limited (< 2 hrs) fasting, and alcoholism.

❑❑ What percentage of patients with acute calculous cholecystitis develop complications?

1) Gallbladder empyema 2% to 12%
2) Perforation 3% to 15%
3) Gangrenous cholecystitis < 2%
4) Bleeding or hemiperitoneum very rare
5) Emphysematous cholecystitis (usually due to *Clostridium* species) occurs rarely. The incidence of gangrenous gallbladder in these patients is as high as 75%.
6) Septic metastases rare

❑❑ What percentage of all cases of acute cholecystitis is due to acalculous disease?

Acute acalculous cholecystitis accounts for approximately 6% to 17%.

❑❑ What factors are involved in the development of acute acalculous cholecystitis?

Obstruction of the cystic duct by sludge, inspissation of bile with associated reduced flow, mechanical obstruction of the cystic duct by other diseases such as tumors or nodes, decreased gallbladder motility, systemic volume depletion, ischemia and possibly infectious agents.

❑❑ T/F: Infections may cause acute acalculous cholecystitis.

True. Infections are particularly important in patients with AIDS, where cytomegalovirus and *Cryptosporidium* play an important role. Typhoid fever is also associated with acalculous cholecystitis.

❑❑ What diseases are associated with the development of acute acalculous cholecystitis?

Diseases associated with mesenteric vascular compromise (vasculitis), sepsis, prolonged use of total parenteral nutrition, severe burns and intra-abdominal surgery.

❑❑ What patient group is more commonly associated with acute acalculous cholecystitis?

Contrary to calculous disease, acalculous cholecystitis is more common in men, especially the elderly.

❑❑ What is the main complication that may occur in acute acalculous cholecystitis?

Perforation may occur in as many as 60% of these patients.

❑❑ What is the overall mortality in acute acalculous cholecystitis?

Approximately 50%.

❑❑ T/F: Computed tomography is useful in diagnosing choledocholithiasis.

True. Abdominal computed tomography (CT) can aid in the diagnosis of both cholelithiasis and choledocholithiasis. In a recent study utilizing CT scan immediately before endoscopic retrograde cholangiopancreatography in patients with suspected choledocholithiasis, the CT sensitivity was 88%, the specificity was 97%, with an accuracy of 94%.

❏❏ **What is the current gold-standard test for the diagnosis of choledocholithiasis?**

Endoscopic retrograde cholangiography (ERC) remains the gold standard in the diagnosis of choledocholithiasis. In expert hands, ERC is successful in completely visualizing the biliary tree in almost 100% of the patients. The stones may also be removed using this technique.

❏❏ **What is the most common cholangiographic pattern of primary sclerosing cholangitis (PSC)?**

While it may affect both intra- and extra-hepatic ducts, PSC more commonly presents as multiple short strictures found throughout the liver with characteristic beading and pruning and isolated dilations of the intrahepatic ducts

❏❏ **What other conditions can mimick the cholangiographic appearance of PSC?**

Cirrhosis and metastatic disease to the liver may give a similar appearance.

❏❏ **T/F: Endobiliary stents are the non-surgical treatment of choice for PSC-related bile duct strictures.**

False. Unless absolutely necessary, less is more when it comes to endoscopic therapy in PSC.

❏❏ **T/F: Cholangiocarcinoma is usually easily detected in the setting of PSC.**

False.

❏❏ **What is the most common cause of acute suppurative cholangitis?**

Intrahepatic or extrahepatic stones are the cause of almost all cases. Patients with a biliary endoprosthesis and/or previous biliary manipulation are also at risk.

❏❏ **What is the classic clinical triad of acute suppurative cholangitis?**

Charcot's triad consists of right upper quadrant abdominal pain, jaundice and fever. Hypotension and full blown septic shock (Reynold's pentad) may subsequently ensue very quickly.

❏❏ **What is the treatment of choice in acute suppurative cholangitis?**

Endoscopic decompression along with systemic antibiotics.

❏❏ **What biliary tract disease is associated with the acquired immunodeficiency sydrome (AIDS)?**

AIDS can produce a sclerosing cholangitis-like picture associated with upper abdominal pain and elevated liver function tests, especially alkaline phosphatase. The cholangitis may be associated with the AIDS virus alone or with other infections such as CMV, *Cryptosporidium*, or *microsporidia*. A causative organism is found in about 60% of cases.

❏❏ **At what T lymphocyte count is AIDS cholangiopathy more likely to occur?**

When the T-cell count is below 200.

❏❏ **What is the most likely diagnosis in a patient with AIDS who complains of severe abdominal pain and has an elevated alkaline phosphatase?**

Papillary stenosis. AIDS may produce severe abdominal pain associated with elevated alkaline phosphatase due to papillary stenosis. The pain may improve dramatically after endoscopic sphincterotomy.

❑❑ **T/F: AIDS cholangiopathy adversely affects the overall outcome of AIDS patients.**

False. AIDS cholangiopathy does not appear to have any influence on the progression of the underlying disease.

❑❑ **What patient group is at high risk for infectious and parasitic cholangiopathies?**

Patients from Southeast Asia are particularly at risk for parasite-related bile duct disease.

❑❑ **What are the most common parasites implicated in biliary obstruction?**

Clonorchis sinensis and *Ascaris lumbricoides* are the most frequently found parasites causing biliary disease. More frequent than stricturing is the presence of undulating and elongated filling defects of the bile ducts.

❑❑ **What is Oriental cholangitis?**

Oriental cholangitis is characterized by the development of pigmented stones, diffuse biliary strictures and chronic, recurrent episodes of cholangitis. This is particularly common in people from southeast Asia.

❑❑ **What is autoimmune cholangitis?**

The clinical expression of autoimmune cholangitis is very similar to that of primary biliary cirrhosis except it is not associated with antimitochondrial antibodies.

❑❑ **What type of cholangiographic injury has been associated with intra-arterial infusion of 5-fluorodeoxyuridine?**

An intra-hepatic sclerosing cholangits-type picture.

❑❑ **What other conditions are associated with the development of bile duct disease causing stricture formation?**

1) Surgical trauma.
2) Anastomotic arterial strictures.
3) Hepatic artery thrombosis.

❑❑ **What autoimmune diseases may have pancreatic involvement?**

Systemic lupus erythematosis, rheumatoid arthritis, polyarteritis nodosa and Bechet's Syndrome.

❑❑ **What etiologic factors have been proposed in systemic autoimmune-related pancreatic inflammation?**

Presumed causes include vasculitis, systemic steroid use and circulating antibodies to acinar cells.

❑❑ **What is the most common hereditary disease involving the exocrine pancreas?**

Cystic fibrosis (CF) , which affects 1 in every 2000 live births.

❑❑ **Describe the inheritance pattern of CF.**

Autosomal recessive with a gene frequency of approximately 5% among caucasians.

❑❑ **What are pancreatic manifestations of cystic fibrosis (CF)?**

In the early stages, the pancreas may appear normal or there may be a deposition of eosinophilic concretions within ductules. Larger ductular involvement may lead to dilatation and acinar disruption.

Later on, the pancreas may appear indistinguishable from chronic pancreatitis as cyst development may occur and fat and scar replace pancreatic lobules.

❑❑ **What percentage of patients with CF do not have clinically evident pancreatic exocrine insufficiency?**

15%.

❑❑ **What percentage of patients with CF have diabetes mellitus?**

One percent of children and 13% of adults.

❑❑ **T/F: Gallstones are more common in CF and can lead to acute inflammatory exacerbations.**

True. Gallstones develop in 10% to 15% of CF patients.

❑❑ **T/F: Laparoscopic cholecystectomy should be considered for CF patients with asymptomatic gallstones detected during screening radiography.**

False.

❑❑ **Describe the pathophysiology of pancreatic endocrine insufficiency that may occur in CF.**

Replacement of pancreatic tissue with fibrosis and fat in severe disease leads to disruption of normal islets by autodigestion and dimunition of the number of islets.

❑❑ **T/F: Microscopic pancreatic involvement is seen in the majority of patients with sarcoidosis.**

False. Pancreatic involvement occurs in only 1% to 6% of all affected individuals and is rarely seen before the diagnosis is made from the upper aerodigestive tract.

❑❑ **T/F: Microscopic gastrointestinal involvement is seen in the majority of patients with sarcoidosis.**

True. Granulomas are seen in nearly 100% of patients with known sarcoidosis, although symptoms are described in less than 1%.

❑❑ **Briefly describe the pathophysiology of sarcoidosis.**

Non-caseating granulomata occur in sarcoidosis. Enlarged lymph nodes may cause pressure-related symptoms and granulomatous infiltration may cause dysfunction or dysmotility in the gastrointestinal tract.

❑❑ **T/F: Involvement of the pancreas in Crohn's Disease is not seen in the absence of duodenal involvement.**

False.

❑❑ **What are the suggested mechanisms of Crohn's disease involvement of the pancreas?**

There are four suggested mechanisms: ampullary involvement, cholelithiasis secondary to ileal disease, immunologic injury and drug therapy.

❑❑ **Describe the usual, albeit rare, manifestation of Wegener's granulomatosis involving the pancreas.**

Pancreatic mass.

❑❑ **What is the classic triad of Wegener's granulomatosis?**

Focal glomerulonephritis, vasculitis and necrotizing granulomas.

❏❏ Classically, Wegener's granulomatosis affects what part of the alimentary tract?

The intestine. The associated vasculitis can lead to intestinal or colonic bleeding, ischemia or perforation.

❏❏ What is the most common cause of pancreatitis in childhood?

Trauma (child abuse must be considered). In one recent study, 42% of cases resulted from bicycle accidents. Drugs and infections are the other two major causes in children.

❏❏ What is Shwachman's Syndrome?

A disorder of pancreatic exocrine insufficiency and hematologic abnormalities with normal sweat electrolytes. This autosomal recessive disorder is the second most common cause of pancreatic insufficiency in children.

❏❏ A patient recovering from gallstone pancreatitis develops multiple painful, erythematous subcutaneous nodules. What is the diagnosis?

Pancreatic panniculitis. Subcutaneous fat necrosis occurs in 2% to 3% of patients with acute pancreatitis or pancreatic cancer. The lesions may resemble erythema nodosum.

❏❏ What are the effects of end-stage renal disease on the pancreas?

Morphologically, multiple abnormalities (acinar dilation, interlobular fibrosis) may be seen. Functionally, an elevated trypsin with a normal output of lipase and impaired bicarbonate secretion may be seen. Clinically, the frequency of acute pancreatitis may be increased in these patients but the mechanisms are unclear.

❏❏ What are the pancreatic effects of hereditary hemochromatosis?

Selective accumulation of excess iron in islet beta-cells results in a loss of endocrine granules and subsequent glucose intolerance or frank diabetes.

❏❏ T/F: Diabetics have an increased risk of exocrine pancreatic insufficiency.

True. Nearly 30% of diabetics will have impaired pancreatic secretion. This is thought to be due to the inhibitory effects of excess glucagon and lack of stimulatory effects of insulin on the pancreas, vagal neuropathy, and nutritional wasting.

MOTILITY DISORDERS

Nyingi Kemmer, M.D., Robin D. Rothstein, M.D., Edy E. Soffer, M.D.
Roger D. Soloway, M.D., Gervais Tougas, M.D. and Richard A. Wright, M.D.

❏❏ **What is the most common cause of chronic intermittent solid dysphagia in an otherwise healthy adult?**

Lower esophageal (Schatzki's) ring.

❏❏ **A 46 year-old man develops solid food dysphagia 2 months following laparoscopic Nissen fundoplication. What is the most appropriate initial investigation?**

Barium esophagography with a marshmallow challenge is the best initial study. Endoscopy and manometry may subsequently be required.

❏❏ **What is the prevalence of esophageal dysmotility in systemic sclerosis (scleroderma)?**

As many as 70% of patients with scleroderma will have involvement of the esophagus.

❏❏ **What two major manometric abnormalities are associated with systemic sclerosis?**

Diminished lower esophageal sphincter tone and decreased or absent contraction wave amplitude in the smooth muscle (distal) portion of the esophagus. Proximal esophageal peristalsis remains normal as only smooth muscle is involved.

❏❏ **A 48 year-old woman with severe reflux symptoms is being considered for laparoscopic fundoplication. She is found to have facial telangiectasia and Raynaud's phenomenon. What further investigation(s) would be absolutely essential prior to surgery?**

Esophageal manometry. A diagnosis of scleroderma would be a major contraindication to a 360° fundoplication.

❏❏ **What is the most common abnormality observed during esophageal manometry in patients with non-cardiac chest pain?**

While esophageal manometry is usually normal in patients with non-cardiac chest pain, high amplitude contractions (> 180 mmHg) of prolonged duration (> 6 seconds) and associated with pain constitute the most common manometric abnormality observed in these patients. This constitutes the Nutcracker Esophagus.

❏❏ **What is the most common esophageal motility abnormality associated with gastroesophageal reflux disease?**

An increased frequency of transient lower esophageal sphincter relaxation is the primary abnormality observed in most patients with reflux. It can typically be seen only during prolonged studies using a manometry catheter incorporating a sleeve sensor.

❏❏ **A 76 year-old patient with progressive solid and liquid dysphagia is found to have an absence of lower esophageal relaxation and esophageal peristalsis on manometry and a bird beak deformity of the gastroesophageal junction on barium swallow. What condition should be considered besides achalasia?**

Cancer of the cardia with pseudoachalasia. Carcinoma-induced achalasia is responsible for 2% - 5% of all cases of achalasia. Gastric cardia cancer is most commonly implicated.

❑❑ **When is an ambulatory esophageal pH study indicated in a patient with non-cardiac chest pain?**

Recent data would suggest that an ambulatory esophageal pH study is only indicated in patients who have no response to a trial of a proton pump inhibitors. In those not responding to acid inhibition, a pH study should be done while the patient is receiving acid suppression in order to document the persistence of acid reflux and its association with symptoms.

❑❑ **What is the most common upper gastrointestinal symptom in the elderly?**

Dysphagia is present in 16% of the elderly population living in the community and swallowing dysfunction is present in as much as 50% of residents living in nursing homes.

❑❑ **Which segment of the esophagus is commonly affected in dermatomyositis or polymyositis?**

The wall of the proximal one-third of the esophagus is composed of striated muscle whereas the distal two-thirds consists of smooth muscle. The proximal one-third can be affected by any condition affecting striated muscle function.

❑❑ **Esophageal propulsion of swallowed food involves coordinated peristaltic activity within the longitudinal and circular muscle layers. What structure must relax in synchrony with the peristaltic wave to allow passage of the food bolus?**

Relaxation of the lower esophageal sphincter is coordinated with the peristaltic activity in the esophageal body through a vagally-mediated reflex pathway.

❑❑ **What are the 5 manometric features of achalasia?**

1)   Absence of complete LES relaxation with swallowing.
2)   Simultaneous contractions within the esophageal body (loss of peristaltic activity).
3)   Low amplitude of esophageal contractions.
4)   Increased tone of the LES (present in about 60% of cases).
5)   Resting intraesophageal pressure greater than intragastric pressure.

❑❑ **A 73 year-old woman with Parkinson's disease develops liquid dysphagia with frequent coughing and choking. What is the most appropriate initial test?**

A videoesophagram is the best test for the initial investigation of oropharyngeal dysphagia.

❑❑ **A 43 year-old woman with scleroderma and severe gastroesophageal reflux experiences a recent worsening of regurgitation. What is the most likely cause?**

Worsening regurgitation is frequently associated with the development of gastroparesis in patients with scleroderma.

❑❑ **A 23 year-old man presents with odynophagia of three months duration. How would you investigate this?**

Odynophagia typically is associated with mucosal damage. An endoscopy would be the best initial investigation. GERD, esophageal candidiasis and viral ulceration are the most common causes of odynophagia in this age group.

❑❑ **A 47 year-old diabetic man develops solid food dysphagia without odynophagia one month following renal transplantation. He has no signs of rejection and has complied with his immunosuppressive therapy. What is the most likely cause of the dysphagia?**

Esophageal candidiasis is very likely in this setting and would be best treated using oral antifungal therapy such as fluconazole.

❑❑ A 40 year-old woman complains of a constant feeling of a lump in her throat. What is the likely diagnosis?

She describes the typical globus sensation. It is differentiated from oropharyngeal dysphagia by being present continuously regardless of whether the patient is swallowing or not. The etiology of this condition is controversial. Gastroesophageal reflux, hypertensive upper esophageal sphincter and anxiety have all been suggested as possible causes.

❑❑ Why do patients with scleroderma develop dysphagia?

Dysphagia usually occurs as a consequence of poor peristalsis; however, it can also be due to a stricture resulting from severe reflux that occurs in many of these patients secondary to atony of the lower esophageal sphincterand poor esophageal acid clearance.

❑❑ What are two common radiological signs seen in scleroderma patients with esophageal involvement?

Moderately dilated aperistaltic distal esophagus and free reflux. Peptic strictures can also be seen in as much as 30% of patients.

❑❑ What is the pathognomonic manometric feature of diffuse esophageal spasm?

Simultaneous esophageal contractions occurring after more than 50% (controversial) of 5 mL water bolus swallows. Associated findings include repetitive or prolonged (> 6 seconds) contractions, frequently of high (> 180 mmHg) amplitude. The more abnormalities present, the more specific the diagnosis.

❑❑ What is the most effective therapeutic option for achalasia?

The best results (80% - 90% success) have been reported following Heller myotomy. Alternative approaches include pneumatic dilation (70% - 80% success) and botulinum toxin injection (40% - 60% success).

❑❑ A 50 year-old man has classical achalasia. He is considering either pneumatic dilation or laparoscopic Heller myotomy. He would rather not have surgery and would like to know the risks associated with pneumatic dilation. Describe the risks.

Esophageal perforation is the main complication associated with pneumatic dilation. It occurs in 3% - 5% of cases. There are no absolute risk factors associated with an increased occurrence of perforation.

❑❑ A patient with severe gastroesophageal reflux disease is being considered for laparoscopic fundoplication. What is the most important test to be performed to rule out gastrointestinal contraindications to the procedure?

Esophageal manometry to confirm good esophageal peristaltic activity and rule out scleroderma. While controversial, weak esophageal peristalsis is thought to be a predictor of postoperative dysphagia.

❑❑ What cancer is associated with idiopathic achalasia?

The incidence of squamous cell cancer of the esophagus is 0.15 %. The risk of esophageal cancer in achalasics is 17 times greater than in the normal population. It typically occurs in those with long-standing, ineffectively treated (i.e., dilated esophagus) disease.

❑❑ A 59 year-old man is referred for esophageal manometry because of chest pain and solid dysphagia. He is found to have a high resting lower esophageal sphincter tone (45 mmHg), 90% relaxation with deglutition and normal peristaltic activity. What is the diagnosis?

Hypertensive lower esophageal sphincter is diagnosed by the finding of elevated lower esophageal sphincter pressure with normal relaxation and normal peristalsis. The clinical significance of this finding is unclear.

❑❑ **A 50 year-old man is referred from cardiology for evaluation of non-cardiac chest pain. He only gets chest pain when swallowing crusty bread and baked potatoes. He has no associated dysphagia and has had a normal barium esophagram recently. What is the most likely diagnosis?**

Nutcracker esophagus is characterized by hypertensive (> 180 mmHg) esophageal contractions of prolonged (> 6 seconds) duration with normal peristalsis and lower esophageal sphincter relaxation.

❑❑ **An elderly smoker develops progressive solid food dysphagia over a month. What is your initial investigation?**

Endoscopy. The history is more suggestive of esophageal carcinoma rather than a motility disorder. Alternatively, a barium esophagram could be done but would not provide the opportunity for tissue biopsy and dilatation.

❑❑ **A 35 year-old woman complains of severe heartburn that has not responded to twice-daily proton pump inhibitor therapy. What diagnostic test would be most useful at this point?**

Ambulatory esophago-gastric pH-metry while continuing to take the proton pump inhibitor. This will determine if her symptoms are associated with acid reflux and if the drug has successfully suppressed acid secretion and reflux.

❑❑ **A 45 year-old man with portal hypertension and esophageal varices develops dysphagia following sclerotherapy for a variceal bleed. What is the most likely cause of the dysphagia?**

The most common cause of dysphagia in this setting is the development of a stricture following healing of the local ulceration that almost invariably occurs with sclerotherapy. This complication is almost never seen following band ligation of varices.

❑❑ **A 68 year-old woman with metastatic esophageal cancer develops solid dysphagia and rapid weight loss. She is not anorectic. What would you recommend to help her maintain nutrition?**

Endoscopic stent placement should help restore her ability to eat solid food. Alternatively, laser therapy could be considered. Esophageal resection is not advisable as the procedure has high mortality and morbidity in a patient with a very short life expectancy. Chemotherapy and radiotherapy are unlikely to be of any benefit in advanced cases.

❑❑ **Below what ring diameter does dysphagia develop in patients with Schatzki rings?**

As with any esophageal luminal stricture, dysphagia regularly occurs with a ring diameter of less than 13 mm. It is less common with rings between 13 and 20 mm and almost never seen if the diameter exceeds 20 mm.

❑❑ **In patients with a hypertensive lower esophageal sphincter, what is often seen on barium swallow?**

A lower esophageal muscular ring at the level of the cephalad part of the lower esophageal sphincter.

❑❑ **How are a hypertensive lower esophageal sphincter and its accompanying muscular ring treated?**

Esophageal dilatation with a large (17mm - 20 mm) bougie is temporarily effective. Alternatively, botulinum toxin injection has been reported to be effective in some patients.

❑❑ **An 83 year-old man is referred because of regurgitation of undigested food, recurrent aspiration pneumonia and chronic halitosis. He admits to frequent choking while eating, to a sense of difficulty initiating swallows and to food getting stuck in his throat? A barium swallow shows a large pharyngoesophageal diverticulum. What is the diagnosis?**

Zenker's diverticulum.

❏❏ How is Zenker's diverticulum formed?

Zenker's diverticula are pulsion diverticula formed in the hypopharyngeal region by high intraswallowing pressures resulting from a poorly compliant upper esophageal sphincter.

❏❏ What is the effect of a hiatus hernia on lower esophageal sphincter tone?

None. Lower esophageal sphincter tone is related to the myogenic and neurogenic properties of the sphincter, not its location relative to the diaphragmatic hiatus. However, competence of the antireflux barrier at the lower esophageal sphincter is, in part, maintained by contraction of the diaphragm.

❏❏ What location of a cerebrovascular accident (stroke) most commonly results in swallowing difficulties?

Brainstem strokes are commonly associated with acute oropharyngeal dysphagia, which often persists. This is much less common with cortical strokes.

❏❏ What is the mechanism of dysphagia in amyotrophic lateral sclerosis (ALS)?

ALS is characterized by motor neuron degeneration. Dysphagia is common in the later phases of the disease. The tongue is first involved followed by the pharynx and the larynx. Aspiration is common.

❏❏ What is the main manometric abnormality seen in Parkinson's patients with dysphagia?

Diminished pharyngeal propulsive forces are almost always present. Incomplete upper esophageal relaxation is seen in 21% of dysphagic Parkinson's patients.

❏❏ A 47 year-old man with ptosis develops progressive dysphagia and aspiration. What is the diagnosis?

Oculopharyngeal dystrophy, a syndrome characterized by progressive dysphagia and palpebral ptosis. This type of muscular dystrophy is linked to chromosome 14 abnormalities and is more common in, but not limited to, patients of French-Canadian lineage. Failure of pharyngeal motility leads to aspiration.

❏❏ What symptoms besides dysphagia and regurgitation occur commonly in patients with achalasia?

Chest pain and weight loss are reported in as many as 50% of patients.

❏❏ What is the frequency of pulmonary complications in achalasia?

As many as 10% of patients with achalasia will present with bronchopulmonary complications including aspiration pneumonia.

❏❏ What is the most common cancer associated with manometrically-determined achalasia (pseudoachalasia)?

Adenocarcinomas of the gastroesophageal junction account for more than 50% of cases of pseudoachalasia. Pancreatic, oat cell, pulmonary and hepatic cancers account for most of the rest.

❏❏ What infectious disease can mimic achalasia?

Chagas disease can produce a clinical picture identical to classical achalasia. Usually other tubular organs are also involved in Chagas disease. The presence of antibodies to *Trypanosoma cruzi* is diagnostic. Treatment is identical.

❏❏ What pathways mediate the control of gastric emptying?

Gastric motor activity is governed by extrinsic neural control from the parasympathetic nervous system, intrinsically by the enteric nervous system, and at the level of the smooth muscle by depolarization of the smooth muscle membrane.

❑❑ What neural transmitters are involved in peristalsis?

The excitatory neurotransmitters are acetylcholine, serotonin and tachykinins while the inhibitory neurotransmitters include nitric oxide and vasoactive intestinal peptide.

❑❑ What are the major components of the enteric nervous system?

The enteric nervous system consists of the myenteric (Auerbach's) plexus, which lies between the circular and longitudinal muscle layers, and the submucosal (Meissner's) plexus, which lies between the circular muscle layer and the mucosa.

❑❑ What are the two functional motor components of the stomach?

The stomach consists of two discrete functional segments. The proximal stomach/fundus represents the accommodating portion of the stomach. It is able to expand to allow large volumes of material to accumulate without causing a resultant increase in gastric pressure. It also receptively relaxes upon deglutition. The second functional portion of the stomach consists of the distal body and antrum. The distal stomach is responsible for trituration and emptying of gastric contents into the duodenum. This portion is governed by the gastric pacemaker which is located on the greater curvature of the stomach in the mid body. The pacemaker generates electrical potentials that sweep circumferentially and distally and correspond to peristaltic contractions during the appropriate stage of digestion.

❑❑ What are the interstitial cells of Cajal?

These are specialized nonmuscular pacemaker cells that account for the inherent rhythmicity of gut smooth muscle.

❑❑ What receptors are present in the prepyloric region?

Size and osmole receptors are present in the prepyloric mucosa. Size receptors will not allow particles greater than 1 mm to pass through the pylorus in the two hour postprandial period. Osmole receptors prevent the passage of hyperosmolar solutions into the duodenum. Hypertonic solutions must be diluted by gastric secretions to isotonicity before they are allowed to pass into the duodenum.

❑❑ What is trituration?

Trituration is the process of breaking down solid food to a size less than 1 mm by an antral grinding action. Large particles are repetitively propelled and retropulsed in the antrum, breaking them down to a size compatible with digestion and absorption.

❑❑ What duodenal mechanisms cause feedback inhibition of gastric emptying?

Acid stimulates the release of secretin from the duodenal mucosa which causes a decrease in gastric emptying. Lipids and amino acids cause release of cholecystokinin-pancreazymin from the duodenal mucosa, also resulting in the inhibition of gastric emptying.

❑❑ What is the effect of vagotomy on the gastric fundus?

Both the receptive relaxation response to deglutition and accommodation are abolished. This may be partially responsible for the accelerated emptying that occurs after vagotomy (dumping syndrome). This is also the proposed mechanism for rapid gastric emptying that is sometimes seen in patients with diabetes mellitus.

❑❑ What abnormalities in gastric motor function have been described in patients with non-ulcer (functional) dyspepsia?

Decreased fundal compliance, gastric dysrhythmias, antral hypomotility and gastroparesis have all been described. Studies have reported that between 30% and 80% of patients with non-ulcer dyspepsia have delayed gastric emptying of solids. This occurs most commonly in middle-aged females with postprandial bloating and vomiting.

❑❑ What is the effect of hyperglycemia on gastric emptying?

Hyperglycemia delays gastric emptying in healthy individuals and patients with diabetes. The mechanism is multifactorial.

❑❑ What is the most common gastric defect in patients with diabetes mellitus.

Autonomic neuropathy with "autovagotomy" results from long-standing diabetes mellitus. The clinical result is usually a delay in gastric emptying with the potential for bezoar formation; however, occasionally rapid emptying, especially of liquids, occurs and results in a dumping syndrome.

❑❑ What connective tissue diseases are associated with gastroparesis?

Scleroderma and systemic lupus erythematosis are most commonly implicated.

❑❑ T/F: Patients with bulimia or anorexia nervosa and chronic vomiting frequently have gastric emptying abnormalities.

True. In patients with anorexia nervosa or bulimia, impaired gastric emptying of solid foods has been reported, whereas liquid emptying is usually normal. Promotility drugs have been found to be helpful in alleviating gastroparetic symptoms in some of these patients.

❑❑ How can gastric emptying be measured?

Currently, the most common technique is scintigraphy using radionuclide-labeled meals. Abdominal ultrasonography can be used to measure gastric emptying by determining serial measurements of antral size before and after a standard liquid meal. Magnetic resonance imaging is able to determine gastric emptying rates and the regional distribution of a meal within the stomach. Finally, breath tests utilizing octanoic acid, which do not contain radioactivity, are being developed to measure gastric emptying.

❑❑ What is the role of electrogastrography (EGG) in the evaluation of patients with dysmotility-like symptoms?

The exact role of EGG remains controversial. While certain dysrhythmias have been described in patients with these symptoms, there remains no consistent correlation between EGG findings, gastric emptying study results and symptomatic response to promotility agents. Electrogastrography has been suggested to be complementary to the more conventional testing of gastric emptying.

❑❑ What is the normal residual fasting gastric volume?

Less than 100 ml.

❑❑ What is the most common finding on physical examination in a patient with delayed gastric emptying?

While most of these patients will have a normal examination, a succussion splash may occasionally be appreciated.

❑❑ What infectious diseases have been associated with delayed gastric emptying?

Acute infection with Norwalk agent, a parvovirus, has been associated with a delay in gastric emptying. *Trypanosoma cruzi* causes delayed gastric emptying by damaging the myenteric plexus. Temporary delays in gastric emptying have also been noted in patients with varicella zoster, Epstein-Barr virus, cytomegalovirus and *Clostridium botulinum* poisoning. While delayed gastric emptying has been described in patients with HIV infection, the mechanism is not clear. Patients with *Helicobacter pylori* infection have normal gastric emptying.

❑❑ T/F: Gastroparesis occurs commonly in patients with gastroesophageal reflux disease.

True. Some studies have reported the presence of gastroparesis in up to one-half of these patients. The clinical significance of this delay in most patients remains disputed, however. Gastroparesis is not more prevalent in patients with Barrett's esophagus than in patients with erosive disease.

❑❑ What is the mechanism of action of cisapride?

Cisapride is a $5\text{-}HT_4$ (serotonin) receptor agonist which facilitates the release of acetylcholine from the myenteric plexus. It is also an antagonist of the $5\text{-}HT_3$ receptor, causing a direct stimulatory effect on smooth muscle.

❑❑ What is the mechanism of action of metoclopramide?

Metoclopramide is a centrally- and peripherally-acting dopamine (D_2 receptor) antagonist which enhances myenteric cholinergic transmission.

❑❑ What is the mechanism of action of erythromycin?

Erythromycin is a motilin receptor agonist which results in stimulation of gastric smooth muscle directly and *via* cholinergic myenteric neural pathways.

❑❑ Name the abnormalities of the gastric pacemaker?

The normal discharge (normogastria) from the gastric pacemaker is 3 cycles per minute (cpm). Bradygastria is said to exist when the discharge rate is less than 2 cpm. Tachygastria is defined as a discharge rate of greater than 4 cpm.

❑❑ What are the major subtypes of non-ulcer (functional) dyspepsia?

Ulcer-like, dysmotility-like and unspecified. There is considerable overlap among these groups and the subtypes are not based upon pathophysiological differences. Patients with ulcer-like dyspepsia typically experience pain relieved by food and antacids, often awakening them from a sound sleep, but have no evidence of ulcer disease by radiography or endoscopy. Dysmotility-like dyspepsia consists of nausea, vomiting, bloating, distention, anorexia and pain made worse by eating. Nonspecific dyspepsia consists of a combination of symptoms of ulcer-like dyspepsia and dysmotility-like dyspepsia and, occasionally, symptoms of GERD.

❑❑ T/F: *Helicobacter pylori* plays a central role in the pathophysiology of non-ulcer dyspepsia.

False. While controversial, most investigators believe that *Helicobacter pylori* plays no role in non-ulcer dyspepsia.

❑❑ What is an appropriate treatment approach for patients with non-ulcer dyspepsia?

After an appropriate evaluation to exclude other potential causes, treatment should be focused on the patient's dominant symptom(s). For example, a patient with ulcer-like dyspepsia should receive a therapeutic trial with an acid-reducing agent; a patients with dysmotility-like dyspepsia should be given a trial of prokinetic agents; and, an individual with suspected visceral hyperalgesia may be treated with a low dose of a tricyclic antidepressant.

❑❑ What is the migrating motor complex (MMC)?

The migrating motor complex is a cyclical pattern of gastrointestinal motility occurring during the fasting period that consists of three phases that repeat every 90 to120 minutes. Phase I is a period of absent motor activity (motor quiescence) lasting 40 to 70 minutes. Phase II lasts 20 to 30 minutes and is characterized by irregular motor activity. Phase III consists of a 5 to 10 minute period of intense lumen-occluding contractions that begin in the body of the stomach and sequentially propagate aborally through the small intestine.

❏❏ **T/F: The esophagus is the most common gastrointestinal organ involved in scleroderma.**

True.

❏❏ **What physical finding is usually present in a scleroderma patient with esophageal involvement?**

Raynaud's phenomenon.

❏❏ **What complications may occur in a scleroderma patient with small bowel involvement?**

Malabsorption, pseudo-obstruction, pneumatosis cystoides intestinalis, bacterial overgrowth and malnutrition

❏❏ **T/F: The abnormalities in small bowel motility that may occur in scleroderma occur secondary to a myopathic process.**

False. Both myopathic and neuropathic abnormalities are responsible. The neurologic changes typically occur first followed by myopathic alterations.

❏❏ **Subcutaneous octreotide has been used to manage small bowel motor complications of scleroderma. What is a common long-term complication of this therapy?**

The development of biliary sludge and gallstones.

❏❏ **What developmental abnormality of the gastrointestinal tract may occur in children with familial pseudo-obstruction syndromes.**

Intestinal malrotation or nonrotation.

❏❏ **In general, surgery is not performed in patients with chronic idiopathic intestinal pseudoobstruction; however, surgery may be considered in certain circustances. What surgical procedures are occassionally performed in these patients?**

Placement of venting gastrostomy and/or jejunostomy tubes and intestinal transplantation (most commonly performed in children).

❏❏ **What complication of gut dysmotility is associated with an increased risk of spontaneous bacterial peritonitis in patients with end-stage liver disease.**

Small bowel dysmotility is associated with bacterial overgrowth which is postulated to translocate across the bowel wall and into the lymphatics and ascitic fluid.

❏❏ **A 36 year-old man with short bowel syndrome as a result of vascular injury during a cholecystectomy presents with persistent diarrhea despite various dietary maneuvers and anti-diarrheals. What small intestinal condition is likely to be responsible for the diarrhea?**

Small intestinal bacterial overgrowth.

❏❏ **The use of proton pump inhibitors may further increase what complication in patients with chronic intestinal pseudo-obstruction?**

Small intestinal bacterial overgrowth. While the hypochlorhydria caused by potent antisecretory agents does not generally result in clinically significant bacterial overgrowth (with clinically significant types of bacteria) in otherwise healthy individuals, it may in patients with chronic intestinal pseudo-obstruction.

❑❑ **List some causes of mechanical obstruction that may occur in patients with chronic intestinal pseudo-obstruction.**

Adhesions from prior surgery, Ladd's bands or bezoars related to hypomotility.

❑❑ **What endocrine conditions may cause small intestinal dysmotility?**

Diabetes mellitus, hypothyroidism and hyper- and hypoparathyroidism.

❑❑ **What non-gastrointestinal developmental abnormalities are associated with familial visceral myopathy?**

Megacystis/megaureters, ophthalmoplegia, peripheral neuropathy, deafness and mydriasis.

❑❑ **What non-gastrointestinal developmental abnormalities are associated with familial visceral neuropathy?**

Patent ductus arteriosus and malformations of the central nervous system.

❑❑ **What medications are associated with the development of chronic intestinal pseudo-obstruction?**

Narcotics, tricyclic antidepressants, phenothiazines, ganglionic blockers, calcium-channel blockers and anti-parkinson medications are a few of the more common medications associated with this condition.

❑❑ **What effect does low doses of octreotide have on small bowel motility as detected by intestinal manometry?**

Stimulates phase III of the migrating motor complex. However, higher doses of octreotide actually inhibit gastrointestinal motility.

❑❑ **What features suggestive of mechanical obstruction may be seen on intestinal manometry?**

Simultaneous or rapidly propagating clustered contractions and/or high amplitude, prolonged or giant contractions.

❑❑ **If intestinal manometry is unavailable, what other manometric test might be helpful in the diagnosis of pseudo-obstruction? What abnormalities might this test show?**

Esophageal manometry usually demonstrates nonspecific motility abnormalities such as a hypotensive lower esophageal sphincter and/or low amplitude esophageal contractions. Alternatively, patients may have findings consistent with diffuse esophageal spasm or achalasia.

❑❑ **What features on small bowel manometry suggest myopathic or neuropathic causes of pseudo-obstruction?**

In myopathic conditions, there is a decrease in the amplitude of contraction waves, during both fed and fasting phases. The phase III component of the MMC, while usually present, may be reduced in amplitude. Neuropathic conditions typically result in disorganized and uncoordinated activity. The direction of propagation of contractile activity may be altered or the duration shortened. In addition, there may not be conversion of the fasting phase to the fed pattern following the ingestion of a meal.

❑❑ **What small bowel manometry features distinguish an extrinsic from an intrinsic intestinal neuropathy?**

The most common feature suggestive of an extrinsic (autonomic) neuropathy is an absence of conversion of the fasting phase to the fed pattern following the ingestion of a meal. Other testing which is supportive of autonomic dysfunction include formal autonomic function testing such as pancreatic polypeptide response to hypoglycemia and tests to assess sweat and thermoregulation and hemodynamic responses to various maneuvers. Abnormalities that occur during fasting and at night, particularly involving the phase III component of the MMC, are suggestive of intrinsic (enteric nervous system) dysfunction.

❑❑ Why is it important to differentiate mechanical obstruction from pseudo-obstruction and how is this best accomplished?

Treatment of the two conditions is significantly different. Barium contrast studies, including small bowel follow-through or enteroclysis, may indicate a transition point. The latter is the more sensitive of the two. Computed tomography scans may also be useful in this situation.

❑❑ What tumors and associated autoantibodies occur with paraneoplastic visceral neuropathies?

The most common tumor causing paraneoplastic visceral neuropathy is small cell cancer of the lung, which may also be associated with a generalized sensory neuropathy. Histologically, there may be degeneration of neurons and infiltration with plasma cells in the bowel, but no evidence of tumor. Associated antibodies that can be detected in the serum are anti-Hu or ANNA (anti-neuronal nuclear antibody).

❑❑ What tests are useful for the diagnosis of bacterial overgrowth and what are their potential shortcomings?

Culture of a sterilly-collected small intestinal aspirate is the gold standard in the diagnosis of bacterial overgrowth. However, both false positives (contamination by mouth flora) and false negatives (difficulties in culturing anerobes) may occur. Alternatively, a 14C-xylose breath test, which measures expired CO_2 production, can be used. However, it requires the use of radiolabeled material and is not widely available. Hydrogen breath testing for either glucose or lactulose may also be used; however, its utility is limited in patients who do not have hydrogen generating bacteria (8% - 20%).

❑❑ What findings are suggestive of small bowel bacterial overgrowth on the breath hydrogen test?

A significant increase in breath hydrogen expired during the first two hours of ingestion of substrate. Sometimes, a high fasting breath hydrogen may also be found.

❑❑ What disturbances in small bowel motility may be seen in amyloidosis?

Dysmotility seems to correlate with the degree of amyloid deposition in the gut. Small bowel loops may be dilated and transit can be delayed. Small bowel motility studies may reveal findings consistent with either a myopathic or a neuropathic disturbance.

❑❑ What small bowel motility abnormalities have been described in irritable bowel syndrome?

Most studies do not indicate any specific abnormality. However, some patients have discrete clustered contractions in the duodenum and jejunum that are associated with symptoms. Recent studies have suggested that these occur more commonly than in controls. Other motor abnormalities described in these patients includes ileal high-pressure waves and a disturbed postprandial motor response.

❑❑ What is the utility of a full-thickness intestinal biopsy in a patient with suspected pseudo-obstruction?

To completely evaluate the neuromuscular apparatus of the gut, a full-thickness intestinal biopsy with special stains for muscle, nerves and connective tissue is needed. Unfortunately, opportunities to obtain such tissue specimens rarely arise.

❑❑ What is the pathophysiology of ileus?

The lack of intestinal activity is most likely related to increased sympathetic inhibitory activity (imbalance of autonomic nervous system) and a resultant loss of normal coordination of activity.

❑❑ What segments of the colon are usually involved in volvulus?

Sigmoid volvulus accounts for approximately 70% of all cases of colonic volvulus followed by the cecum.

❑❑ How helpful are abdominal x-rays in making the diagnosis of colonic volvulus?

Classic radiological features of sigmoid or cecal volvulus are observed in approximately 50% of patients. Water soluble enemas and computed tomography scans are indicated when the diagnosis is unclear.

❑❑ How effective is endoscopic decompression in the management of colonic volvulus?

Flexible sigmoidoscopy and rectal decompression tube placement for sigmoid volvulus is effective in 60% to 80% of cases. In the case of cecal volvulus, non-operative decompression is usually not successful.

❑❑ What is the recurrence rate of colonic volvulus after endoscopic decompression?

Sigmoid volvulus recurs in approximately 50%. Therefore, surgical correction is often subsequently performed on an elective basis. Primary surgical correction of cecal volvulus is the treatment of choice.

❑❑ T/F: Hirschprung's disease can occur in adults.

True. Hirschprung's disease may be diagnosed in adolescence and adults. Diagnosis should be suspected in patients who have history of constipation dating back to early childhood.

❑❑ T/F: Anorectal manometry can exclude Hirschprung's disease.

True. The presence of a rectoanal inhibitory reflex (RAIR) - reflex relaxation of the anal sphincter with distention of the rectum - excludes Hirschprung's disease. On the other hand, the absence of the RAIR does not necessarily prove the diagnosis of Hirschprung's as, occasionally, the RAIR is absent in patients with normal innervation of the colon.

❑❑ T/F: A full thickness colon biopsy is always needed to confirm the diagnosis of Hirschprung's disease.

False. Colonic mucosal biopsy using either a large forceps or suction biopsy technique is the first step. If taken from the appropriate segment of the rectum and ganglion cells are present in the submucosa, Hirschprung's is excluded. The absence of ganglion cells using these techniques, on the other hand, mandates a full thickness biopsy.

❑❑ What are the predisposing factors for acute colonic pseudo-obstruction?

This condition is typically seen in the elderly following trauma or recovery from surgery, particularly, orthopaedic, obstetric or abdominal surgery. It can also occur in the setting of any severe medical illness.

❑❑ What is the most effective drug therapy for acute colonic pseudo-obstruction?

While several mostly uncontrolled clinical trials have suggested that a number of medications may be effective, a recent report from a randomized and double-blinded study suggests a high rate of success using parenteral administration of neostigmine.

❑❑ When should colonoscopic decompression be attempted in the management of acute colonic pseudo-obstruction?

In a patient without evidence of compromised bowel, if initial measures such as nasogastric decompression, discontinuation of narcotics/anticholinergic medications, correction of electrolytes and hypoxemia and pharmacological therapy are unsuccessful, colonoscopic decompression should be attempted. Standard recommendations suggest colonoscopy when the diameter of the cecum is greater than 11 or 12 cm. A colonic decompression tube may be left in place.

❑❑ T/F: A gender difference exists in the irritable bowel syndrome.

True. Irritable bowel syndrome is twice as common in females.

☐☐ **T/F: There is an association between irritable bowel syndrome and physical and sexual abuse.**

True. A history of previous abuse has been reported in up to 40% of these patients. These patients tend to be seen in tertiary referral centers. This is far higher than in patients with organic disorders.

☐☐ **T/F: Irritable bowel syndrome is associated with other gastrointestinal symptoms and non-gastrointestinal conditions.**

True. Upper gastrointestinal symptoms such as heartburn, nausea and vomiting are reported in up to 50% of patients with irritable bowel syndrome. Urinary symptoms, dyspareunia and fibromylagia are also more common in patients with irritable bowel syndrome compared to patients with organic gastrointestinal diseases.

☐☐ **T/F: Irritable bowel syndrome is associated with an identifiable motor abnormality.**

False. While a number of motor changes have been described in patients with irritable bowel syndrome, no pathognomonic motor abnormality has been defined thus far.

☐☐ **Which laxatives are associated with melanosis coli?**

Anthranoid laxatives such as senna, cascara and aloe.

☐☐ **Where in the gut is melanosis seen?**

Melanosis can be seen throughout the colon; however, the proximal colon is usually more affected.

☐☐ **How soon does melanosis coli appear and how quickly does it resolve following use and discontinuation of anthranoid laxatives, respectively?**

It can be seen within months of starting and will usually disappear within months after discontinuation.

☐☐ **What is the most common reason for fecal incontinence in children and institutionalized elderly?**

Fecal retention resulting in overflow soiling.

☐☐ **What is the most common etiology of constipation?**

Idiopathic.

☐☐ **What subtypes are included in idiopathic constipation?**

Slow transit, pelvic floor dyssynergia and functional.

☐☐ **What is pelvic floor dyssynergia?**

In this condition also referred to as anismus, pelvic floor dysfunction or obstructed defecation, there is contraction rather than relaxation of the external sphincter and puborectalis in response to straining.

☐☐ **How can pelvic floor dyssynergia be diagnosed?**

Several tests are available. The more of these tests that are abnormal, the stronger the diagnosis of pelvic floor dyssynergia. Digital exam of the anal canal may show contraction of the sphincter apparatus rather than relaxation when the patient is asked to bear down. Anorectal manometry and electromyography may show contraction rather than relaxation of the muscles. Evacuation proctography (defecography) may show that the anorectal angle narrows rather than widens during attempted defecation. Finally, a balloon expulsion test may demonstrate difficulty expelling the balloon from the rectum.

❏❏ **What is the most appropriate treatment for this condition?**

Pelvic floor retraining (biofeedback). Successful results following biofeedback methods have been reported in 50% to 80% of patients with pelvic floor dyssynergia.

❏❏ **What medications can cause or aggravate constipation?**

Opiate derivatives, anti-cholinergics, calcium- or aluminum-containing antacids, calcium channel blockers and clonidine are a few.

❏❏ **T/F: Surgery is indicated if both a rectocele and difficult evacuation are present.**

False. Rectoceles are common, even in non-constipated women. A history of applying digital pressure on the posterior wall of the vagina to help evacuation and a defecogram showing a large rectocele with residual barium at the end of defecation suggest that surgical repair may be helpful.

❏❏ **T/F: Surgery is often helpful in the management of pelvic floor dyssynergia.**

False. Operations, such as division of the internal anal sphincter and puborectalis are usually not successful and may result in fecal incontinence.

❏❏ **How is colonic transit measured?**

Both radiology (radio-opaque markers) and scintigraphy can be used. In clinical practice, radio- opaque markers are more commonly used.

❏❏ **When should a colonic transit study be used?**

In patients with severe intractable constipation. A normal colonic transit in such patients is associated with a higher prevalence of psychological distress when compared to patients with slow transit.

❏❏ **T/F: Exercise is helpful in the treatment of constipation.**

False. While constipation is associated with inactivity, there is no convincing data to suggest that, in active subjects, bowel habits are affected by exercise.

❏❏ **What is the recommended daily dose of fiber per day?**

Between 20 to 30 grams.

❏❏ **T/F: Fiber is effective in patients with severe constipation.**

False. Fiber comes from different sources and its effect on colonic transit is variable. All patients with constipation should have an appropriate amount of fiber in their diet; however, while patients with mild constipation may improve with additional fiber, those with significant slow transit constipation tend not to improve on fiber alone.

❏❏ **What are the potential complications of mineral oil?**

Lipoid pneumonia, if aspirated. It can also cause anal seepage and there is a potential risk of malabsorption of lipid soluble vitamins.

❏❏ **How do stimulant laxatives work?**

Both anthranoid laxatives, such as senna and aloe, and the diphenylmethanes, such as phenolphthalein and bisacodyl, act by increasing colonic motility and by inducing secretion. Phenolphthalein compounds have been withdrawn from the market.

❏❏ **How do osmotic laxatives work?**

Osmotic laxatives contain poorly absorbable ions such as magnesium.

❏❏ **What are potential side effects of osmotic laxatives?**

Hypermagnesmia.

❏❏ **T/F: Polyethylene glycol solution is useful for chronic constipation.**

True. Polyethylene glycol is a non-absorbable electrolyte solution. While normally given for bowel cleansing prior to colonoscopy, when taken in smaller amounts (250 ml to 750 ml per day), it can be extremely helpful in the treatment of chronic constipation.

❏❏ **What is the most common operation for patients with severe constipation and slow colonic transit?**

Subtotal colectomy with ileorectal anastomosis.

❏❏ **T/F: Prior to consideration of surgery for refractory slow transit constipation, an evaluation to exclude a more diffuse gut dysmotility syndrome (intestinal pseudo-obstruction) should be performed.**

True. In particular, an evaluation of gastric and small bowel motility, usually accomplished by antroduodenal manometry, should be considered prior to surgery. Similarly, testing to evaluate for the presence of pelvic floor dyssynergia should be performed.

❏❏ **What are the three components of the Sphincter of Oddi?**

The three components are the Sphincter choledochus, Sphincter pancreaticus and sphincter ampulla which surround the distal common bile duct, duct of Wirsung and common channel, respectively.

❏❏ **What is the role of the Sphincter of Oddi?**

It regulates flow of pancreatic and biliary secretions into the duodenum by its basal pressure and prevents the reflux of material from the duodenum into the duct by its phasic contractions.

❏❏ **What is the normal basal Sphincter of Oddi (SO) pressure?**

The normal mean basal SO pressure is less than 35 mmHg.

❏❏ **What are the features of the normal phasic contractions of the Sphincter of Oddi?**

The phasic contractions consist of three components: amplitude, duration and frequency. The amplitude is less than 220 mmHg with a duration less than 8 seconds and a frequency of less than 10 per minute.

❏❏ **What drugs relax the Sphincter of Oddi?**

Anticholinergics, nitrates, calcium channel blockers and glucagon.

❏❏ **What is the gold standard for the diagnosis of Sphincter of Oddi dysfunction?**

Sphincter of Oddi manometry.

❏❏ **What manometric findings are typical in patients with of Sphincter of Oddi dysfunction?**

Manometric criteria include 1) elevated basal sphincter pressure, 2) increased frequency of phasic contractions, 3) increased proportion of phasic contractions propagated in the retrograde direction, and 4) paradoxical sphincter response to CCK-OP (cholecystokinin-octapeptide) injection. In clinical practice, a basal sphincter pressure > 40 mmHg is the single most useful parameter in which to make this diagnosis.

❏❏ **What type of catheter is used in biliary manometry?**

A triple lumen, water-perfused catheter. The use of one lumen for aspiration may reduce the risk of procedure-related pancreatitis.

❏❏ **T/F: Glucagon affects Sphincter of Oddi manometry.**

True. Glucagon causes relaxation of the sphincter and so a waiting period of 8 to 10 minutes is required before measuring the basal sphincter pressure if glucagon was used to aid in cannulation.

❏❏ **T/F: Benzodiazepines affect Sphincter of Oddi manometry.**

False. Benzodiazepines do not affect the sphincter and can be used as a sedative for patients undergoing Sphincter of Oddi manometry.

❏❏ **What are indications for Sphincter of Oddi manometry?**

Patients with idiopathic pancreatitis and patients with unexplained pancreaticobiliary pain with or without abnormal liver or pancreatic enzymes.

❏❏ **T/F: Endoscopic retrograde cholangiopancreatography (ERCP) is required in the evaluation of Sphincter of Oddi dysfunction (SOD).**

True. ERCP is required in order to exclude other causes of biliary obstruction such as retained stones and anatomical lesions.

❏❏ **What are the four clinical criteria for the diagnosis of SOD type I?**

1) Typical biliary-type pain, 2) elevated aspartate aminotransferase or alkaline phosphatase > 2 times normal and measured on more than two occasions, 3) delayed drainage of contrast more than 45 minutes at the time of ERCP, and 4) dilated common bile duct more than 12 mm. The third criteria is seldomly used in routine clinical practice.

❏❏ **What is SOD type II?**

Patients with typical biliary-type pain and one or two of the previously mentioned criteria .

❏❏ **What is SOD type III?**

Patients with typical biliary-type pain and no other abnormalities.

❏❏ **T/F: Sphincter of Oddi manometry is always indicated in type I SOD.**

False. It is not essential before endoscopic sphincterotomy since these patients benefit from sphincterotomy regardless of findings on manometry.

❏❏ **T/F: Sphichter of Oddi manometry is always indicated in type II or III SOD.**

True. Sphincter of Oddi manometry is mandatory in these patients to confirm the presence of SOD and to predict the subset that will benefit from sphincterotomy. Those with elevated basal pressures more predictably experience improvement of pain after sphincterotomy.

❏❏ **How does SOD cause pain?**

It is postulated that, by impeding the flow of pancreatic and biliary secretions, there is a resulting increase in the ductal pressure (ductal hypertension) causing pain.

❏❏ What is the estimated frequency of SOD in patients with biliary-type pain following cholecystectomy?

9% to 11%.

❏❏ What is the best predictor of pain relief in patients with SOD after sphincterotomy ?

Elevated basal sphincter pressure (> 40 mmHg).

❏❏ What are indications for surgical Sphincter of Oddi ablation?

1) Recurrent stenoses after repeated endoscopic sphincterotomies, 2) when an experienced therapeutic endoscopist is not available and 3) when endoscopic sphincterotomy is not technically feasible.

❏❏ What pharmacological agents have been used in the treatment of SOD?

Nitrates and nifedipine. There has also been recent interest in the use of botulinum toxin injections into the Sphincter of Oddi.

❏❏ What is the Nardi test?

A positive result occurs when the injection of morphine, 10mg subcutaneously, or neostigmine, 1mg subcutaneously, causes typical biliary-type pain with an associated four-fold increase in aminotransferases, alkaline phosphatase, amylase or lipase. A positive test may occur in patients with SOD; however, it can also occur in patients with choledocholelithiasis. This test is neither sensitive nor specific. Morphine causes Sphincter of Oddi contraction while neostigmine increases the pancreatic flow of secretions.

❏❏ What is a positive secretin stimulation test?

A positive result occurs when secretin administration leads to dilatation of the common bile duct and main pancreatic duct, as detected by ultrasound. This may occur when the Sphincter of Oddi is dysfunctional causing obstruction. Secretin normally results in Sphincter of Oddi relaxation.

❏❏ What is a positive hepatobiliary scintigraphy test?

This test assesses bile flow through the biliary tract and into the duodenum. A positive test is defined as a duodenal arrival time greater than 20 minutes and a hilum to duodenal time greater than 10 minutes.

❏❏ T/F: The gallbladder empties during fasting.

True. During fasting, 25% of gallbladder contents empty approximately every 120 minutes. This coincides with the migrating motor complex seen in the intestine.

❏❏ What happens to the gallbladder in the fed state?

Eating initiates gallbladder contraction through both neural (cephalic and local gastroduodenal reflexes) and hormonal (cholecystokinin) influences. This results in the emptying of over 75% of the gallbladder contents.

❏❏ What are the phases of gallbladder emptying?

Gallbladder emptying after meals consists of three phases: 1) Cephalic phase - stimulated by sham feeding; 2) Gastric phase - stimulated by distension of the stomach and the gastroduodenal reflex; and, 3) Intestinal phase - stimulated by hormones. The bulk of the contractions occur during the gastric and intestinal phases.

❏❏ T/F: Fat, protein and carbohydrate lead to gallbladder contraction.

True. Meal composition determines cholecystokinin release and, hence, gallbladder contraction. Protein and fat result in gallbladder contraction via cholecystokinin release while carbohydrate also causes gallbladder contraction but via an unknown mechanism.

❑❑ **How does motilin affect the gallbladder?**

Motilin induces gallbladder contraction indirectly via cholinergic nerves.

❑❑ **T/F: Patients with gallstones have reduced gallbladder emptying.**

True. This impairment results from depression of gallbladder contractility and not the gallstones themselves.

❑❑ **What tests are available for the measurement of gallbladder emptying?**

Cholescintigraphy, which measures radioisotope distribution and output into the intestine over time, and ultrasonography, which measures volume changes over time. The gold standard for measuring gallbladder emptying is cholecystokinin-cholescintigraphy.

❑❑ **Why is cholecystokinin used?**

Cholecystokinin is the most potent stimulus of gallbladder emptying and, in addition, causes relaxation of the Sphincter of Oddi via inhibitory nerves.

❑❑ **What radiopharmaceutical agent is commonly used in cholescintigraphy?**

Hepatoiminodiacetic acid (HIDA).

❑❑ **What drugs cause impaired gallbladder emptying?**

The most common drugs that cause impaired gallbladder emptying are narcotics and anticholinergic agents.

❑❑ **What is gallbladder dyskinesia?**

Gallbladder dyskinesia refers to abnormal gallbladder function which may be either hypokinetic (depressed) or hyperkinetic (excessive).

❑❑ **What is the gallbladder ejection fraction?**

Quantitative measurement of gallbladder emptying. The normal gallbladder ejection fraction is over 35%.

❑❑ **T/F: A diminished gallbladder ejection fraction is a characteristic finding in patients with chronic acalculous cholecystitis.**

While controversial, the demonstration of a low gallbladder ejection fraction is the most reliable indicator of chronic cholecystitis and is the best prognosticator of a good response to cholecystectomy.

NUTRITION, OBESITY AND EATING DISORDERS

Deborah Cohen, MMSc, RD, CNSD, Douglas A. Drossman, M.D. and Tamar Ringel-Kulka, M.D.

❑❑ **T/F: Anorexia nervosa and bulimia are best understood as psychiatric diseases with secondary physiologic manifestations.**

False. Anorexia nervosa and bulimia are multifactorial disorders that result from biologic, psychological and social influence.

❑❑ **What is the incidence and prevalence of anorexia nervosa in the United States? Has it changed over the years?**

Incidence rates for females 16 to 25 years of age range from 30 per 100,000 to 156 per 100,000. The incidence has increased two- to four-fold in the last decade. The prevalence is thought to be 0.5% to 1%.

❑❑ **How common is anorexia nervosa in female adolescents and young adults?**

Anorexia nervosa ranks as the third most common illness after obesity and asthma.

❑❑ **What is the male to female ratio in anorexia nervosa?**

Incidence in males is 1/10 to 1/50 that of females.

❑❑ **How do persons with an eating disorder perceive their body size?**

In a recent study, 50% to 67% of female adolescents perceived themselves as too fat while only about 15% were, in fact, overweight. In addition, 50% of female adolescents and 15% of male adolescents were found to engage in dieting behavior. Forty percent of them where dissatisfied with their body image. Hips, waist and thighs are the common sites of dissatisfaction.

❑❑ **T/F: Increased risk of anorexia nervosa is equal in developed and developing countries.**

False. Common risk factors for developing anorexia nervosa include: being from a western-culture or developed country, age 15 to 25 years, female gender, engagement in dieting, sports and activities associated with appearance, presence of physical illness that results in initial weight loss, low self-esteem, obsessive personality, eating disorder in first degree relatives, and being a monozygotic twin.

❑❑ **T/F: Anorectic patients will engage in self-induced vomiting or take purgatives.**

True. In bulimic-type anorexia nervosa, weight loss is accomplished in these ways 50% of the time rather than with restriction and exercise.

❑❑ **T/F: Anorectic patients don't feel hunger.**

False. Anorectic patients do feel hunger; however, in their pursuit of thinness, they struggle against hunger to achieve an unrealistic degree of weight loss.

❑❑ **What physiologic measures are decreased in anorectic patients?**

Core temperature, blood pressure, pulse rate and gastric emptying rate.

❏❏ **T/F: Erythrocyte sedimentation rate is increased in anorexia nervosa.**

False. The sedimentation rate is usually decreased in anorexia nervosa.

❏❏ **What is the most common endocrine abnormality in anorexia nervosa?**

Amenorrhea is the most common endocrine abnormality in anorectic patients. The origin of amenorrhea is due to hypothalamic-pituitary dysfunction. Serum levels of estradiol, follicle-stimulating hormone and luteinizing hormone are lower than in normal controls.

❏❏ **T/F: Amenorrhea may precede weight loss.**

True. In about one-third of the patients, amenorrhea precedes weight loss. Stress appears to cause psychogenic amenorrhea prior to the onset of weight loss.

❏❏ **T/F: Amenorrhea always resolves after achieving ideal body weight.**

False.

❏❏ **What is the lower limit of weight under which hospitalization is recommended?**

Hospitalization is recommended for patients with loss of 25% to 30% of ideal body weight over a few months. Other indications considered include hemodynamic disturbances, electrocardiographic abnormalities, dehydration, electrolyte abnormalities and failure to gain weight with intensive outpatient management.

❏❏ **T/F: The most common cause of death in anorexia nervosa is cardiac arrhythmia.**

False. The most common cause of death in anorexia nervosa is suicide followed by cardiac arrhythmia.

❏❏ **T/F: Electrocardiographic abnormalities are common in anorexia nervosa.**

False. Although various electrocardiographic abnormalities have been described in anorexia nervosa, most patients who are not chronically vomiting or abusing laxatives will have a normal electrocardiogram. Prolongation of the QTc interval is the main predictor for risk of sudden death.

❏❏ **T/F: The primary goal of nutritional intervention in anorexia nervosa is to slowly get the patient to a body weight out of the range of medical risk.**

True.

❏❏ **T/F: Carotene can be a helpful diagnostic biochemical test in anorexia nervosa.**

True. High levels of carotene can be seen in anorexia nervosa while low levels of carotene are seen in patients with starvation. Carotenemia in anorexia nervosa causes a yellow discoloration of the skin.

❏❏ **What is a common long-term morbidity acssociated with anorexia nervosa?**

Osteoporosis is the most common morbidity and is due to hypoestrogenemia along with nutritional deficiencies.

❏❏ **T/F: Constipation is one of the acute gastrointestinal complications in patients with bulimia.**

False. Constipation is a chronic complication of anorexia nervosa. Mallory-Weiss tears and Boerhaave's syndrome are potential acute gut complications of bulimia.

❏❏ **What is the most common metabolic complication in bulimic patients?**

Hypochloremic, hypokalemic, metabolic alkalosis.

❏❏ What are common/typical signs that can be recognized on physical examination in bulimic patients?

Russell sign (excoriation on the dorsum of hands or fingers), loss of dentine on the lingual and occlusal surface of the teeth and parotid gland hypertrophy.

❏❏ T/F: The incidence and prevalence of bulimia are lower than that of anorexia nervosa.

False. The incidence and prevalence of bulimia are higher than that of anorexia nervosa. The incidence is estimated at 2% to 5% in high school and college-aged females while the prevalence is estimated at 1% to 3%.

❏❏ T/F: Unlike anorectic patients, bulimic patients have normal body size.

True. Bulimic patients have normal body size, less body image distortion, greater awareness that their secret compulsive behaviors are aberrant and greater acceptance of treatment compared to anorectic patients.

❏❏ T/F: Satiety interrupts binging episodes in bulimic patients.

False. The binge-purge cycle is an eating compulsion associated with failure to achieve or respond to normal satiety. The episodes occur secretly, are planned and are terminated by a feeling of guilt or physical discomfort.

❏❏ What is the leading cause of death in bulimia nervosa?

Cardiac arrhythmia.

❏❏ T/F: More than half of anorexia nervosa or bulimia patients will not improve following treatment.

False. Full recovery will occur in 50% of the patients. Of the remainder, about 30% will have partial recovery and 20% will experience no improvement.

❏❏ What proportion of adults in the United States is obese?

Approximately 33%.

❏❏ T/F: Fifty percent of people who lose weight on a well-designed program of diet and exercise will maintain their achieved weight.

False. Ninety to 95% of persons who lose weight subsequently regain it within 5 years.

❏❏ What measure is commonly used to define obesity?

Body-mass index: weight in kilograms divided by the square of the height in meters.

❏❏ What are the definitions of overweight and obesity?

The World Health Organization definitions of obesity and overweight are: Overweight - body mass index (BMI) > 25; Obesity - BMI > 30; Moderate obesity - BMI over 30 - 34.9: Severe obesity - BMI 35 - 39.9; and, Very severe obesity - BMI > 40.

❏❏ What health risks are associated with obesity?

Stroke, ischemic heart disease and diabetes mellitus occur at three to four times the risk of the general population in patients with a BMI > 28.

❏❏ **T/F: The distribution of fat over the body is important with respect to morbidity and mortality.**

True. A higher risk of morbidity and mortality is associated more with a central distribution rather than a peripheral distribution of body fat.

❏❏ **What is the role of leptin in the pathogenesis of obesity?**

The role of leptin in humans is still unclear. It is thought to be an indicator of sufficient fat stores for growth and fertility. Reduction in plasma leptin concentrations may cause hyperphagia, low energy output and infertility.

❏❏ **T/F: The goal when treating obesity is to achieve normal body weight.**

False. The goal is reduction of health risks. Even modest weight loss can alleviate symptoms from obesity-related comorbidities.

❏❏ **T/F: Caloric and fat reduction diet is the most successful treatment for obesity.**

False. A combination of reduced caloric and fat intake, regular activity and reinforcement of behavioral modification is the most successful approach.

❏❏ **What is the role of cholecystokinin (CCK) in the satiety mechanism?**

While CCK is secreted both from the duodenum and the brain, it cannot cross the blood brain barrier. The presumed primary site of action for CCK is peripheral. CCK has been shown to induce satiety and reduce food intake in rats.

❏❏ **T/F: Pharmacotherapy is recommended for all patients with obesity.**

False. Drug treatment can be useful in combination with diet and exercise. It is recommended for people with BMI > 30 and no comorbidities or BMI > 27 with comorbidity.

❏❏ **Which neuropeptide plays a major role in the central control of appetite?**

Neuropeptide Y - a potent appetite stimulant.

❏❏ **T/F: Gastroplasty is the most common surgical procedure recommended in the treatment of obesity.**

True. Gastroplasty, with or without bypass, is the most common surgical procedure used in severely obese patients.

❏❏ **T/F: Jejunoileal bypass for morbid obesity is rarely performed because of a high incidence of serious intestinal and liver complications.**

True. In addition, a characteristic arthropathy may complicate the post-operative course.

❏❏ **Individuals with achlorhydria may need regular injections of which vitamin?**

Vitamin B12.

❏❏ **A patient who takes megadoses of which vitamin is at risk for developing iron overload?**

Vitamin C.

❏❏ **What vitamin deficiency does the Schilling test indicate?**

Vitamin B12.

❑❑ **Macrocytic anemia can result from deficiencies in what two B vitamins?**

Folate and Vitamin B12.

❑❑ **What biliary factors may contribute to calcium malabsorption?**

Decreased bile flow and decreased bile salt excretion.

❑❑ **What nutritional therapy is prescribed for metabolic bone disease due to calcium malabsorption?**

25-hydroxyvitamin D3 and low fat diet.

❑❑ **Why does a patient with an ileal resection develop Vitamin D deficiency?**

Disrupted enterohepatic cycling of bile acids leads to its relative deficiency.

❑❑ **How long is the half-life of albumin? Prealbumin?**

Twenty-one days (albumin) versus three days (prealbumin).

❑❑ **What conditions, other than malnutrition, may result in hypoalbuminemia?**

Renal disease, liver disease, hydration, chemotherapy, post-operative setting and blood loss.

❑❑ **T/F: All patients receiving mechanical ventilation require a specialized pulmonary enteral formula.**

False.

❑❑ **What are the macronutrient characteristics that make a pulmonary enteral formula unique?**

High fat and low carbohydrate.

❑❑ **What is an acceptable level of gastric residual for a patient receiving gastric enteral tube feeding?**

Twice the current rate or 100 to 150 ml.

❑❑ **List factors that may contribute to aspiration in a tube fed patient.**

Feeding tube in the stomach, lying flat during formula infusion, delayed gastric motility, depressed gag reflex and a high fat formula.

❑❑ **What classical electrolyte disturbances occur with the refeeding syndrome?**

Low serum levels of magnesium, potassium and phosphorus.

❑❑ **How much fat is required in the diet to prevent essential fatty acid deficiency?**

Three to 4% of the total calories.

❑❑ **How much fat is required in the diet in order to have adequate absorption of fat-soluble vitamins?**

10%.

❑❑ **What are clinical implications of providing excess parenteral dextrose?**

Exacerbation of hyperglycemia, hepatic steatosis and elevated liver tests.

❑❑ **How many days after the initiation of total parenteral nutrition will a rise in liver tests typically occur?**

Ten to twelve days.

❑❑ **A patient has been receiving nothing by mouth and total parenteral nutrition for three weeks after a surgical resection for Crohn's disease. A J-tube was placed during surgery in anticipation of long-term enteral nutrition support and now the patient is ready to begin enteral feeds. What type of formula would you utilize and why?**

In this situation, a semi-elemental formula is usually tolerated best because of gut mucosal atrophy that developed during the prolonged period when nothing was given by mouth.

❑❑ **In the previous patient, why is it important to increase the tube feeds slowly?**

In order to allow adequate time for mucosal regeneration.

❑❑ **At what point would you discontinue the total parenteral nutrition?**

When the patient is tolerating approximately 50% of the goal tube feed.

❑❑ **Why is it inappropriate to bolus feed into the small intestine?**

The small intestine is very sensitive to volume/distension.

❑❑ **What nutritional factors, other than enteral feeding itself, contribute to diarrhea in critically ill patients?**

Bowel wall edema secondary to severely low serum albumin levels and gut mucosal atrophy resulting from prolonged periods of receiving nothing by mouth or chronic malnutrition.

❑❑ **Which vitamin is produced in the gut on a daily basis?**

Vitamin K.

❑❑ **Medium chain triglyceride (MCT) oil is given to patients with severe fat malabsorption as a calorie supplement. What are gastrointestinal side effects of an excess of MCT oil in the diet?**

Excess gas, bloating, diarrhea and anal seepage.

❑❑ **How long does it take to develop biochemical evidence of an essential fatty acid deficiency on a fat free diet, either enteral or parenteral?**

Three weeks.

❑❑ **What two organs are storage sites for Vitamin A?**

Adipose tissue and liver.

❑❑ **What can result from megadoses of Vitamin D?**

Soft tissue calcium deposition.

❑❑ **T/F: Residuals should be checked in a patient receiving nasoduodenal feedings.**

False.

❑❑ **What specific nutritional characteristics of a renal enteral formula make it clinically useful in a patient with-end stage renal disease?**

Low protein/nitrogen; lower amounts of electrolytes such as potassium, magnesium and phosphorus; and, calorie dense to provide more calories in less volume.

❑❑ **T/F: It is preferable to enterally, rather than parenterally, feed a patient with acute pancreatitis.**

True – as long as the feeding tube is placed into the jejunum.

❑❑ **What nutritional laboratory parameters need to be monitored closely in a patient with pancreatitis who is receiving total parenteral nutrition and lipids?**

Serum triglycerides and blood glucose levels.

❑❑ **Why is the total amount of calcium and phosphorus limited in a parenteral nutrition solution?**

An excess in the total calcium/phosphate product will cause precipitate formation in the solution.

❑❑ **T/F: A patient has been tolerating tube feeding for three weeks and suddenly develops a stool output of 950 cc per day. The tube feeding is the most likely cause of the sudden increase in stool output.**

False. In this situation, especially if tolerance had been good, an investigation for other causes of diarrhea should be initiated. Potential causes include gut infections, particularly *Clostridium difficile*, and the use of medications given through the feeding tube that contain sorbitol.

❑❑ **In the meantime, what changes could you make to the tube feeding regimen in the previous patient without compromising his/her nutritional status?**

Decrease the rate, change to a semi-elemental formula or try a fiber-containing formula.

❑❑ **What types of individuals are at risk for developing a refeeding syndrome?**

Malnourished patients with recent involuntary weight loss.

❑❑ **List advantages of continuous enteral feeding into the jejunum compared to the stomach.**

Potentially lower risk of aspiration and useful for patients with poor gastric motility.

❑❑ **What are formula restrictions of jejunal feedings?**

Low fat (< 35%), low fiber, not nutrient dense (1.5 to 2.0 calories/ml) and isotonic. High fat, high fiber, nutrient dense formulas can clog the small caliber tubes used for jejunal feeds and, in addition, hypertonic formulas are usually not well tolerated when given directly into the jejunum.

❑❑ **What are potential complications of a surgical jejunostomy?**

Infection, obstruction, torsion, dislodgement, leakage, bowel necrosis and the general risks of surgery and anesthesia.

❑❑ **T/F: Whenever possible, all medications administered through a feeding tube should be given as solutions or elixirs.**

True. Crushed medications have the potential to clog the feeding tube.

❑❑ **A patient has a total bilirubin of 17.8 mg/dl and is receiving total parenteral nutrition. What two trace elements should be removed from the solution to avoid toxicity?**

Copper and manganese. Both are excreted via the biliary tract. The standard trace elements should be discontinued and the zinc and chromium added back separately.

❑❑ **How many calories are there in a 500 cc container of 20% lipids? How much protein is in the bottle?**

One thousand calories. There is no protein.

❑❑ **T/F: A 20% lipid emulsion can be given through a peripheral intravenous line.**

True. All intravenous lipids are isotonic.

PEDIATRIC GASTROINTESTINAL DISEASES

Jon A. Vanderhoof, M.D.

❑❑ **Formula fed and human milk fed infants have different patterns of gut flora colonization. The stools of breast fed infants have a predominance of which bacterial genus?**

Bifidobacterium.

❑❑ **What is the coefficient of fat absorption in a normal individual?**

In a normal individual, 93% of fat is absorbed. In newborn infants, the number drops to a level of 90% and even less in premature infants. Nevertheless, its caloric density (9 kcal/g) makes it an excellent source of calories, even in premature infants.

❑❑ **Absent responses to which gastrointestinal hormones occur in gluten-sensitive enteropathy prior to treatment?**

Cholecystokinin, secretin and glucose-dependent insulin trophic peptide.

❑❑ **In the medical evaluation of anorexia nervosa, laboratory studies to screen for pregnancy, inflammatory bowel disease, thyroid disease, central nervous system disorders, drug abuse and metabolic disorders are routinely done. What additional serum study may be useful in this scenario?**

Serum carotene.

❑❑ **What disorder should be suspected in a patient with a history of caustic ingestion who develops a late onset or worsening of dysphagia?**

Esophageal carcinoma.

❑❑ **What percentage of school-age children have chronic abdominal pain to the extent that it interferes with normal daily activity?**

10%.

❑❑ **What is the most useful diagnostic tool to identify the cause of chronic recurrent abdominal pain of childhood?**

Careful history and physical examination.

❑❑ **Chronic, nonspecific diarrhea or toddler diarrhea, the most common cause of chronic diarrhea in this age group, is best treated utilizing what dietary maneuvers?**

High fat, low carbohydrate diet.

❑❑ **Constipation in school age children has recently been identified as a possible consequence of intolerance to what dietary component?**

Cow's milk protein.

❑❑ **What is the most common cause of acute abdomen in the infant age group?**

Intussusception.

❑❑ **What is the most common cause of painless, lower gastrointestinal bleeding in school age children?**

Colonic polyps.

❑❑ **Infantile failure to thrive is a serious condition requiring early identification and treatment. What is responsible for nearly all the mortality in this condition?**

Abused or seriously neglected infants.

❑❑ **What is the most common malignant tumor of the gastrointestinal tract in children and presents most frequently in the distal ileum?**

Lymphoma.

❑❑ **What is the drug of choice if sedation is required for esophageal manometry?**

Chloral hydrate, 50 mg/kg. It does not effect lower esophageal sphincter pressure or the amplitude of esophageal contractions.

❑❑ **What is the most common type of tracheoesophageal fistula?**

Proximal esophageal atresia with a fistula between the trachea and the distal esophagus accounts for 85%.

❑❑ **What is the major value of an upper gastrointestinal x-ray in an infant with frequent emesis?**

An upper gastrointestinal barium-contrast x-ray excludes anatomical lesions, gastric outlet obstruction and proximal small bowel anomalies. It does not diagnose or exclude gastroesophageal reflux.

❑❑ **What is the most common cause of idiopathic portal hypertension in a child without liver disease?**

Portal vein thrombosis. Further history may reveal that a venous umbilical catheter was placed during the newborn period.

❑❑ **T/F: Newborn infants are achlorhydric.**

False. Newborn infants have high serum gastrin levels and normal stimulated gastric acid production has been demonstrated in the first few days of life.

❑❑ **How long does an infant need to receive nothing by mouth after a pyloromyotomy for pyloric stenosis?**

They can eat as soon as they wake up.

❑❑ **What is the most common cause of erosive gastritis associated with eosinophilic infiltrates on biopsy in a 6 week-old infant?**

Cow's milk protein allergy. Eosinophilia, more common in small bowel and rectal biopsies, may be seen in esophageal and gastric biopsies as well.

❑❑ **An institutionalized child with Down's syndrome presents with abdominal pain and is found to have an iron deficiency anemia. What is the most likely cause?**

The child needs an upper gastrointestinal endoscopy as children with Down's syndrome have a high incidence of celiac disease. It should also be kept in mind that institutionalized children also have a high incidence of symptomatic *Helicobacter pylori* disease.

❏❏ **Why is cow's milk allergy so common in infants?**

The infant's gut is more permeable to macromolecules in the first month of life permitting greater antigen exposure. Since cow's milk is the only antigen utilized in infants under a month of age, allergy to this protein is more common than other dietary protein allergies.

❏❏ **When should gut malrotation be surgically repaired?**

Only if symptomatic; however, it is often difficult to determine if the symptoms, such as abdominal pain, are directly related to the malrotation.

❏❏ **How do you differentiate between gastroschisis and omphalocele?**

An omphalocele involves the umbilicus and a gastroschisis does not. An omphalocele is also covered by peritoneal membrane, which may or may not be apparent, but a gastroschisis is not covered by this membrane.

❏❏ **What is a common cause of lactase deficiency in infants less than 6 months of age?**

Infection or enteropathy due to cow's milk protein intolerance. Primary acquired lactose intolerance does not occur until after age 5 years.

❏❏ **Bacterial proliferation in small bowel bacterial overgrowth is diminished by an increase in which macronutrient and concurrent decrease in which nutrient?**

Increase in fat and a decrease in carbohydrate.

❏❏ **How many children with celiac disease present with chronic diarrhea and failure to thrive?**

This is unknown. However, as the child ages, classic symptoms become less apparent and he/she may present merely with abdominal pain and short stature.

❏❏ **What is the most common non-IgE-mediated food-related immunologic reaction?**

Milk protein. Although IgE-mediated food allergies occur, they are manifested by gastrointestinal symptoms and, oftentimes, respiratory symptoms and/or skin reactions occurring within 2 hours after food ingestion.

❏❏ **What is the safest, most effective drug therapy for eosinophilic gastroenteritis in a child who does not respond completely to dietary restrictions?**

Oral cromolyn sodium. Although prednisone therapy is highly efficacious, long-term therapy is often associated with numerous side effects.

❏❏ **What is the definition of short bowel syndrome?**

The presence of malabsorption and malnutrition following massive small bowel resection. It is not based on the length of remaining bowel.

❏❏ **What is the most common and frequently unrecognized complication in a child with short bowel syndrome?**

Chronic small bowel bacterial overgrowth.

❏❏ **What type of triglyceride has the most potent effect on enhancement of intestinal adaptation after resection?**

Long-chain triglycerides.

❑❑ **What would characteristically be found on upper endoscopy in a child who presents with stool lymphocytes, lymphopenia, hypoalbuminemia and hyperlipidemia?**

Scattered milky white spots with a snowflake-like appearance. These represent markedly dilated lymphatics in the lamina propria and/or the submucosa (lymphangiectasia).

❑❑ **Currant jelly stools in an infant with severe irritability and a palpable sausage-shaped abdominal mass is the classic description of what disorder?**

Intussusception. This classic presentation is seen in only about 15%. More commonly, emesis and abdominal pain with various forms of rectal bleeding is seen.

❑❑ **What is the most likely consideration in a pediatric patient carrying the tentative diagnosis of pseudo-obstruction who never demonstrates ileus or air fluid levels?**

Munchausen-by-proxy.

❑❑ **Children presenting with significant abdominal pain may warrant screening by stool microscopy for what particular infectious agents?**

Parasitic infections may present solely with abdominal pain in the absence of other gastrointestinal symptoms.

❑❑ **What is the most common anomaly of an omphalomesenteric duct remnant?**

Meckel's diverticulum.

❑❑ **What are the most common tumors of the lower gastrointestinal tract in children?**

Benign polyps including the juvenile polyp, hamartomatous polyp, inflammatory fibroid polyp and lymphoid polyp. Malignant adenomas of the colon are usually seen in conjunction with familial polyposis syndromes.

❑❑ **What is the most common cause of abdominal pain in children who present to the Emergency Room?**

Gastroenteritis. The most common error is to diagnose gastroenteritis in a child who actually has a retrocecal appendicitis.

❑❑ **What single most important factor reduces the morbidity and mortality of Hirschsprung's disease in children?**

Enterocolitis is a major cause of mortality in infants with Hirschsprung's disease. Therefore, the recognition of Hirschsprung's disease before enterocolitis develops is important.

❑❑ **What is the most likely cause of acute diarrhea in school-age children who present with watery stools, vomiting and a low grade fever that spontaneously resolves within 24 hours?**

Norwalk virus.

❑❑ **Continuing oral feedings in patients with acute infectious enteritis is done primarily to avoid what complication?**

Weight loss.

❑❑ **A 6 year-old boy treated with amoxicillin-clavulanic acid for otitis media develops *Clostridium difficile* diarrhea requiring treatment with metronidazole. After successful treatment, he experiences a recurrence of *C. difficile* three weeks later. What would be the most beneficial course of action to prevent recurrence again?**

Retreat with metronidazole and initiate and maintain a probiotic such as Lactobacillus GG for 2 to 3 months.

❑❑ **What fat soluble vitamin is least well-absorbed in patients with cholestatic liver disease?**

Vitamin E.

PEPTIC ULCER DISEASE

Joseph Cullen, M.D. and Michael S Fedotin, M.D.

❑❑ **Peptic disease involving the duodenum occurs in what percentage of patients with mastocytosis?**

30% to 50%.

❑❑ **What non-invasive tests are available for *Helicobacter pylori* diagnosis?**

^{13}C- and ^{14}C-urea breath tests, whole blood rapid test kits, serology for IgG antibody and fecal antigen test.

❑❑ **In what part of the pancreas are gastrinomas usually found?**

Ninety percent are discovered in the head of the pancreas.

❑❑ **Where is the most frequent location of a Dieulafoy's lesion?**

Proximal stomach on the lesser curve.

❑❑ **What are some causes of false-negative tests for *Helicobacter pylori*?**

Among the more common causes are recent use of proton pump inhibitors and antibiotics.

❑❑ **What are causes of recurrent ulcer disease after gastric surgery?**

Incomplete vagotomy, retained antrum, Zollinger-Ellison syndrome and nonsteroidal anti-inflammatory drug use.

❑❑ **What is the most common complication of peptic ulcer disease?**

Gastrointestinal bleeding which occurs in 10% to 20%.

❑❑ **What endoscopic sign is most useful in predicting rebleeding from an ulcer?**

The presence of a visible vessel in the ulcer base.

❑❑ **What is the mechanism of gastric ulcer formation associated with nonsteroidal anti-inflammatory drugs?**

Decreased production of cyclooxygenase (COX) with a resultant decrease in production of prostaglandins E1 and E2.

❑❑ **What type of nonsteroidal anti-inflammatory drugs are the safest and produce the fewest ulcers?**

Those that selectively inhibit the COX-2 isoform.

❑❑ **What is the peak age of incidence of a duodenal ulcer?**

Fifty. Over the years, the age has decreased in men but remains the same in women.

❑❑ **What are complications of a duodenal ulcer?**

Bleeding, perforation, gastric outlet obstruction and penetration into the pancreas.

❏❏ **What effect on gastrin levels occurs with infection by *Helicobacter pylori*?**

A rise in basal and stimulated serum gastrin.

❏❏ **What is antral gastrin cell hyperplasia and how can it be differentiated from a gastrinoma?**

Like gastrinoma, it is associated with hypergastrinemia and the development of duodenal ulcers. However, it can be differentiated from a gastrinoma on the basis of a negative secretin test.

❏❏ **What mucosal effects do bismuth salts have on the stomach?**

The putative actions of bismuth salts are many. Bismuth forms a glycoprotein-bismuth complex and creates a protective layer over ulcers. It also stimulates prostaglandin E2 and bicarbonate secretions. Recent evidence also suggests a role of bismuth in decreasing free radical production in the stomach. Bismuth has no effect on gastric acid production.

❏❏ **How do bismuth salts affect *Helicobacter pylori*?**

They cause detachment of *H. pylori* from the mucosa which leads to bacterial lysis by gastric luminal contents.

❏❏ **What are adverse effects of misoprostol?**

Diarrhea (dose-related), increased uterine smooth muscles contractions and subsequent abortion.

❏❏ **What is the reinfection rate of *Helicobacter pylori* treatment after eradication?**

Less than 1% per year.

❏❏ **What factor is most important in determining the successful eradication of *Helicobacter pylori*?**

Compliance with the regimen. At a compliance rate of 60%, the eradication rate has been reported to be 96% using a proton pump inhibitor and two antibiotics for two weeks.

❏❏ **What role does gastric acidity play in infections of the stomach?**

It inhibits bacterial growth and decreases the potential for infection.

❏❏ **Where in the small intestine would you expect to find ulcers that occur secondary to Zollinger-Ellison syndrome?**

Seventy-five percent occur in the first portion of the duodenum, 15% in the distal duodenum and 1% in the jejunum.

❏❏ **Why is monotherapy treatment for *Helicobacter pylori* ineffective?**

Resistance develops very quickly.

❏❏ **In what diseases has *Helicobacter pylori* been implicated as a possible etiology?**

Chronic gastritis, peptic ulcer disease, non-ulcer dyspepsia, gastric cancer and low-grade MALT lymphoma.

❏❏ **T/F: The presence of *Helicobacter pylori* in the corpus of the stomach is associated with a lower gastric pH and a higher incidence of gastroesophageal reflux disease.**

False. Diffuse gastritis with *Helicobacter pylori* in this location is associated with an increase in gastric pH and may serve as a protective mechanism against reflux. In this situation, the eradication of *H. pylori* may result in a decrease in gastric pH and an increase in gastroesophageal reflux symptoms in susceptible individuals.

❏❏ **What is the most likely route of infection of *Helicobacter pylori*?**

The fecal-oral contamination route seems most likely. In Peru, where the rate of infection is the highest in the world, DNA consistent with *H. pylori* has been found in the water supply.

❏❏ **What effect does bile have on *Helicobacter pylori*?**

Helicobacter pylori is inhibited by bile.

❏❏ **What percentage of *Helicobacter pylori* isolates express the highly immunogenic CagA?**

At least 60%. The presence of CagA is associated with more virulent strains of *H. pylori*.

❏❏ **What is the difference between the Carbon-13 and Carbon-14 labeling used in urea breath tests?**

Carbon-13 does not involve a radioactive isotope but needs a mass spectrometer. The Carbon-14 test exposes the patient to radiation but can be more readily analyzed.

❏❏ **What is the best non-invasive method for assessing the effectiveness of therapy for *Helicobacter pylori*?**

Currently, the urea breath test is the best noninvasive test. Studies are currently ongoing to evaluate the use of the fecal antigen test for this indication.

❏❏ **How does amoxicillin destroy *Helicobacter pylori*?**

Amoxicillin binds specific proteins within the bacterial cell walls and disrupts the cell cycle at the time of cell division.

❏❏ **How do clarithromycin and tetracycline destroy *Helicobacter pylori*?**

Clarithromycin and tetracycline inhibit bacterial protein synthesis by entering the bacterial cell and binding to receptors on ribosomal subunits. This inhibits RNA-dependent protein synthesis.

❏❏ **How does metronidazole eliminate *Helicobacter pylori*?**

Metronidazole generates intracellular products that damage DNA. Metronidazole is insensitive to pH.

❏❏ **T/F: Duodenal ulcers are more likely than gastric ulcers to rebleed after endoscopic treatment.**

False. Gastric ulcers are three times as likely to rebleed.

❏❏ **In what locations of the stomach and duodenum are ulcers more likely to bleed?**

Ulcers located high on the lesser curve of the stomach or on the posterior inferior wall of the duodenal bulb are more likely to bleed.

❏❏ **What are side effects of metronidazole?**

Metronidazole can interact with alcohol, causing a disulfiram-like reaction. It can also cause a peripheral neuropathy and leukopenia.

❏❏ **What is the overall life-time risk of developing a peptic ulcer?**

10%. The mortality related to gastrointestinal bleeding is also about 10%.

❑❑ **What effect does smoking have on peptic ulcer disease?**

Smoking doubles the risk of peptic ulcer disease.

❑❑ **What effect does *Helicobacter pylori* infection have on interleukin-8 in the gastric epithelium?**

Helicobacter pylori infection stimulates production of interleukin-8.

❑❑ **What are the three phases of gastric secretion?**

1) The cephalic phase results from the response to the sight, smell and taste of food and is mediated by the vagus nerve.
2) The gastric phase results from mechanical stimulation and distension.
3) The intestinal phase is initiated by food entering the intestine.

❑❑ **What are the two distinct motor functions of the stomach?**

The proximal stomach functions primarily to accommodate in response to ingested material (reservoir/storage function) and then transfer it to the distal stomach; the distal stomach functions to triturate and empty the material into the duodenum in a controlled manner. Both functions are vagally-mediated.

❑❑ **T/F: The incidence of duodenal ulcer has declined over the past 30 years.**

True. This decline is only partially explained by the introduction of potent antisecretory agents as it predated their availability. It may be partly explained by a decrease in smoking or possibly by an increase in antibiotic use.

❑❑ **What are the major factors that disrupt gastric mucosal resistance resulting in ulcer development?**

Nonsteroidal anti-inflammatory drugs, *Helicobacter pylori*, cigarette smoking and an imbalance between gastric mucosal bicarbonate and acid secretion.

❑❑ **What are some underlying medical illnesses that appear to be important in the development of ulcers?**

Cirrhosis and chronic obstructive pulmonary disease.

❑❑ **What percentage of the world population is colonized with *Helicobacter pylori*?**

Approximately 50%.

❑❑ **Chronic nonsteroidal anti-inflammatory drug (NSAID) use is associated with mucosal ulceration in what percentage of patients?**

20%. There is an estimated 40-fold increase in gastric ulcers and 8-fold increase in duodenal ulcers in daily NSAID users.

❑❑ **What is the mechanism responsible for chronic NSAID-induced mucosal injury?**

Inhibition of, predominantly, cyclooxygenase-1, resulting in decreased mucosal prostaglandin synthesis and impaired mucosal defense.

❑❑ **What diagnostic modality is most accurate in diagnosing ulceration of the stomach and duodenum?**

Endoscopy is greater than 95% accurate and also allows for biopsy and determination of bleeding risk. It also allows for treatment of ulcers with bleeding stigmata.

❑❑ Currently, what are the main indications for gastric analysis?

1)   Patients who have suspected Zollinger-Ellison syndrome.
2)   Patients who have recurrent ulceration following a previous ulcer operation.

❑❑ What class of pharmacologic agent is most efficacious in the treatment of NSAID-associated gastric ulcers?

Proton pump inhibitors are more effective than H_2-receptor antagonists or prostaglandin analogues. Although the mechanism of NSAID-associated ulceration is an alteration in mucosal defense, the marked acid inhibition provided by proton pump inhibitors permits healing of these ulcers.

❑❑ Bismuth compounds enhance mucosal defense by what mechanisms?

1) Bismuth crystals bind preferentially to ulcer craters, creating a protective barrier; 2) bismuth enhances mucosal production of prostaglandin E_2 and bicarbonate secretion; and, 3) bismuth compounds have direct antibacterial action against *H. pylori.*

❑❑ What are indications for the operative treatment of duodenal ulcer?

Perforation, obstruction, and bleeding. Traditionally, intractability was included but with the decrease in the incidence of peptic ulceration, the development of potent antisecretory medications and an increase in information regarding the role of *H. pylori* and NSAIDs, intractability occurs rarely.

❑❑ Chest radiographs demonstrate pneumoperitoneum in what percentage of patients with perforated duodenal ulcer?

75%. In a minority of patient, omentum or liver seals the perforation.

❑❑ What is the principal cause of death from peptic ulcer disease?

Hemorrhage, even though the vast majority of patients who have acute hemorrhage from duodenal ulcers stop bleeding spontaneously.

❑❑ A 62 year-old man who is postoperative day 5 after antrectomy, vagotomy and Billroth II gastrojejunostomy for an obstructing duodenal ulcer acutely develops severe abdominal pain and fever. What is the diagnosis?

Patients who have leakage from a duodenal stump have an acute exacerbation of abdominal pain, typically on the fifth to seventh postoperative day. When the leak is sizable, symptoms of an acute abdomen result.

❑❑ What is the mortality rate for duodenal stump blowout after an antrectomy and gastrojejunostomy for peptic ulcer disease?

50%.

❑❑ T/F: Recurrent ulcers are more common after an operation for "intractable" duodenal ulcer than after an operation for gastric ulcer?

True.

❑❑ What percentage of postgastrectomy patients are free of *H. pylori*?

Up to 90%.

❑❑ What is the first symptom of postoperative recurrent ulcer?

Usually there are no symptoms and upper gastrointestinal bleeding is frequently the first sign of postoperative recurrent ulcer, occurring in 40% to 60% of patients.

❑❑ T/F: Perforation is a common presentation of recurrent ulcer in a postgastrectomy patient?

False.

❑❑ Where do postoperative recurrent ulcers occur?

Recurrent ulcers nearly always occur within 1 to 2 cm of the gastrointestinal anastomosis.

❑❑ A postgastrectomy patient presents with recurrent ulceration. Serum gastrin levels are elevated. What are some of the possible causes?

Gastrinoma, retained antrum, G-cell hyperplasia or administration of antisecretory medications.

❑❑ What are the characteristic endoscopic findings of stress ulceration?

The lesions of stress ulceration are generally superficial rather than deep, multiple rather than single, gastric rather than duodenal, fundic rather than antral, and usually bleed and do not perforate.

❑❑ A 57 year-old woman who recently underwent an antrectomy, vagotomy and gastrojejunostomy for peptic ulcer disease complains of crampy abdominal pain, diaphoresis, dizziness and palpitations 25 minutes after a meal. What is the diagnosis?

The patient has the early dumping syndrome, which occurs in response to the ingestion of a hyperosmolar carbohydrate-rich meal.

❑❑ What are the mechanisms that lead to the dumping syndrome?

Loss of the gastric reservoir function and rapid emptying of hyperosmolar carbohydrates into the small intestine.

❑❑ Which enteric hormones are released and contribute to the vasomotor symptoms of early dumping?

Serotonin, gastric inhibitory peptide, vasoactive intestinal peptide and neurotensin.

❑❑ After the Billroth II gastric resection, what is the incidence of the dumping syndrome?

The incidence of the dumping syndrome may exceed 50% because the operation bypasses both pyloric control and duodenal inhibiting mechanisms.

❑❑ T/F: Octreotide acetate, a long-acting somatostatin analogue, is effective in improving the symptoms of early dumping in patients unresponsive to other medical therapy.

True. Octreotide improves the symptoms in 90% of patients with dumping.

❑❑ What type of vagotomy is responsible for the highest incidence of postvagotomy diarrhea: truncal, selective or proximal?

Truncal vagotomy has the highest incidence (20%), followed by selective vagotomy (5%) and proximal (highly selective) gastric vagotomy (4%).

❑❑ What percentage of postgastrectomy patients exhibit histologic gastritis?

Over 60% exhibit histologic gastritis; however, the vast majority remain asymptomatic.

❑❑ **The highest incidence of alkaline gastritis occurs after which operation for peptic ulcer disease?**

Billroth II gastrojejunostomy has the highest incidence, followed by loop gastrojejunostomy, Billroth I gastroduodenostomy and the pyloroplasty.

❑❑ **What medical disorders increase the risk of gastric atony following ulcer surgery?**

Preoperative gastric outlet obstruction, diabetes mellitus, hypothyroidism and autonomic neurologic disorders increase the risk of gastric atony.

❑❑ **What percentage of patients who have the combination of vagotomy, antrectomy and Roux-en-Y gastrojejunostomy develop epigastric fullness, abdominal pain, nausea and vomiting - the so-called Roux stasis syndrome?**

Up to 50% of patients who have a Roux-en-Y gastrojejunostomy develop the Roux stasis syndrome.

❑❑ **A 76 year-old man who had an unknown gastric operation for peptic ulcer disease in the remote past presents with epigastric fullness, nausea and vomiting. Upper gastrointestinal barium radiographs demonstrate a mass in the gastric remnant. What is the most likely diagnosis?**

A bezoar is the most likely diagnosis; however, endoscopy is needed to distinguish the bezoar from a neoplasm.

❑❑ **What percentage of the total gastric carcinomas develop in patients who have had a gastrectomy?**

1%.

❑❑ **What percentage of patients have abnormal bone loss following gastric resection?**

25%.

❑❑ **What are some of the side effects of metoclopramide for the treatment of chronic gastric atony?**

Dystonic reactions and dyskinesia.

❑❑ **T/F: The majority of patients who require treatment for perforation or bleeding due to duodenal ulcer do not have an antecedent history of ulcer pain?**

False. Only about 20% of patients who require treatment for bleeding or perforation do not have a history of ulcer pain.

❑❑ **In what area do the majority of duodenal ulcers occur?**

About 95% of duodenal ulcers occur in the duodenal bulb and 5% are postbulbar.

❑❑ **Which factor does not predict death in perforated duodenal ulcer: preoperative shock, perforation for longer than 24 hours, concomitant medical illness, or age?**

Age. Preoperative shock, perforation for longer than 24 hours and concomitant medical illness are three factors that predict death in perforated duodenal ulcer patients.

❑❑ **What endoscopic findings are indications for endoscopic hemostatic treatment?**

An actively bleeding visible vessel, oozing from an ulcer base and a nonbleeding visible vessel or sentinel clot in the ulcer base are indications for endoscopic hemostatic treatment.

❑❑ **T/F: A second hospitalization for ulcer hemorrhage is an indication for operation in the treatment of bleeding from duodenal ulcer.**

True, depending upon the treatment and prevention recommendations performed previously.

❏❏ Which artery is primarily responsible for bleeding duodenal ulcers?

Gastroduodenal artery. During operation for bleeding from duodenal ulcer, the gastroduodenal artery is ligated proximally and distally. Additionally, the transverse pancreatic branch, which enters posteriorly is also ligated.

❏❏ What is the primary factor responsible for the symptoms of late dumping?

After the hyperosmolar carbohydrate is absorbed, the hyperinsulinemia causing hypoglycemia is the primary factor responsible for the symptoms.

RADIATION AND ISCHEMIC GI INJURY AND VASCULAR GUT ABNORMALITIES

Yvonne Renée Lee, M.D., FACP

❑❑ **What component of radiation exposure determines cell survival?**

The dose. Doses greater than 4000 rads (4000 centigray) usually cause some form of injury depending upon the region irradiated.

❑❑ **What radiation factors determine cellular damage?**

Dose rate, type of radiation, division of rate exposure, field size and linear energy transfer.

❑❑ **During which period of the cell cycle is the cell at most risk for radiation damage?**

Mitosis.

❑❑ **What type of intestinal cell is affected during acute radiation injury?**

Crypt cell.

❑❑ **What type of cellular damage occurs with chronic radiation toxicity?**

Degeneration of the endothelial cells, obliteration of the vasculature and fibrosis of the connective tissue.

❑❑ **How long is cellular turnover in the rectum?**

Four to six days.

❑❑ **What develops as a result of chronic radiation vascular and endothelial injury?**

Obliterative endarteritis and endophlebitis.

❑❑ **When does recanalization of the exposed cells occur?**

During the subacute and chronic period.

❑❑ **What are the most common locations for radiation-induced colitis?**

Sigmoid and rectum.

❑❑ **What type of receptor antagonist can control radiation-induced emesis?**

5-HT$_3$ receptor antagonist. Endotoxins and free radicals from radiation injury stimulate these receptors.

❑❑ **What is the most common late manifestation of radiation-induced small bowel injury?**

Partial small bowel obstruction.

❑❑ **What substances may lead to radiation-induced malabsorption and diarrhea?**

Lactose, bile salts, fat and vitamin B12.

❑❑ **What is the most common location for radiation-induced rectal ulcers?**

Anterior wall. Approximately 6 to 8 cm from anal verge.

❑❑ **What barium radiographic findings are seen in late or chronic radiation injury?**

Mucosal edema, separation of intestinal loops and floculations resulting from excessive secretions.

❑❑ **What are the most radiosensitive cells in the small bowel?**

Crypts of Langerhans.

❑❑ **What factors are responsible for acute radiation damage?**

Rate and duration of applied radiation.

❑❑ **What factors are responsible for chronic radiation damage?**

Total dose and volume of tissue irradiated.

❑❑ **What is the most common complication of chronic, non-gangrenous ischemic colitis?**

Stricture formation.

❑❑ **What percentage of cases of ischemic colitis are gangrenous?**

15% to 20%.

❑❑ **What segment of the colon is most affected by hypotension?**

Right colon.

❑❑ **In which arterial location do emboli lodge to cause a "major" embolic event?**

Proximal to the ileocolic artery.

❑❑ **What percentage of patients have right-sided colonic ischemia?**

10%. Involvement of the right side of the colon seems to increase the risk of an unfavorable outcome.

❑❑ **Up to what percentage of decreased blood flow is tolerated by the bowel for 24 hours or less?**

Up to 75%.

❑❑ **What is the pathogenesis of the initial intestinal ischemic injury?**

Reperfusion injury and release of endotoxins.

❑❑ **What is the most common cause of acute mesenteric ischemia?**

Superior mesenteric artery emboli.

❑❑ **What are common causes of acute venous mesenteric ischemia?**

Mesenteric vein thrombus and focal segmental ischemia. These processes are typically related to an underlying hypercoagulable state.

❑❑ **What percentage of patients with non-obstructive mesenteric ischemia present with painless hematochezia?**

25%.

❑❑ **What percentage of patients with acute mesenteric ischemia develop a metabolic acidosis?**

50%.

❑❑ **What is the best test to diagnose mesenteric ischemia?**

Selective mesenteric angiography. Of note, in most instances of colonic ischemia, angiography is not necessary.

❑❑ **What is the most common site of a superior mesenteric artery thrombus?**

At the origin of the artery.

❑❑ **What is the test of choice to diagnose a mesenteric vein thrombosis?**

Abdominal CT scan with intravenous contrast.

❑❑ **What vasculitis is associated with aneurysms that can be identified on mesenteric angiography?**

Polyarteritis nodosa.

❑❑ **What is the triad seen in Henoch-Schonlein Purpura?**

Abdominal pain, arthritis and palpable purpura.

❑❑ **What percentage of patients with colonic arteriovenous malformations have concomitant small bowel vascular ectasias?**

10%.

❑❑ **What is the most likely cause of the formation of an arteriovenous malformation?**

Intermittent, low-grade obstruction of the submucosal veins.

❑❑ **What are angiographic abnormalities diagnostic of arteriovenous malformations?**

A vascular tuft and an early-filling vein during the arterial phase and a dilated, slow-emptying vein during the venous phase.

❑❑ **What is the most common site for colonic vascular ectasias to bleed?**

The right side of the colon. About 80% of colonic vascular ectasias that bleed are right-sided.

❑❑ **At what age do patients with Hereditary Hemorrhagic Telangiectasia (Osler-Weber-Rendu) usually present with gastrointestinal bleeding?**

Fourth decade of life.

❑❑ **What conditions are associated with gastric antral vascular ectasia ("Watermelon stomach")?**

Achlorhydria, atrophic gastritis and cirrhosis. Nearly all of these patients develop an iron deficiency anemia.

❏❏ What is the classic location of a Dieulafoy's lesion?

Six centimeters distal to the gastroesophageal junction along the lesser curvature.

❏❏ What is the second most common vascular lesion in the colon?

Hemangioma.

❏❏ What diseases are associated with cutaneous vascular nevi and intestinal bleeding?

Blue rubber bleb nevus syndrome and Klippel-Trenaunay-Weber Syndrome.

❏❏ What is the best study to identify an aortoenteric fistula?

Abdominal CT scan with oral and intravenous contrast.

SHORT BOWEL SYNDROME AND ITS COMPLICATIONS

Saeed Zamani, M.D. and Anthony J. DiMarino, Jr., M.D.

❑❑ **T/F: The length of small bowel is different in men and women.**

True. The length of small intestine is approximately 630 cm in men and approximately 590 cm in women. The length of colon is about 150 cm in both sexes.

❑❑ **Where is the border between the jejunum and ileum?**

In general, the proximal two-fifths (about 240 cm) of small bowel is called the jejunum and the distal three-fifths (about 360 cm) the ileum.

❑❑ **What are major factors responsible for the development of short bowel syndrome?**

Extent of the resection, the site of resected intestine, the presence of an ileocecal valve, the condition of the residual intestine and the degree of intestinal adaptation.

❑❑ **Resection of which part of small intestine has only a limited effect on absorption?**

Jejunum. The ileum has the greatest capacity for adaptation and is able to compensate for and takeover almost all of the jejunum's absorptive function.

❑❑ **What is the leading cause of short bowel syndrome in adults?**

Crohn's Disease. Two large studies reported Crohn's disease as the cause of short bowel syndrome in 58% to 77% of patients.

❑❑ **Patients with short bowel syndrome will have compromised nutrition if the remaining length is less than:**

Approximately 200 cm (6.5 feet). This length can be used as an anatomic guideline for definition of short bowel syndrome.

❑❑ **What are other major causes of short bowel syndrome?**

Mesenteric infarction, radiation enteritis and volvulus.

❑❑ **What is the leading cause of short bowel syndrome in pediatrics?**

Congenital abnormalities such as intestinal atresia, gastroschisis, malrotation with midgut volvulus and aganglionosis.

❑❑ **What is the difference in villi shape in different parts of small intestine?**

The villi are taller and crypts deeper in the jejunum than ileum. The activity of microvillus enzymes and nutrient absorptive capacity per unit length of intestine is several-fold higher in the proximal than in distal small bowel.

❑❑ **The digestion and absorption of most nutrients in normal humans occurs in:**

The first 100 centimeters of jejunum. Therefore, patients with short bowel syndrome in general can maintain nutritional balance on oral feeding if more than 100 cm of jejunum is left intact. Conversely, most patients with a jejunal length of less than 100 cm will require long-term parenteral nutrition.

❏❏ **Where is the site of absorption of macronutrients (fat, protein, carbohydrate) and micronutrients (calcium, magnesium, iron)?**

Proximal jejunum. Bile acids and vitamin B12 are only absorbed in the ileum. Electrolytes and water are absorbed in both the small and large intestines.

❏❏ **What is the absorptive efficiency of fluids received by the small intestine?**

The proximal small intestine receives about 9 liters per day of water and electrolytes from food and secretions. About 8 liters of this is absorbed in the small intestine.

❏❏ **What is the minimum required length of jejunum to maintain a positive water and electrolyte balance?**

One hundred centimeters of intact jejunum.

❏❏ **What should be the appropriate content of sodium and glucose in oral solutions to achieve net sodium and water absorption in jejunum?**

A mixture of 120 mmole sodium chloride and 50 mmole glucose.

❏❏ **What is the effect of a low fat diet on the absorption of calcium and magnesium in patients with short bowel syndrome?**

Low fat diet improves absorption of calcium and magnesium.

❏❏ **What length of ileum should be resected to cause moderate bile acid malabsorption?**

Less than 100 cm. More extensive resection causes severe bile acid and fat malabsorption resulting in a decreased bile acid pool and eventually steatorrhea.

❏❏ **What degree of ileal resection will cause vitamin B12 deficiency?**

More than 60 cm.

❏❏ **Unabsorbed hydroxylated fatty acids in patients with extensive ileal resection can cause more diarrhea by:**

Stimulating colonic electroloytes and water secretion.

❏❏ **What are major regulatory hormones in the proximal gastrointestinal tract?**

Gastrin, cholecystokinin, secretin, motilin and gastrin inhibitory peptide.

❏❏ **What is the effect of extensive small intestinal resection on the serum gastrin level?**

Hypergastrinemia. This may lead to gastric acid hypersecretion.

❏❏ **Why do some patients with short bowel syndrome have rapid gastric emptying of liquids and rapid intestinal transit time?**

Lack of enteroglucagon and polypeptide YY secretion by the resected ileum (ileal brake).

❏❏ **How is the gastric emptying of solids in patients with short bowel syndrome?**

Same as normal controls.

❑❑ What part of small intestine has the highest adaptive capability?

Ileum.

❑❑ What is the most prominent clinical symptom in patients with short bowel syndrome?

Diarrhea, steatorrhea or both.

❑❑ T/F: The estimated length of short bowel from a small bowel radiograph correlates with the measured length at surgery.

True.

❑❑ What type of solution should be started postoperatively in patients with high jejunostomy output?

Isotonic glucose-saline solutions. Low sodium solutions may result in jejunal sodium and water secretion.

❑❑ A patient with ischemic bowel disease underwent intestinal resection and the total length of jejunum now is 180 cm with an intact colon. What type of diet can be started for this patient?

Liquid polymeric diet.

❑❑ What is the treatment of diarrhea in a patient with limited ileal resection (less than 100 cm resection)?

Cholestyramine to bind unabsorbed bile salts.

❑❑ What is the treatment of diarrhea in a patient with extensive ileal resection (more than 100 cm resection)?

Low fat, high carbohydrate diet and cholestyramine.

❑❑ What is the effect of resection of the ileocecal valve on absorption of nutrients?

Loss of the ileocecal valve promotes small bowel bacterial overgrowth leading to maldigestion.

❑❑ T/F: A patient with jejunal length of 150 cm can tolerate an oral intake.

True. Patients with a jejunal length of less than 200 cm but more than 100 cm in continuity with the colon can usually be managed by oral intake alone.

❑❑ What is the most critical determinant of severe malabsorption in a patient with extensive small bowel resection and colectomy?

Length of remaining jejunum. Patients with jejunal length of less than 100 cm cannot maintain adequate nutrient absorption. These patients will usually require long-term parenteral nutrition.

❑❑ What is your recommendation in a patient with extensive small bowel resection whose stomal losses exceed liquid intake?

Use of H_2 receptor antagonists, proton pump inhibitors or somatostatin analogues.

❑❑ What are the major electrolyte losses in a patient with jejunostomy and colectomy?

Sodium, potassium, calcium, magnesium, iron, zinc and copper.

❑❑ **Why are patients with short bowel syndrome prone to develop cholesterol gallstones?**

Decreased hepatic bile secretion, supersaturation of bile with cholesterol, gallbladder hypomotility and formation of gallbladder sludge.

❑❑ **What is the prevalence of oxalate kidney stones in patients with short bowel syndrome and colectomy?**

None. An intact colon is required for absorption of oxalate.

❑❑ **How do you treat hyperoxaluria in patients with short bowel syndrome and preserved colon?**

Restrict oxalate-containing food products such as tea, chocolate, cola beverages, certain fruits and vegetables. If hyperoxaluria persists, then oral calcium citrate should be tried.

❑❑ **A patient with short bowel syndrome and a preserved colon presents with episodes of confusion, ataxia and inappropriate behavior. What is the most likely diagnosis?**

D-lactic acidosis is a rare complication of short bowel syndrome observed only in patients with an intact colon. The episodes of acidosis are usually precipitated by an increased oral intake of refined carbohydrate. Malabsorbed carbohydrates are metabolized by colonic bacteria to short chain fatty acids and lactate.

❑❑ **How do you manage a patient with D-lactic acidosis?**

Treatment consists of correction of acidosis by sodium bicarbonate and stopping oral carbohydrate intake. The potential benefit of oral antibiotics is debated.

❑❑ **What is the reason for gastric hypersecretion after extensive jejunal resection?**

Cholecystokinin, vasoactive intestinal peptide, gastrin inhibitory peptide and serotonin secreted by jejunum inhibit gastric secretion.

❑❑ **How is the adaptive capability of the colon to prevent fluid loss in patients with extensive ileal resection?**

Very poor.

❑❑ **What is the mechanism of secretory diarrhea in a patient with an ileal resection?**

Unabsorbed bile acids spill into the colon and are deconjugated by colonic bacteria. The deconjugated bile acids directly stimulate the colon to secrete fluid and electrolytes.

❑❑ **What is the cause of diarrhea in a patient with a more than 100 centimeter ileal resection?**

Steatorrhea secondary to fat malabsorption which occurs as a result of bile acid deficiency.

❑❑ **Why do patients have rapid transit time after an ileal resection?**

Loss of ileal brake phenomenon controlled by polypeptide YY.

❑❑ **In a patient with an ileal resection, preservation of the colon improves fluid and electrolyte absorption but has consequences such as:**

Secretory diarrhea induced by bile acids, calcium oxalate kidney stones and D-lactic acidosis.

❑❑ **What are the adaptive responses to a major small intestinal resection?**

Luminal dilation, thickening and lengthening of gastrointestinal tract and hyperplasia of the crypt-villus axis leading to increased surface area.

❑❑ How long does it take for maximal small intestinal adaptive response in humans after major small intestinal resection?

One year.

❑❑ What are the major mechanisms by which enteral nutrients stimulate intestinal adaptation?

Direct contact of epithelial cells, stimulation of trophic gastrointestinal hormone secretion and stimulation of pancreatic and biliary secretions.

❑❑ Which hormones have a trophic effect on the small intestine?

Gastrin, secretin, cholecystokinin, epidermal growth factor, corticosteroids, enteroglucagon, prostaglandins and growth hormone releasing factor.

❑❑ How soon after small intestinal resection does gastric hypersecretion occur?

Twenty-four hours.

❑❑ What effect does short bowel syndrome have on lipase activity?

Lipase decreases due to acid hypersecretion.

❑❑ What is the best magnesium supplement in patients with short bowel syndrome?

Magnesium gluconate is less likely to cause an osmotic diarrhea than other magnesium-containing compounds.

❑❑ What are the major vitamin deficiencies in a patient with extensive jejunal resection?

The fat-soluble vitamins A, D, E and K.

❑❑ What is the ideal caloric intake in a patient with short bowel syndrome?

The caloric intake should be increased slowly and progressively until it reaches to a target of 32 kcal/kg/day.

❑❑ What percentage of patients with short bowel syndrome require total parenteral nutrition in the immediate postoperative period?

100%.

❑❑ When can you start an oral balanced solution containing carbohydrates and electrolytes?

Once stool output is less than 2 liters per day.

❑❑ What is the nutritional value of a clear liquid diet in patients with short bowel syndrome?

Useless due to inadequate nutritional value. In addition, they are hyperosmolar and can provoke osmotic diarrhea.

❑❑ What is the value of a full liquid diet in patients with short bowel syndrome?

A full liquid diet is poorly tolerated because it contains lactose. Most patients with short bowel syndrome are lactose intolerant.

❑❑   What is the main indication for small bowel transplantation in a patient with severe short bowel syndrome?

Severe short bowel syndrome complicated by progressive liver disease. Other indications include loss of vascular access, recurrent episodes of central venous catheter sepsis and severe impact on quality of life. Small intestinal transplantation is currently a technically feasible but impractical alternative to conservative treatment of patients with severe short bowel syndrome.

❑❑   What are future potential therapeutic options to promote mucosal growth in patients with short bowel syndrome?

Growth hormone and glutamine.

TUMORS

Gowri Balachandar, M.D., Randall E. Brand, M.D., John K. DiBaise, M.D.,
Eric B. Goosenberg, M.D., David S. Hodges, M.D., Terrence Jackson, M.D.,
A. Steven McIntosh, M.D., Bola Olusola, M.D. and Hemant K. Roy, M.D.

❑❑ What are risk factors for squamous cell carcinoma of the esophagus?

Use of hard liquor, smoking or chewing tobacco, pre-existing head and neck cancer, history of lye-induced esophageal strictures, achalasia, Plummer-Vinson syndrome and tylosis. Tobacco and alcohol increase the risk in a dose-dependent manner. Use of both is associated with a much higher incidence than with either substance alone. For unknown reasons, neither smoking nor alcohol is associated with esophageal cancer outside of the United States.

❑❑ What demographic factors are associated with esophageal cancer in Americans?

Males are more often affected than are females (ratio 3:1), African-Americans more often than Caucasians (ratio 4:1) and individuals of lower socioeconomic status have a greater incidence.

❑❑ T/F: The incidence and mortality related to esophageal cancer are highest in portions of China, Iran and Africa.

True. Environmental risk factors are assumed but not proven to be responsible.

❑❑ T/F: People with tylosis have approximately a 50% likelihood of developing esophageal cancer.

False. This rare condition presents with hyperkeratosis of the skin on the palms and soles and papillomas of the esophagus that progress to squamous cell cancer in virtually 100% of cases.

❑❑ T/F: The most common location of squamous cell carcinoma is the distal esophagus.

False. Squamous cell carcinomas are most often located in the mid-esophagus. Adenocarcinomas are most often located in the distal esophagus and are frequently associated with Barrett's esophagus.

❑❑ How does achalasia influence the age of onset of esophageal cancer?

It occurs 10 to 20 years earlier (mean age 52 years) than in patients without achalasia. The esophageal malignancy is squamous cell carcinoma in over 90% of achalasia patients and typically occurs about 20 years after the diagnosis of achalasia is made. The risk of squamous cell carcinoma in achalasia is about 10- to 30-fold greater than in the general population.

❑❑ When squamous cell esophageal cancer is diagnosed due to related symptoms, what can be predicted about its stage?

Distant metastases will be present in 25% to 30% of cases, peri-esophageal lymph nodes will be affected in up to 2/3 of cases and it will be limited to the mucosa in only 2% of cases.

❑❑ What are the most common causes of hematemesis in patients with esophageal cancer?

Tumor ulceration or aorto-esophageal fistulization.

❑❑ T/F: The incidence of squamous cell carcinoma of the esophagus has fallen dramatically over the past several decades, such that squamous cell carcinoma and adenocarcinoma are now equally common in the United States.

False. While it is true that these two cancers of the esophagus are now of roughly equal frequency, the incidence of squamous cell carcinoma has remained steady while adenocarcinoma has increased markedly.

❏❏ What can be done to distinguish benign esophageal masses from esophageal cancer?

Endoscopic biopsies and brush cytology are the most commonly used techniques for confirmation of cancer. Endoscopically applied vital stains such as toluidine blue and endoscopic ultrasound with or without fine needle aspiration are also useful. Balloon cytology is used as a screening strategy in the Orient where squamous cell esophageal cancer is very common.

❏❏ What are the roles of endoscopic ultrasound (EUS) in esophageal cancer?

Radial endosonography can determine the depth of esophageal wall invasion of cancer (T stage in the TNM system), the presence or absence of malignant peri-esophageal lymph nodes (N stage) and to evaluate for celiac adenopathy (part of the M stage). Newer linear array instruments can be used to perform fine needle aspirates of submucosal lesions and adenopathy. The role of EUS to evaluate for evidence of malignancy in Barrett's esophagus is controversial. It does not seem to be an effective technique in evaluating the esophagus after radiation therapy, however, because fibrosis can be difficult to distinguish from recurrent or residual cancer.

❏❏ What are the histologic equivalents of the five esophageal layers found by endoscopic ultrasonography?

Layer 1 (white, hyperechoic) – superficial mucosa
Layer 2 (dark, hypoechoic) – deep mucosa
Layer 3 (white, hyperechoic) - submucosa
Layer 4 (dark, hypoechoic) – muscularis propria
Layer 5 (white, hyperechoic) – adventitia and peri-esophageal fat

❏❏ What is the likely ultrasound T stage of stenotic esophageal cancers?

These tumors are usually locally advanced - either T3 (invading the adventitia and peri-esophageal fat) or T4 (invading adjacent organs).

❏❏ What should be done in the initial diagnosis and staging of esophageal cancer?

Initial evaluation should include a barium esophagram, endoscopy with biopsies and possibly cytologic brushings, endoscopic ultrasound, a chest x-ray and CT scanning of the chest and upper abdomen to include the liver and adrenals. Laparoscopy and either thoracotomy or thoracoscopy may have a role in selected cases. Bronchoscopy should also be done in tumors occurring in the proximal or middle third of the esophagus.

❏❏ How do squamous cell carcinomas and adenocarcinomas of the esophagus differ in terms of their natural history?

Squamous cell carcinoma is more likely to be widespread at the time of diagnosis. Adenocarcinoma tends to progress by local extension. Accordingly, surgery has a much more limited role in squamous cell carcinoma than in adenocarcinoma.

❏❏ Which form of endoscopic palliation, laser or BICAP, would be more useful in the management of a friable, exophytic and partially-obstructing esophageal cancer encompassing two-thirds of the lumen?

Endoscopic laser therapy. It can be targeted directly to the tumor, as opposed to the BICAP tumor probe which is only useful with circumferential tumors.

❏❏ Which form of endoscopic palliation would be most useful in the management of a tight stricture due to a leiomyosarcoma of the mid-esophagus?

Stent placement is the only treatment mode that is useful in extrinsic stenoses due to submucosal or extrinsic tumors (such as lung cancer). Dilatation is usually ineffective, typically providing only transient relief of symptoms. Thermal devices have no role.

❑❑ **Which form of endoscopic palliation would be most useful in the management of an esophageal carcinoma causing severe dysphagia before initiation of neoadjuvant chemotherapy and radiation?**

Dilatation with either Savary or hydrostatic balloon dilators often provides effective palliation before and during therapy. Laser or BICAP tumor probes may be used if there is a significant volume of exophytic tumor causing luminal stenosis.

❑❑ **How should tracheo-esophageal fistulae in esophageal cancer be managed?**

Cuffed plastic stents or newer cellophane-coated self-expanding metal stents are probably the best intervention in this setting. Low doses of radiation may be effective, although larger doses may result in enlargement of a fistula.

❑❑ **What are the most common complications of radiation therapy to the esophagus?**

Esophagitis (early) and esophageal strictures (late).

❑❑ **What potentially curative endoscopic treatment options are available for early but not late stage esophageal cancer?**

Endoscopic mucosal resection and photodynamic therapy

❑❑ **Which esophageal tumors are most amenable to endoscopic laser therapy?**

Tumors should be in a straight segment (as opposed to the esophago-gastric junction), should be exophytic and should be located at least a few centimeters distal to the cricopharyngeus muscle.

❑❑ **How should nutritional support be provided to a patient with a resectable esophageal cancer?**

In patients who cannot eat, a feeding jejunostomy tube is preferable to a gastrostomy tube because it will not affect the segment of the gut that needs to be mobilized (e.g., gastric pull-up) after esophagectomy.

❑❑ **T/F: Of the three common subtypes of Barrett's esophagus (cardiac, fundic and specialized intestinal metaplasia), only the specialized intestinal type is associated with an increased risk of adenocarcinoma.**

True. This type of metaplastic mucosa is characterized histologically by the presence of goblet cells.

❑❑ **T/F: Short-segment Barrett's esophagus is not associated with an increased risk of adenocarcinoma.**

False. Short-segment Barrett's esophagus has recently been shown to be a risk factor for adenocarcinoma; although, it is unclear how the relative risk compares to longer-segment Barrett's.

❑❑ **What is the initial appropriate approach to a patient who has Barrett's esophagus and low-grade dysplasia?**

Biopsies should be reviewed by a second expert pathologist and then, if the finding of low-grade dysplasia is confirmed, endoscopy with multiple biopies should be repeated within 6 months.

❑❑ **What is an appropriate approach to a patient who has Barrett's esophagus and high-grade dysplasia?**

Confirmation of the diagnosis by a second expert pathologist is the first step. Because of the strong possibility that adenocarcinoma will already be present in patients whose biopsies show only high-grade dysplasia, many experts advocate that patients who are surgical candidates should undergo esophagectomy. Patients who cannot tolerate surgery should either be surveyed endoscopically every 3 months or have ablation with photodynamic therapy, laser, BICAP or argon plasma coagulator therapy. The potential limitation of ablative therapy is that non-neoplastic mucosa may be restored over submucosal neoplasia.

❏❏ **What is the likelihood that endoscopic biopsies showing Barrett's esophagus and high-grade dysplasia but no cancer will contain cancer in an esophagectomy specimen?**

Up to 40%.

❏❏ **What should be offered to a patient with non-dysplastic Barrett's esophagus to reduce the likelihood of developing cancer?**

Only periodic endoscopic surveillance, every 2 to 3 years, can be offered. Currently, there is no proof that any anti-reflux therapy will eliminate Barrett's esophagus or the risk of adenocarcinoma.

❏❏ **What is the EUS appearance (echogenicity, layer or layers) of esophageal varices?**

Anechoic lesion of the submucosa (3rd ultrasonic layer).

❏❏ **What is the EUS appearance (echogenicity, layer or layers) of an esophageal lipoma?**

Hyperechoic lesion of the submucosa (3rd layer).

❏❏ **What is the EUS appearance (echogenicity, layer or layers) of an esophageal leiomyoma or leiomyosarcoma?**

Hypoechoic lesion of the muscularis propria (4th layer).

❏❏ **What tumors are most likely to metastasize to the esophagus?**

Melanoma and breast cancer. Metastases account for less than 1% of esophageal tumors.

❏❏ **T/F: Smooth muscle tumors of the esophagus that cause dysphagia and bleeding are virtually always malignant (leiomyosarcomas).**

False. These symptoms, as well as chest pain, are indicators of a large tumor, but not necessarily of malignancy. Large leiomyomas may be difficult to distinguish from sarcomas.

❏❏ **What is the most common type of malignant tumor of the stomach?**

Adenocarcinoma comprises 90% of all cases. Less common tumor types include lymphoma, stromal tumor, carcinoid, adenosquamous and metastases.

❏❏ **T/F: *Helicobacter pylori* plays a role in the etiology of gastric cancer.**

True. *H. Pylori* results in chronic gastritis which, presumably, may proceed to metaplasia, dysplasia and cancer. It has been classified as a class A carcinogen by the World Health Organization.

❏❏ **What percentage of patients with early gastric cancer are symptomatic?**

Less than 10%; however, about 90% of patients with advanced disease are symptomatic.

❏❏ **What is a Krukenberg tumor?**

Gastric cancer metastatic to the ovary.

❏❏ **What are the two most common sites of gastric cancer metastasis?**

The liver and lungs constitute about 40% of total cases.

❑❑ What is most sensitive and specific diagnostic modality for gastric adenocarcinoma?

Upper endoscopy with biopsy is 96% sensitive and 99% specific.

❑❑ T/F: Gastric ulcers require endoscopic follow-up to document healing.

True. However, it has been suggested that extensive biopsies from the ulcer taken at the time of the initial endosocopy may obviate the need for follow-up endoscopy, if the biopsies were negative/not suspicious for malignancy.

❑❑ A 64 year-old man with gastric cancer presents with velvety, pigmented lesion in the axilla. What is the diagnosis?

Acanthosis nigricans is considered a paraneoplastic manifestation.

❑❑ T/F: Screening of the general western population for gastric cancer is recommended.

False. Screening is done in Japan with good results but this is not recommended in low risk areas, such as the United States, except in patients with high-risk conditions such as pernicious anemia, adenomatous polyps and chronic atrophic gastritis.

❑❑ What is the best modality to assess the extent of local disease in gastric cancer?

Endoscopic ultrasound. This can be combined with a CT scan to allow for complete staging.

❑❑ What is the best prognostic factor in gastric cancer?

The TNM (Tumor, Node, Metastasis) stage at the time of diagnosis.

❑❑ What treatment has the best curative potential for gastric adenocarcinoma?

Surgical resection. Unfortunately, two-thirds of western patients present with advanced disease and are not surgical candidates for cure.

❑❑ What is the most common type of gastric malignancy after adenocarcinoma?

Primary gastric lymphoma.

❑❑ What is the most common extranodal site for occurrence of lymphoma?

Gastrointestinal tract. About 50% involve the stomach.

❑❑ What are the two most common types of gastric lymphoma?

Diffuse large B cell lymphoma and low-grade B cell mucosa-associated lymphoid tissue (MALT) lymphoma.

❑❑ T/F: Patients with acquired immune deficiency syndrome (AIDS) have a reduced risk of gastric lymphoma.

False. AIDS patients have five-fold increased risk of gastrointestinal lymphoma.

❑❑ T/F: *Helicobacter pylori* is associated with gastric lymphoma.

True. Ninety percent of low-grade MALT lymphomas are positive for *H. pylori*. Additionally, tumor remission has been documented after eradication of *H. pylori* in a number of cases.

❑❑ **Where are the majority of gastrointestinal stromal tumors located?**

Fifty percent are in the stomach. Smooth muscle tumors are now preferably called stromal tumors.

❑❑ **What is Carney's triad?**

Gastric stromal tumor, extra-adrenal paraganglioma and pulmonary chondroma.

❑❑ **What is the best indicator of malignancy in a gastric stromal tumor specimen?**

The mitotic index. Ten or more mitoses per 10 high-power fields suggests malignancy.

❑❑ **Which patients have a higher incidence of gastric carcinoid?**

Patients with hypergastrinemia as occurs in pernicious anemia, atrophic gastritis with achlorhydria and Zollinger-Ellison syndrome.

❑❑ **T/F: All patients with Zollinger-Ellison syndrome have an increased risk of developing gastric carcinoids.**

False. Only the 20% associated with multiple endocrine neoplasia (MEN) type 1.

❑❑ **A 73 year-old woman with a history of melanoma undergoes upper endoscopy and a brownish-black nodule is present in the stomach. What is the diagnosis?**

Metastatic melanoma involving the stomach.

❑❑ **What is the most common location for a gastric lipoma?**

The antrum. These are benign submucosal tumors. Endoscopic ultrasound is very useful for differentiation from other tumors.

❑❑ **What is the most common type of gastric polyp?**

Hyperplastic polyps represent about 75% of gastric polyps.

❑❑ **T/F: There is an association between fundic gland polyps and familial adenomatous polyposis (FAP).**

True. One-third of fundic gland polyps are found in patients with FAP.

❑❑ **What conditions are associated with hyperplastic polyps of the stomach?**

Atrophic gastritis, megaloblastic anemia and intestinalization of the gastric mucosa.

❑❑ **What are the most common benign gastric neoplasms?**

Leiomyomas represent 90% of benign gastric neoplasms.

❑❑ **T/F: Operative treatment of a gastric polyp is indicated for a sessile lesion of 3 cm in diameter.**

True. Operative treatment is indicated for sessile lesions over 2 cm in diameter, when tissue removed endoscopically arouses a question of malignancy, or when definitive treatment cannot be completed endoscopically.

❑❑ **What fraction of hyperplastic polyps coexist in a stomach that is the site of a synchronous invasive carcinoma?**

In approximately one-third of cases, hyperplastic polyps coexist in a stomach that is the site of a synchronous invasive carcinoma.

❐❐ **What is the most likely diagnosis of a 2 cm antral nodule with a central dimple?**

Pancreatic rest. This constitutes about 1% of gastric polyps.

❐❐ **What is the only benign gastric polyp with significant malignant potential?**

Adenomatous polyp.

❐❐ **What endoscopic test is most useful diagnosing small bowel tumors?**

Intraoperative small bowel endoscopy. Its yield is much higher than either push enteroscopy or Sonde enteroscopy.

❐❐ **What radiologic studies are helpful in the diagnosis of small bowel tumors?**

Barium contrast small bowel follow-through and enteroclysis. The yield of enteroclysis is higher than the small bowel follow-through; 90% versus 65%, respectively.

❐❐ **What is the most appropriate treatment of small bowel adenomas that cannot be resected endoscopically?**

Laparotomy with segmental resection. As in the colon, adenomas of the small bowel are considered premalignant.

❐❐ **What non-gastrointestinal malignancy has the highest rate of metastasis to the small intestine?**

Melanoma.

❐❐ **Which benign small bowel tumors have the highest propensity for malignant change?**

Villous adenomas. They are often sessile, located in the second portion of the duodenum and 40% to 45% have undergone malignant degeneration at the time of diagnosis.

❐❐ **Where are lipomas of the small intestine most often located?**

Ileum.

❐❐ **What is the most common cause of intussusception in adults?**

Benign small bowel tumors. Lipomas are the leading cause.

❐❐ **What percentage of intestinal tract malignancies arise from the small bowel?**

2%.

❐❐ **What is the leading cause of cancer death in patients who have undergone proctocolectomy for familial adenomatous polyposis?**

Adenocarcinoma of the proximal small bowel.

❐❐ **When do patients with small bowel carcinoid tumors develop the carcinoid syndrome?**

Typically only when hepatic metastasis is present. Even with hepatic lesions, 30% to 50% of patients with carcinoid tumors do not develop the carcinoid syndrome.

❏❏ **Which benign small bowel tumor has the highest predilection for severe gastrointestinal bleeding?**

Leiomyoma. As these tumors grow, they can undergo necrosis and bleeding which is sometimes severe.

❏❏ **What is the most important factor that influences whether a carcinoid tumor is metastatic?**

Size of the primary lesion. Metastasis is found in only 6% of tumors less than 1 cm in diameter. Conversely, tumors over 2 cm have metastases in over 80% of cases.

❏❏ **What are the most common symptoms of carcinoid syndrome?**

Flushing, diarrhea and abdominal pain. Asthma, pellagra and cardiac valvular lesions are uncommon.

❏❏ **When do 5-HIAA (hydroxyindoleacetic acid) levels elevate in carcinoid tumors?**

5-HIAA is cleared by the liver after the first pass from the primary tumor. Thus, it is not elevated until hepatic metastases are extensive.

❏❏ **What laboratory test can be used to diagnose carcinoid syndrome?**

Urinary 5-HIAA level. Levels greater than 20 mg in 24 hours are diagnostic .

❏❏ **What serotonin-containing foods should be avoided when collecting urine for 24-hour 5-HIAA?**

Walnuts, bananas, pecans, butternuts, pineapples and tomatoes.

❏❏ **What is the most common clinical presentation of benign small bowel tumors?**

While most remain asymptomatic, mechanical small bowel obstruction, usually related to intussusception, is the most common clinical presentation.

❏❏ **T/F: Peutz-Jeghers syndrome affects the small bowel.**

True. Patients with this syndrome develop hamartomatous polyps throughout the gut. These polyps are especially common in the jejunum. Malignant degeneration can occur but is rare.

❏❏ **What cell type is present in the majority of primary gastrointestinal lymphomas?**

B-cell.

❏❏ **What are criteria for the diagnosis of a primary gastrointestinal lymphoma?**

1)   Absence of palpable peripheral lymphadenopathy on initial presentation.
2)   Absence of mediastinal lymphadenopathy on chest radiography.
3)   A normal peripheral blood smear.
4)   At laparotomy, involvement of only the gut and regional lymphadenopathy.
5)   Absence of liver and spleen involvement except by direct spread from a contiguous focus.

❏❏ **What organs are most frequently involved by metastases from small bowel carcinoid tumors?**

Liver, bone (especially bones of the orbit and the eye itself), female breast and ovary.

❏❏ **How do small bowel carcinoid tumors lead to intestinal ischemia?**

Spread of disease into mesenteric and celiac lymph nodes produces encasement of the mesenteric artery causing ischemia and eventually small bowel infarction. This is a surprisingly frequent cause of death with small bowel carcinoids.

❑❑ **What is the most common clinical presentation of small bowel carcinoids?**

Intermittent abdominal pain simulating bowel obstruction. Gastrointestinal bleeding is uncommon as these lesions ulcerate rarely. Presentation with the carcinoid syndrome is much less common than obstruction.

❑❑ **Which small bowel malignancy has the slowest rate of growth and metastasis?**

Carcinoid. The average time from onset of symptoms to death from metastases is 9 years.

❑❑ **What radiographic or endoscopic feature is common of leiomyomas/sarcomas?**

Central ulceration of the lesion may be obvious as umbilication on barium radiograph and at endoscopy.

❑❑ **What should be suspected in a patient with long-standing celiac sprue who develops a relapse of symptoms despite compliance with a gluten-free diet?**

Intestinal lymphoma, which occurs in 7% to 12% of patients with long-standing celiac disease. The cells of this secondary lymphoma are of T-cell origin.

❑❑ **T/F: Endoscopic surveillance of the upper gastrointestinal tract is indicated in individuals with familial adenomatous polyposis.**

True. About 5% of these patients develop invasive upper gastrointestinal adenocarcinoma and more than 90% of these tumors are in the duodenum or at the ampulla of Vater. An upper endoscopy should be performed prior to a prophylactic colectomy, again at age 30 and every 5 years thereafter.

❑❑ **What clinical conditions are associated with an increased risk of small bowel tumors?**

1) Crohn's disease of the small intestine (adenocarcinoma).
2) Familial adenomatous polyposis (adenoma and adenocarcinoma, particularly periampullary).
3) Celiac sprue (lymphoma and adenocarcinoma).
4) AIDS (non-Hodgkin's lymphoma and Kaposi's sarcoma).
5) Neurofibromatosis (leiomyoma and adenocarcinoma).
6) Ileal conduit or ileocystoplasty (adenocarcinoma).
7) Ileostomy after colectomy (adenocarcinoma at ileocutaneous junction).
8) Immunoproliferative small intestine disease (non-Hodgkin's lymphoma).
9) Nodular lymphoid hyperplasia (non-Hodgkin's lymphoma).

❑❑ **What is the angiographic appearance of adenocarcinoma of the small bowel?**

Hypovascular mass with arteries that are occluded or encased. Conversely, leiomyomas, leiomyosarcomas and carcinoids tend to be hypervascular.

❑❑ **What are the radiologic features of small bowel carcinoids?**

Narrowing and kinking of the small bowel with dilated proximal bowel is seen on small bowel follow-through and enteroclysis. This occurs as a result of intense fibroplastic or desmoplastic response in the adjacent mesentery.

❑❑ **What nuclear medicine scans can be used to diagnose carcinoid tumor?**

Scanning with ^{123}I-labeled Tyr3-octreotide (TOCT, a somatostatin analog) or ^{123}I-labeled metaiodobenzylguanidine. These scans take advantage of the large numbers of somatostatin receptors expressed by most carcinoid tumors.

❑❑ **What is the significance of the development of carcinoid syndrome as opposed to having asymptomatic carcinoid tumors?**

Patients with the carcinoid syndrome already have widespread metastases. Liver involvement is usually diffuse and fewer than 10% of patients with the carcinoid syndrome have resectable hepatic metastases.

❏❏ What medical therapy is available for treating the symptoms of carcinoid syndrome?

Octreotide, a synthetic somatostatin analog, injected subcutaneously in doses of 50 to 250 µg BID-TID. Symptoms improve in more than 90% of patients; however, disease progression is not altered.

❏❏ What small bowel lymphoma is seen exclusively in underdeveloped countries?

Immunoproliferative small intestinal diasease (IPSID), also known as alpha-chain disease and Mediterranean lymphoma. Microbial colonization of the small bowel is of major etiologic significance in IPSID.

❏❏ T/F: After complete removal of a small bowel tubular adenoma, long-term endoscopic surveillance should be done.

True.

❏❏ What is the best therapy for patients with villous adenomas of the small bowel?

Surgical resection is usually indicated for the treatment of small bowel villous adenomas. The size and sessile nature of most villous adenomas make complete resection by endoscopic methods almost impossible. High rates of cancerous transformation also make surgery a preferred option.

❏❏ What symptoms are most commonly produced by duodenal villous adenomas?

Most symptomatic duodenal villous adenomas are 3 cm or more in diameter. The usual clinical presentations include partial gastric outlet obstruction, pancreatitis, bleeding and obstructive jaundice.

❏❏ What is the most common malignant small bowel tumor?

Adenocarcinoma. Followed in descending order by carcinoid, lymphoma and leiomyosarcoma

❏❏ What malignant small bowel tumor often remains asymptomatic?

Carcinoid.

❏❏ What is the most common benign small bowel tumor?

Adenoma. Followed in descending order by leiomyoma, Brunner's gland hamartoma and lipoma.

❏❏ Malignant carcinoids are most commonly found in which portion of the small bowel?

Ileum. Although 70% of all carcinoids are found in the appendix, metastases from appendiceal carcinoids are so rare that they are usually regarded as benign.

❏❏ Weight loss is usually most severe in what type of malignant small bowel tumor?

Lymphoma.

❏❏ What is the most common presentation of malignant periampullary tumors?

Jaundice is seen in up to 80% of cases.

❏❏ A physical finding seen in 40% of malignant small bowel tumors and rarely seen with benign small tumors is:

Palpable abdominal mass.

❑❑ **What part of the gastrointestinal tract is the most common site for a primary gastrointestinal lymphoma?**

The stomach is the site in 70% or more of the cases. The remaining cases are equally divided between the small and large intestine.

❑❑ **T/F: A patient whose parents have familial adenomatous polyposis (FAP) has a normal flexible sigmoidoscopy at age 12. He is unlikely to develop FAP.**

False. Fifty percent of patients with FAP will develop polyps by age 15. In general, screening is accomplished by flexible sigmoidoscopy starting after puberty. For early diagnosis, gene testing is available if a proband is positive. The upper age for screening is unclear given that most patients will develop full-blown FAP by their 30's. Of note, the discovery of attenuated FAP syndromes, which can present later in life, has complicated this.

❑❑ **What are recommended screening options for a patient with a family history of familial adenomatous polyposis (FAP)? With hereditary nonpolyposis colon cancer (HNPCC)?**

FAP: receive genetic counseling and consider genetic testing. A negative test result rules out FAP only if an affected family member has an identified mutation. Gene carriers or indeterminate cases should be offerered flexible sigmoidscopy every 12 months beginning at puberty and, if polyposis is identified, offered colectomy.

HNPCC: receive genetic counseling and consider genetic testing. They should undergo a colonoscopic examination every 1 to 2 years starting between the ages of 20 and 30 and yearly after age 40.

❑❑ **What is recommended for the surveillance interval in patients with an adenomatous polyp?**

According to recent guidelines, patients with large or multiple adenomatous polyps should have repeat colonoscopy 3 years after the initial exam. If this exam is normal or shows only a small tubular adenoma, follow-up colonoscopy can be performed in 5 years. In special circumstances (e.g., polyps with invasive cancer, large sessile adenomas or numerous adenomas), follow-up colonoscopy may be done sooner.

❑❑ **T/F: A 28 year-old woman with no significant family history is found to have thousands of colonic polyps. Based on this, she is given the diagnosis of familial adenomatous polyposis and undergoes colectomy. Genetic testing is negative. The patient's 2 year-old son is also tested for the adenomatous polyposis coli (APC) gene mutation and is negative. No further surveillance is necessary for the child.**

False. Approximately 20% of patients with APC gene mutations will not have a family history of FAP. The IVSP assay that is commercially available only has an 80% sensitivity for APC gene mutations. Therefore, a negative test is not interpretable if no one else in the family is known to be positive for gene mutations by this assay.

❑❑ **T/F: Gastric polyps in patients with FAP occur in the proximal stomach.**

True. Gastric polyposis typically occurs in half the patients with FAP. They generally consist of fundic gland polyps and are most common in the proximal stomach. Rarely, adenomatous polyps can be found in the antrum (5%).

❑❑ **T/F: Gastric cancer is the next most common cause of mortality in patients with FAP following colectomy.**

False. The next most common cause of mortality is from periampullary duodenal carcinomas (lifetime risk 4%). Periodic screening with a side-viewing endoscope is probably cost-effective.

❑❑ **T/F: Retinoblastomas are common in patients with FAP.**

False. Congenital hypertrophy of the retinal epithelium may occur.

❏❏ What is the earliest histological abnormality that occurs during colon carcinogenesis?

Aberrant crypt foci (ACF). ACF are clonal lesions present on macroscopically normal mucosa. They are often seen by examining, under magnification, colons stained with methylene blue. Recent studies have shown that these may be detectable by utilization of a magnifying colonoscope. These lesions typically demonstrate K-*ras* mutations with dysplastic ACF having APC mutations.

❏❏ T/F: Juvenile polyps have no malignant potential.

False. Juvenile polyps are hamartomas characterized by distended mucus-filled glands. They typically occur in children and usually slough off or regress but occasionally may be found in adults. When single they have no malignant potential; however, when part of familial juvenile polyposis syndrome, they are associated with mixed juvenile-adenomatous polyps and have malignant potential.

❏❏ What is the inheritance of juvenile polyposis?

The genetics are unknown. Recent data suggest that mutations may occur in stromal cells leading to a 'landscaper" defect. The gene that has been implicated is PTEN (phosphatase and tensin homologue) on the deleted part of chromosome 10q.

❏❏ A 27 year-old man with mucocutaneous pigmentation presents with abdominal pain. What malignancies are associated with this syndrome?

Peutz-Jeghers polyps are hamartomas that, not uncommonly, cause intussusception. These patients are at higher risk for carcinomas of the colon, duodenum, jejunum and ileum. Ovarian sex cord tumors and testicular cancers have also been described.   Breast and pancreatic cancers have been known to occur at a young age. Approximately half of the patients with this syndrome will develop cancer. The gene, recently discovered (STK 11), is a serine-threonine kinase.

❏❏ A 50 year-old man presents with diffuse gastrointestinal polyposis, dystrophic changes in the fingernails, alopecia, cutaneous hyperpigmentation, diarrhea, weight loss, abdominal pain and complications of malnutrition. Do his children need to be screened?

No. Cronkhite-Canada syndrome is an acquired, nonfamilial syndrome. The polyps are juvenile-type but may have adenomatous epithelium. Carcinomas are quite rare. The malaborption syndrome is progressive and portends a poor prognosis.

❏❏ Which is the best estimate for the risk of colorectal cancer in 1 to 2 cm tubular adenomatous polyps - 3%, 10% or 25%?

10%. With adenomas < 1 cm, the risk is about 1.3%, while the risk for those greater than 2 cm is 46%. These rates are higher in villous compared to tubular adenomas. With regard to high-grade dysplasia, it may be found in 1.1% of polyps < 0.5 cm, 4.6% of polyps between 0.5 and 0.9 cm and 20.6% of those > 1.0 cm.

❏❏ T/F: The earliest mutation in colon carcinogenesis is K-*ras*.

False. In the multi-stage colon cancer genetic model, the adenomatous polyposis coli (APC) tumor suppressor gene is mutated in > 80% in histologically normal mucosa followed by K-*ras* at the small adenoma stage, deleted in colon cancer (DCC) at the large adenoma stage and p53 at the malignancy stage. Often, if APC is not mutated, its downstream effector - β-catenin - is altered.

❏❏ T/F: Microsatellite instability is seen only in patients with hereditary nonpolyposis colon cancer (HNPCC).

False. Microsatellite instability is seen in 15% of all colorectal cancers. Fewer than 20% will have germline mutations in the mismatch repair enzymes.

❑❑ **T/F: Tumors with microsatellite instability have a worse prognosis than standard colon cancers.**

False. While tumors with microsatellite instability are typically less differentiated and mucinous, they tend to have a significantly better prognosis than standard tumors. These tumors, whether sporadic or part of HNPCC, tend to be flat, right-sided and have lymphocyte infiltration. The general recommendations for screening for microsatellite instability in colon cancer (Bethesda criteria) include young patients, right-sided mucinous tumors and family history of colon cancer.

❑❑ **What tumors are commonly associated with HNPCC?**

Endometrial, ovarian, gastric, pancreatic and renal pelvis.

❑❑ **What genetic marker has prognostic implications for Dukes B2 colon cancer?**

Deleted in colon cancer (DCC) status. Adjuvant chemotherapy has not been shown to have a survival advantage for Dukes B2 colon cancer; however, recent evidence suggests that if this tumor supressor gene is mutated, B2 tumors 'behave' more like a C1 tumor. Adjuvant chemotherapy has been shown to provide a survival advantage for Dukes C tumors.

❑❑ **T/F: Nonsteroidal anti-inflammatory drugs (NSAIDs) are helpful in preventing polyp formation in FAP but not sporadic colon cancer.**

False. Epidemiological and experimental studies have demonstrated responsiveness to NSAIDs in both of these conditions. Both conditions are characterized by up-regulation of cyclooxygenase-2 early in carcinogenesis.

❑❑ **What type of gastrointestinal polyps are associated with the basal cell nevus syndrome?**

Multiple gastric hamartomatous polyps

❑❑ **T/F: Colon cancer is common in Cowden's syndrome.**

False. The hallmark of Cowden's syndrome is facial trichilemmomas. It is characterized by multiple oral and dermatological hamartomas, breast disease (both fibrocystic and cancer), thyroid disease (nontoxic goiter and cancer) and hamartomatous polyps of the stomach, small bowel and colon. The colorectal polyps have disorganization and proliferation of the muscularis mucosa with normal overlying colonic epithelium. These rarely cause symptoms or degenerate into colon cancer.

❑❑ **What are the major extracolonic manifestations of Gardner's syndrome?**

Gardner's syndrome is a variant of FAP with a germline mutation in the APC gene. It is characterized by bone disease, especially osteomas of the long bones, skull and mandible. Dental abnormalities including supernumerary teeth, impacted teeth and mandibular cysts have been seen. Congenital hypertrophy of the retinal pigmented epithelium (CHRPE) is commonly seen. Soft tissue tumors including fibromas, lipomas and epidermoid cysts can be seen. Extracolonic malignancies are similar to classic FAP (peri-ampullary and gastric); however, papillary carcinoma of the thyroid and adrenals and tumors of the liver and biliary tree have also been reported.

❑❑ **T/F: Bone cancer is the second leading cause of death in patients with Gardner's syndrome.**

False. Desmoid tumors have been reported in 8% to 13% of patients and are second only to metastatic colon cancer as a cause of death. This diffuse mesenteric fibromatosis is often a reaction to a laparotomy but may appear spontaneously. The progressive growth of mesenteric fibroblasts can cause gastrointestinal obstruction, vascular compromise and ureteral obstruction. While responsive to radiation therapy, this is often impractical because of concerns over mesenteric injury. Nonsteroidal anti-inflammatory drugs and anti-estrogens may have some effect.

❑❑ **T/F: Duodenal polyposis is rare in familial adenomatous polyposis.**

False. Sixty to ninety percent of patients have duodenal polyposis and 50% to 85% have adenomatous changes of the papilla of Vater. Four to twelve percent of these patients develop duodenal/periampullary malignacies.

❒❒ T/F: Turcot's syndrome is associated with HNPCC and FAP.

True, partially. The brain tumors that occur in FAP with Turcot's syndrome are generally medulloblastomas while gliomas are generally found with the HNPCC variant.

❒❒ T/F: Neurofibromatosis predisposes to colon cancer.

False. Neurofibromas may be seen throughout the gut. Malignant tumors can be seen, often from degeneration of neurofibromas; however, colorectal adenocarcinomas are rare.

❒❒ T/F: Liver metastases from colorectal cancer are best treated with intra-arterial 5-FU or floxuridine (FUDR).

False. This therapy remains investigational and is complicated by the development of a sclerosing cholangitis-like picture. If there is no evidence of extrahepatic disease and the tumor(s) involve either one lobe of the liver or are focal and surgically accessible in both lobes, surgical resection should be contemplated. After successful surgery, the 5-year survival rate is 20% to 34%. Unfortunately, only 5% to 6% of patients are considered surgical candidates. Recent data suggests that intraarterial chemotherapy in combination with surgery is superior to surgery alone.

❒❒ T/F: Adjuvant chemotherapy has not been shown to have a survival benefit for Dukes B2 rectal cancer.

False. Dukes B2 rectal cancer should be treated with either preoperative or postoperative chemotherapy accompanied by radiation therapy in order to enhance local therapy. This differs for colon cancer *per se*.

❒❒ T/F: The use of the carcinoembryonic antigen (CEA) level, abdominal CT scan and chest x-ray in addition to colonoscopy as surveillance methods after curative resection for colon cancer has been shown to improve survival.

False. Neither routine CT scanning nor chest x-rays have been shown to improve survival. Obtaining CEA levels annually may have a role, although its cost-effectiveness has been controversial.

❒❒ T/F: Patients with a family history of adenomatous polyps are at a higher risk for colorectal cancer.

True. If diagnosed under age 55, there is a markedly increased risk of colorectal cancer.

❒❒ T/F: Most patients with a positive fecal occult blood test (FOBT) will have a colon cancer or polyp.

False. While the sensitivity of FOBT is approximately 80%, the positive predictive value is only about 10% to 20%.

❒❒ T/F: The risk of colon cancer in patients with inflammatory bowel disease may be affected by certain extraintestinal manifestations.

True. While the predominant risk factors include the amount of bowel involved and duration of the disease, coexisting sclerosing cholangitis is also a significant risk factor.

❒❒ What endocrine disorder carries a higher risk of colonic neoplasia?

Acromegaly. Although the studies are retrospective, the estimates of the prevalence of adenomatous polyps and colon cancer range from 6.3% to 25% and 14% to 35%, respectively. The risk may be higher in younger patients, those with a family history of colon cancer and those with multiple skin tags (acrochordons). While the mechanism is unclear, it is not simply growth hormone-related since the risk of neoplasia may be greater in cured acromegalics than those with active disease.

☐☐ What organisms responsible for bacteremia are associated with the presence of colorectal neoplasia?

Streptococcus bovis bacteremia has been associated with the presence of colorectal adenomas and carcinomas. *Clostridium septicum* bacteremia has also been associated with the colonic neoplasia. Finally, endocarditis associated with *Streptococcus agalactiae* has been reported in several patients with rectal villous adenomas containing small foci of carcinoma.

☐☐ T/F: Patients with breast cancer have an increased risk of colon cancer.

False. There is no evidence in case-control studies that having a personal history of breast cancer is a risk factor for colon cancer. However, patients with familial breast cancer associated with mutations in BRCA 1 or 2 have a 3- to 6-fold increased incidence of colon cancer.

☐☐ What are potential mechanisms in colonic neoplasm-induced diarrhea?

A syndrome of large-volume secretory diarrhea has been observed with large villous adenomas in the rectum and rectosigmoid colon and is associated with dehydration and electrolyte abnormalities, especially hypokalemia. The mechanisms are unclear. Some data suggest that prostaglandins are involved.

☐☐ How common are adenomatous polyps in the general population?

Clinical studies indicate that adenomatous polyps occur in 25% of patients 50 years old and increase with age. By the late 70's, 50% of people have polyps. Autopsy studies suggest an even higher rate with approximately 60% of men and 40% of women having adenomatous polyps at age 50. They are found more commonly in men than women. While data on large polyps (> 1 cm) are limited, one autopsy series suggested that 4.6% of the population at age 54 and 15.6% at age 75 had large polyps.

☐☐ T/F: The risk of colon cancer is lower in patients with Crohn's disease compared to those with ulcerative colitis.

False. Crohn's colitis has the same risk as ulcerative colitis when matched for extent, duration and age of onset of the disease. The cumulative risk for developing colorectal cancer with pancolitis is 30% after 35 years. Surveillance colonoscopy every 1 to 2 years is recommended after 8 years in those with pancolitis and after 15 years in those with left-sided colitis.

☐☐ A 63 year-old man had a 2 cm pedunculated polyp, which contained a focus of malignancy, removed from the sigmoid colon. What surveillance is recommended?

If invasive carcinoma is found and poor prognostic features exist (e.g., malignancy incompletely excised, less than a 2 mm margin from polypectomy, a relatively undifferentiated tumor or lymphatic or venous invasion), then hemicolectomy is recommended. Sessile polyps are also considered to have a worse prognosis. If no poor prognostic features exist, as in this patient, it would be reasonable to consider that the polypectomy is the definitive therapy. Colonoscopy is often recommended within 3 months of polypectomy and then 1 year later to ensure that there is no residual malignant tissue.

☐☐ A 10 year-old girl presents with hematochezia and is found to have two juvenile colonic polyps. Her family history is unremarkable. What is the recommended follow-up?

This patient does not meet the criteria for juvenile polyposis which includes the presence of ten or more juvenile polyps, juvenile polyps throughout the gastrointestinal tract or juvenile polyps in a patient with a family history of polyposis. These non-neoplastic hamartomatous colonic polyps are extremely common occurring in 1% to 2% of all children, usually between the ages of 4 and 14. A solitary polyp is seen in 70% of patients but 30% will have 2 or 3. If a polyposis syndrome is not identified, no other evaluation is necessary.

❑❑ **A 28 year-old patient with Gardner's syndrome is noted to have nodular lymphoid hyperplasia of the terminal ileum. What therapy is necessary?**

Nodular lymphoid hyperplasia is a rare lymphoproliferative disorder associated with a variety of disorders including Gardner's. It is also present in 20% of patients with common variable immunodeficiency and is rarely associated with intestinal lymphoma. Of note, it has also been seen in otherwise healthy children. These hyperplastic lymphoid nodules are often found in the small bowel but may be seen in the stomach and colon. These nodules range in size from 3 to 6 mm. No therapy is required for nodular lymphoid hyperplasia.

❑❑ **What agents are FDA-approved for preventing colon neoplasia?**

While nonsteroidal anti-inflammatory drugs as a class protect against colon cancer, only celecoxib has recently been approved for this indication in patients with familial adenomatous polyposis.

❑❑ **What agents have been shown to inhibit colon cancer?**

Epidemiological studies in humans have demonstrated that NSAIDs, estrogens, calcium and folate inhibit colon cancer. The effect of dietary fiber is controversial. Animal studies suggest that ursodeoxycholic acid, vitamin D analogues, polyethylene glycol and fish oil may also be protective.

❑❑ **T/F: Patients with colorectal cancer who undergo surgical resection require follow-up colonoscopy in one year.**

False. The recommended surveillance interval in this setting, if the preoperative colonoscopy was complete and otherwise normal, is 3 years after resection and, if normal, every 5 years thereafter.

❑❑ **What are the screeening recommendations for a patient with a 53 year-old brother who just had an adenomatous polyp removed?**

According to current guidelines, any person with a first-degree relative with either colon cancer or an adenomatous polyp should be offered the same screening options as average-risk patients, except starting at age 40. The guideline states that if the patient had colorectal cancer before 55 or adenomatous polyp before age 60, special efforts should be made to ensure that screening takes place.

❑❑ **What are the screening recommendations for patients at an average-risk for colon cancer?**

Starting at age 50, colonoscopy every ten years, double-contrast barium enema every 5 years, annual fecal occult blood testing , flexible sigmoidoscopy every 5 years or a combination of fecal occult blood testing and flexible sigmoidoscopy.

❑❑ **T/F: Lack of exercise and obesity are associated with colonic neoplasia.**

True. Epidemiological studies have demonstrated that these are independent risk factors for colon cancer.

❑❑ **What is the most common cancer involving the hepatobiliary tree?**

Gallbladder carcinoma. Gallbladder carcinoma is the fifth most common cancer of the gastrointestinal tract and is responsible for 2% to 4% of all gastrointestinal malignancies. It is most frequent in the sixth and seventh decade and is more common in women and Native Americans.

❑❑ **What are two risk factors for the development of gallbladder carcinoma?**

Gallstones larger than 2.5 cm and calcified or 'porcelain' gallbladders.

❑❑ **What are the most common routes of gallbladder carcinoma metastasis?**

Lymphatic spread and direct invasion.

❑❑ **What size of benign adenomas of the gallbladder are at an increased risk for gallbladder carcinoma?**

Adenomas greater than 15 mm have been observed to have malignant foci.

❑❑ **Name two non-specific tumor markers of the gastrointestinal tract that may be elevated in cholangiocarcinoma.**

CA 19-9 and carcinoembyonic antigen (CEA). Alpha fetoprotein is elevated in < 5% of cases of cholangiocarcinoma.

❑❑ **Name three clinical entities associated with extrahepatic bile duct tumors.**

1) Choledochal cysts or polycystic liver disease; 2) Primary sclerosing cholangitis; and, 3) Chronic infection with *Clonorchis sinensis, Ascaris lumbricoides, Giardia lamblia* and *Opisthorcis viverrini*.

❑❑ **What contrast agent can predispose to cholangiocarcinoma?**

Thorotrast.

❑❑ **What is the second most common tumor of the biliary tract?**

Ampullary carcinoma follows gallbladder carcinoma as the second most common tumor of the biliary tract. It occurs more frequently among men than women who are 50 to 70 years old.

❑❑ **What is the most common operative procedure for treatment of distal bile duct carcinomas?**

Pancreaticoduodenectomy (Whipple's procedure). The operative mortality is less than 5% in experienced centers.

❑❑ **Name two physical exam findings of ampullary carcinoma besides jaundice, pruritis and acholic stools.**

Hepatomegaly and Courvoisier's gallbladder. These findings are found in 25% to 40% of patients with ampullary carcinoma. The 5-year survival of ampullary carcinoma is 20% to 40%.

❑❑ **Alternating jaundice and gastrointestinal bleeding are suggestive of what biliary tumor?**

Ulcerating ampullary carcinomas.

❑❑ **Gallbladder cancer is associated with what two anatomical variants of the biliary tract?**

Choledochal cyst and anomalous pancreaticobiliary ductal union.

❑❑ **What histologic subtype of ampullary carcinoma has the best prognosis?**

Papillary > fungating > ulcerative.

❑❑ **Name two carcinogens associated with the development of gallbladder carcinoma.**

Dimethylnitrosamine and petroleum products.

❑❑ **What missense mutations have been associated with gallbladder carcinoma?**

p53 demonstrates abnormal expression in 90% to 95% of gallbladder carcinoma.

❑❑ **List three risk factors for the development of ampullary carcinoma.**

Ampullary adenoma, familial adenomatous polyposis and Gardner's syndrome.

❑❑ **What hormone receptor may be found in cholangiocarcinomas?**

Somatostatin.

❑❑ **Which side of the intrahepatic biliary tree, the right or left system, is preferentially drained by the presence of only one stent in the setting of a proximal intrahepatic bile duct tumor?**

The left hepatic ductal system can be drained with a single stent. The right hepatic duct bifurcates extensively proximal to the confluence with the left hepatic duct.

❑❑ **What gene mutation is associated with 20% of patients with bile duct carcinoma?**

c-K-*ras* at codon 12. The K-*ras* gene normally regulates intracellular growth signal transduction.

❑❑ **The vast majority of primary malignant tumors of the pancreas are of what histological type?**

Ductal adenocarcinomas and its variants constitute approximately 90% of primary malignant tumors of the pancreas. About 5% of pancreatic tumors are of islet cell origin. The rarer types of primary pancreatic cancer include squamous cell carcinoma, giant cell carcinoma, carcinosarcoma, cystadenocarcinoma, acinar cell carcinolma, sarcoma, malignant fibrous histiocytoma, lymphoma and pancreaticoblastoma.

❑❑ **Adenocarcinomas are derived from what part of the pancreas?**

Pancreatic ductal epithelium.

❑❑ **T/F: Since 1970, the incidence of pancreatic cancer has increased in both men and women.**

False. Incidence rates have declined somewhat among men and increased slightly among women. The male-to-female ratio was estimated to be approximately 1:1.06 in 1998.

❑❑ **T/F: In hereditary pancreatitis, patients with a paternal pattern of inheritance are at a higher risk of developing pancreatic cancer.**

True. At age 70, these patients have an estimated 40% risk of developing pancreatic cancer. For patients with a paternal pattern of inheritance, the risk approaches 75%.

❑❑ **Diabetes mellitus or impaired glucose intolerance occurs in what percentage of patients with pancreatic cancer?**

Sixty percent to 80% of patients with pancreatic cancer have diabetes mellitus or impaired glucose tolerance with the majority of patients found to be diabetic within 2 years of the diagnosis of pancreatic cancer.

❑❑ **What is the most consistent environmental risk factor predisposing to pancreatic cancer?**

Cigarette smoking is the only risk factor consistently found in epidemiological studies to predispose to pancreatic cancer.

❑❑ **What hormone is felt to be responsible for the occurrence of diabetes in patients with pancreatic cancer?**

The overproduction of amylin (islet amyloid polypeptide) has been reported in patients with pancreatic cancer.

❑❑ **Why does CA 19-9 only have a maximum sensitivity of 95% for the diagnosis of pancreatic cancer?**

The carbohydrate antigen, CA 19-9, is not expressed in the 5% of individuals who are sialylated Lewis[a] antigen negative.

❑❑ **What is the most common presenting symptom in patients with pancreatic cancer?**

Pain is observed in 80% of patients.

❑❑ **What is the most common presentation in patients with resectable pancreatic carcinoma?**

Painless jaundice is seen in about 50% of patients with a resectable lesion.

❑❑ **What is the most common genetic alteration detected in pancreatic carcinomas?**

A K-*ras* mutation is detected in 95% of cases.

❑❑ **Approximately what percentage of pancreatic carcinoma cases are related to hereditary factors?**

A genetic predisposition for adenocarcinoma of the pancreas may account for up to 10% of cases.

❑❑ **T/F: The risk of pancreatic cancer is increased in kindreds of familial atypical multiple mole melanoma (FAMMM) syndrome.**

False. Only in those kindreds with a p16 germ-line mutation; however, not all of these p16 germ-line mutated kindreds are at an increased risk.

❑❑ **What other disorders can lead to elevations in serum CA 19-9 levels?**

Most commonly, those disorders that cause biliary tract obstruction such as cholangitis, cholangiocarcinoma, gallbladder carcinoma and benign biliary tract diseases. Additionally, elevations may be seen in acute and chronic pancreatitis and chronic liver disease.

❑❑ **T/F: A mutation at codon 15 of K-*ras* is the most commonly identified gene abnormality in pancreatic cancer.**

False. Mutations of K-*ras* almost uniformly occur at codon 12 in pancreatic cancer.

❑❑ **What imaging techniques can be used to assist in obtaining tissue to make the diagnosis of pancreatic cancer?**

Fine-needle aspiration can be performed under endoscopic ultrasound, CT or transabdominal ultrasound guidance. In addition, brushings can be obtained during endososcopic retrograde cholangiopancreatography.

❑❑ **What imaging modality is generally considered to be the best initial study when evaluating patients presenting with symptoms that suggest pancreatic disease?**

CT scan is recommended since it can detect tumors in the pancreas, stage for resectability and evaluate for liver metastases.

❑❑ **What imaging study is most accurate in the detection of small (< 2 cm) pancreatic neoplasms?**

Endoscopic ultrasound has been found in several studies to be the most accurate imaging study available for the detection of small carcinomas.

❑❑ **What percentage of patients with adenocarcinoma of the pancreas are unresectable at the time of diagnosis?**

Due to the insidious nature of the disease, more than 80% of patients are unresectable at the time of diagnosis.

❑❑ What helical CT scanning criteria are used to define unresectability in pancreatic cancer?

1) Presence of extrapancreatic disease.
2) Obstructed superior mesenteric-portal vein confluence.
3) Evidence of direct tumor extension to the celiac axis and superior mesenteric artery.

❑❑ What is the perioperative mortality rate of pancreatoduodenectomy (Whipple procedure) when performed at experienced centers?

Current perioperative mortality rates are less than 5% at experienced centers.

❑❑ How many long-term survivors of pancreatic cancer die of recurrent or metastatic disease?

Unlike most other types of cancer, 5-year survival with this disease does not ensure that the patient has been cured of the disease. One recent study of long-term survivors (> 5 years) reported that almost half of these patients died of recurrent or metastatic disease.

❑❑ What is the preferable method of non-operative palliative biliary decompression?

For reasons of less morbidity, it is preferable to place the stent by ERCP rather than percutaneously through a transhepatic approach.

❑❑ T/F: Preoperative stenting of the bile duct to relieve jaundice decreases perioperative morbidity and mortality.

False. Recent studies do not support preoperative stenting of the bile duct except in cases of acute cholangitis and, possibly, when bilirubin levels are markedly elevated.

❑❑ What is the double-duct sign?

This sign is caused by a mass in the head of the pancreas causing dilation of both the pancreatic and common bile duct. When this sign is present, the patient should be assumed to have pancreatic cancer until proven otherwise.

❑❑ What is the standard adjuvant therapy recommended to patients following potentially curative resection of a pancreatic adenocarcinoma?

Chemoradiation therapy is recommended following a curative resection based on the results of a pivotal randomized controlled study conducted by the Gastrointestinal Tumor Study Group.

❑❑ What is the advantage of preoperative chemoradiation therapy compared to postoperative chemoradiation therapy in resectable patients?

A recent study demonstrated no change in survival advantage; however, 24% of patients were unable to receive postoperative treatment as a result of delayed recovery after surgery. Therefore, preoperative (neoadjuvant) therapy seems preferable.

❑❑ What options are available for treatment of gastric outlet obstruction caused by a pancreatic adenocarcinoma?

A surgical gastrojejunostomy has been the traditional treatment for an outlet obstruction; however, the use of expandable metallic stents also offers an endoscopic method for palliation of this complication.

❑❑ What pathologic characteristics predict long-term survival following surgical resection for pancreatic cancer?

Negative resection margins, negative nodal status and tumor size < 3 cm are strong predictors of long-term survival.

❑❑ **What are some epidemiologic and etiologic factors that are associated with an increased risk for the development of pancreatic cancer?**

Cigarette smoking, alcohol consumption, animal fat-rich diet, idiopathic chronic pancreatitis, alcoholic chronic pancreatitis, diabetes mellitus and gallstones.

❑❑ **What are some names that describe the entity "serous cystadenoma"?**

Microcystic adenoma, benign serous cystadenoma and glycogen-rich serous adenoma.

❑❑ **T/F: A serous cystadenoma occurs more commonly in females than males.**

True.

❑❑ **T/F: A serous cystadenoma is most commonly diagnosed in patients before the age of 40.**

False. These neoplasms are most commonly detected in the sixth decade of a patient's life.

❑❑ **What are the most common presenting symptoms of a serous cystadenoma?**

Abdominal pain (50%), asymptomatic abdominal mass (33%) and weight loss (20%).

❑❑ **What is the typical ultrasonographic appearance of a serous cystadenoma?**

It appears as a complex echo-lucent cystic structure with septae. The individual cysts are usually small.

❑❑ **What is the classic calcification pattern of a serous cystadenoma seen on abdominal plain films?**

A "sunburst" pattern.

❑❑ **How does a serous cystadenoma usually appear on CT scan?**

A multiloculated cystic mass ranging in size from 4 to 6 cm. A central stellate calcification may be present. The neoplasm can occur anywhere within the pancreas.

❑❑ **T/F: Serous cystadenomas are generally benign.**

True.

❑❑ **T/F: Mucinous cystic neoplasms are more common in women and occur around the age of 50.**

True.

❑❑ **What is the usual appearance of a mucinous cystic neoplasm on either ultrasonography or CT scan?**

A loculated cystic mass usually located in the body or tail of the pancreas. Malignant lesions tend to be larger (8 to 11 cm) and often have rim calcifications identified on CT scan.

❑❑ **What is the treatment of choice for a mucinous neoplasm?**

Surgical resection is the treatment of choice due to difficulties in differentiating a benign versus malignant lesion by biopsy of the cyst wall or by fine needle aspiration of the cyst contents.

❑❑ **What are the classic characteristics of an intraductal papillary mucinous tumor of the pancreas as seen during endoscopic retrograde cholangiopancreatography?**

A dilated and irregular main pancreatic duct with filling defects and extrusion of mucin through the major papilla.

❑❑ **What neuroendocrine tumor is associated with a syndrome of large volume diarrhea, achlorhydria and hypokalemia?**

VIPoma. This syndrome, caused by overproduction of vasoactive intestinal peptide, is characterized by the acronym WDHA (watery diarrhea, hypokalemia and achlorhydria).

❑❑ **What neuorendocrine tumor is associated with a dermatitis, glucose intolerance, weight loss and anemia?**

Glucagonoma. Up to 90% of cases will present with characteristic skin lesions and glucose intolerance.

❑❑ **What is the characteristic skin rash that may be seen in patients with glucagonoma?**

Necrolytic migratory erythema. This rash may wax and wane and occurs in 64% to 90% of cases.

❑❑ **Deficiencies of amino acids are a common occurrence in what pancreatic neuroendocrine tumor?**

Glucagonoma. The severity of the deficiency is correlated with the intensity of the disease.

❑❑ **A 55 year-old white man with a history of diabetes and steatorrhea underwent an emergent cholecystectomy for acute cholecystitis. Intraoperatively, he is found to have a small tumor in the head of the pancreas. The patient most likely has what neuroendocrine tumor?**

Somatostatinoma. Diabetes occurs in 95%, gallstone disease in 94% and steatorrhea is found in 83% of cases of pancreatic somatostatinomas.

❑❑ **The majority of gastrinomas are found in what anatomic area?**

The gastrinoma triangle, which extends superiorly from the confluence of the cystic duct and CBD, inferiorly by the junction of the 2nd and 3rd portion of the duodenum, and medially by the junction of the neck and body of the pancreas.

❑❑ **Gastrinomas are classically associated with what syndrome?**

Multiple endocrine neoplasia (MEN) type 1 is reported in approximately 25% of gastrinoma patients.

❑❑ **Describe Whipple's triad?**

Whipple's triad consists of hypoglycemic symptoms, blood glucose levels of less than 50 mg/dL and symptom relief after glucose ingestion. It may be seen in patients with an insulinoma

❑❑ **Besides a CT scan of the abdomen, what is the best imaging study to evaluate for metastatic gastrinoma?**

An octreotide scan (somatostatin receptor scintigraphy). In most series, it assists in the localization of gastrinomas more than 90% of the time.

❑❑ **Where is the most common extra-pancreatic site for a gastrinoma?**

The duodenal wall.

❑❑ **What is the neuroendocrine tumor with the lowest rate of metastasis?**

Insulinoma, with a rate of < 10%.

❑❑ **T/F: Both endoscopic ultrasound and somatostatin receptor scintigraphy are useful in the localization of insulinomas and gastrinomas.**

False. Although both modalities are useful in the evaluation of gastrinomas, only 10% of insulinomas are detected with an octreotide scan.

❏❏ What type of lymphoma may affect the pancreas?

Non-Hodgkin's lymphoma accounts for 1% to 2% of all pancreatic neoplasms. About 1% of non-Hodgkin lymphomas appear to arise from the pancreas. At autopsy, about one-third of all patients with non-Hodgkin's lymphoma will have some microscopic involvement of the pancreas.

❏❏ What is a typical presentation of pancreatic lymphoma?

Weight loss and jaundice. Some patients may also have night sweats.

❏❏ T/F: Surgical resection is usually required in cases of pancreatic lymphoma.

False. Chemotherapy alone results in over a 50% rate of remission. Surgery may occasionally be performed either for tissue diagnosis or resection of small, localized tumors.

HEPATOLOGY

ACUTE LIVER FAILURE AND LIVER TRANSPLANTATION

Timothy McCashland, M.D.

❑❑ **What are the hallmark diagnostic signs of acute liver failure?**

Encephalopathy and coagulopathy. When the international normalization ratio (INR) is greater than 1.5 and encephalopathy is present within 8 weeks of the beginning of the illness, the diagnosis is secure.

❑❑ **Criteria for poor outcome in cases of acetaminophen-induced acute liver failure include:**

Prothrombin time > 50 seconds, pH < 7.3 and Grade 4 encephalopathy.

❑❑ **A 43 year-old woman with Wilson's disease presents with Grade 3 encephalopathy and jaundice. Family members discover that she has not taken her penicillamine over the last few weeks. What treatment does her current clinical condition require?**

Liver transplantation. Restarting penicillamine has shown little efficacy in this setting.

❑❑ **A 25 year-old woman in her third trimester of pregnancy presents with jaundice, confusion and RUQ pain. Laboratory evaluation reveals marked anemia, severe thrombocytopenia and elevated liver tests. What would be the most appropriate management?**

Rapid delivery of the baby with appropriate clotting factor support. HELLP syndrome (hemolysis, elevated liver enzymes and low platelets) is associated with rapid liver failure, usually in the third trimester of pregnancy, and is a medical emergency.

❑❑ **When should a patient with acute liver failure be transferred to a transplant center?**

Any patient with encephalopathy of Grade 2 or more.

❑❑ **What are the most common causes of acute liver failure in the United States?**

Acetaminophen toxicity, indeterminate, other medications and acute viral hepatitis (types A and B).

❑❑ **What is most common cause of death in acute liver failure while awaiting a liver transplant?**

Cerebral edema. Cerebral edema is reported in 80% of those dying from acute liver failure.

❑❑ **T/F: Survival after liver transplantation for acute liver failure is comparable to transplantation for end-stage liver disease.**

False. Survival after transplantation for acute liver failure ranges from 46% to 89% (66% average). The lower survival is related to the presence of multiple organ failure at the time of transplant.

❑❑ **The neurological exam of a patient with acute liver failure begins to deteriorate. What should you do?**

Sequential management of cerebral edema includes elevation of head of bed 10 to 20 degrees, hyperventilation, mannitol and pentobarbital coma. Intracranial pressure monitoring may be very helpful in this situation.

❑❑ **T/F: Survival of patients with acute liver failure is related to their Grade of encephalopathy at the time of transplantation.**

True. Grade 1 - 90%, Grade 2 - 71% and grade 3 or 4 - 48%.

❑❑ **Poor prognostic variables in non-acetaminophen-induced acute liver failure include:**

An international normalization ratio (INR) > 3.5, age < 10 or > 40, drug-induced, indeterminate cause, duration of jaundice > 7 days and bilirubin > 30 mg/dl.

❑❑ **T/F: A 40 year-old man with acute liver failure of unknown etiology (indeterminate) is febrile and has an elevated leukocyte count. He should immediately be listed for liver transplantation.**

False. Contraindications to liver transplantation include active infection and severe cerebral edema. Infection at the time of transplantation has contributed to death in about 11% of patients. Up to 36% of patients with acute liver failure have been reported to develop bacteremia. Cerebral perfusion pressure of < 40 mmHg for longer than 1 hour makes neurological recovery unlikely.

❑❑ **What are the most common infections in acute liver failure?**

Pneumonia (50%) followed by bacteremia (26%) and urinary tract infection (22%).

❑❑ **A 35 year-old woman with acetaminophen-induced acute liver failure is persistently febrile despite being on broad-spectrum antibiotics. What infectious organism should you suspect?**

Fungal infections are common in acute liver failure (13% to 32%). *Candida albicans* is the most common fungal organism identified.

❑❑ **What is the cause of renal failure associated with acute liver failure?**

Renal failure develops in 43% to 80% of cases, depending upon the etiology of liver failure. Acetaminophen may cause direct injury to the distal tubules of the kidney; however, most cases result from a decrease in renal blood flow as a consequence of vasoconstriction. This is similar to what occurs in hepatorenal syndrome.

❑❑ **The use of what medications/substances, when taken chronically, results in a higher risk of acute liver failure with concomitant acetaminophen use?**

Any medication that induces the cytochrome P450 system in the liver may enhance acute liver failure with acetaminophen. The most common medications in this setting are alcohol, phenytoin and antidepressants.

❑❑ **A 20 year-old male body-builder presents with jaundice, confusion and bruises. What is the most likely cause of acute liver failure in this setting?**

Anabolic steroids, when used in high doses, may result in acute liver failure.

❑❑ **A family of campers that just recently returned from a camping trip presents to their physician with diarrhea and confusion. Liver tests and serum creatinine are elevated. What is your diagnosis, treatment and prognosis?**

Amanita phalloides poisoning presents with diarrhea, neurological changes and signs of hepatorenal failure. Children below the age of 10 have the highest rate of fatality with an overall death rate of 20%. Initial management with high-dose penicillin has shown some benefit.

❏❏ **A 45 year-old woman presents to your office four days following laparoscopic cholecystectomy with nausea, vomiting, fevers and diffuse myalgias. Evaluation reveals the aminotransferases to be over four-times greater than normal. What diagnosis do you suspect?**

Idiosyncratic hepatic injury to anesthetic drugs is reported in up to 1 in 9,000 cases. The usual interval from surgery to presentation is 3 to 5 days but can be up to 15 days. Halothane is considered the classic example of anesthetic-induced liver injury.

❏❏ **What is the single most important factor limiting liver transplantation in the United States?**

The availability of cadaveric donors. Approximately 4,000 liver transplants are performed each year; however, up to 10,000 potential candidates are identified each year. As many as 30% of patients die waiting for a liver transplant.

❏❏ **Liver transplant candidates are matched to the cadaveric donor by what variables?**

Weight (liver size limit) and blood type.

❏❏ **How does a transplant center prioritize who receives a transplant?**

The United Network for Organ Sharing (UNOS) dictates medical urgency for transplantation. Highest priority is for fulminant liver failure and primary nonfunction of a graft followed by hospitalized patients in the intensive care unit, other hospitalized patients and, finally, patients requiring continuous medical care at home.

❏❏ **What are contraindications to liver transplantation?**

HIV seropositivity, extrahepatic malignancy, hemangiosarcoma, sepsis, active alcoholism and advanced cardiorespiratory disease.

❏❏ **For patients with alcoholic liver disease, what is the usual period of abstinence before consideration of liver transplantation?**

Most programs require a period of abstinence of at least 6 months with adequate support systems and compliance with medical care.

❏❏ **T/F: Spontaneous bacterial peritonitis is a contraindication to liver transplantation.**

False. Antibiotic treatment for 2 to 5 days is associated with high bacteriologic cure.

❏❏ **T/F: Hepatorenal syndrome is a contraindication to liver transplantation.**

False. Hepatorenal syndrome is reversed by liver transplantation.

❏❏ **What two diseases have a prognostic model index to help in the decision to list for liver transplantation?**

Primary biliary cirrhosis and primary sclerosing cholangitis have a natural history that allows a model to predict the optimal timing of transplantation. The Mayo Model prognostic index incorporates many variables and provides a risk score that predicts 1- and 5-year survival with and without transplant.

❏❏ **T/F: Waiting times for liver transplantation are equal throughout the United States.**

False. There is great variability in waiting times due to availability of donors. Patients with blood type O have the longest waiting times.

❏❏ **What are the most common medications used for immunosuppression after liver transplantation?**

Cyclosporine, tacrolimus (FK 506), azathioprine and prednisone.

❏❏ **What is the mechanism of action of cyclosporine and tacrolimus (FK 506)?**

Both inhibit early T-cell signal pathways and interleukin-2 production and release.

❏❏ **What are the most common side effects of cyclosporine?**

Hypertension, renal toxicity, diabetes mellitus, hirsutism and gingivitis.

❏❏ **What medications can increase the serum levels of cyclosporine?**

Diltiazem, nicardipine, verapamil, erythromycin, clarithromycin and ketoconozole.

❏❏ **What medications can increase the serum levels of tacrolimus (FK 506)?**

Bromocriptine, cimetidine, ciprofloxacin, diltiazem, erythromycin and metoclopramide.

❏❏ **What diseases for which transplantation is performed may recur following liver transplantation?**

Hepatitis C is the most common recurrent disease. Hepatitis B can recur if not adequately treated post transplant. It has also been suggested that autoimmune diseases, such as primary biliary cirrhosis and primary sclerosing cholangitis, may recur after transplant.

❏❏ **Currently, what liver disease is most commonly transplanted?**

Chronic hepatitis C followed by alcoholic liver disease, cholestatic liver disease, cryptogenic liver disease, metabolic liver disease and malignancy.

❏❏ **How is recurrent hepatitis B prevented following liver transplantation?**

Excellent patient and graft survival is now possible with long-term hepatitis B immune globulin (HBIG) and lamivudine prophylaxis. The goal is keep the anti-HBs level greater than 500 IU/L.

❏❏ **T/F: Survival following liver transplant for chronic hepatitis C is poor.**

False. One- and five-year survival after transplantation is generally good and comparable to other diseases (5-year survival 70%). Primary biliary cirhosis has the highest survival with a > 90% 5-year survival.

❏❏ **T/F: A 50 year-old man with chronic hepatitis C presents with worsening ascites. Ultrasound reveals a single 3 cm lesion in the right lobe of the liver. Alpha-fetoprotein level is considerably elevated. This patient is still a liver transplant candidate.**

True. The following variables have been found to correlate with poor prognosis: single tumor size greater than 5 cm, multiple lesions (> 3), vascular invasion and noncircumscribed shape. Nevertheless, survival remains poor with a reported 9% 2-year survival. In contrast, incidental hepatomas found at the time of transplantation do not seem to be associated with a worse prognosis.

❏❏ **T/F: Survival is worse after liver transplantation in patients with hemochromatosis.**

True. The survival for patients with hemochromatosis after transplantation is disappointing low (50% 1-year, 43% 5-year) compared to other liver diseases. The most likely reasons include unsuspected hepatocellular carcinoma, infection and coexistent cardiac disease.

❑❑ **What are the two biliary anastomosis methods used in liver transplantation and when are they used?**

Choledochocholedochostomy (CDC) and Roux-en-Y choledochojejunostomy. Roux-en-Y choledochojejunostomy is commonly employed when the recipient has biliary tract disease (e.g., primary sclerosing cholangitis) and in retransplants.

❑❑ **A 45 year-old woman presents with fever, shortness of breath and increased liver tests twenty days following liver transplantation. She had steroid resistant rejection one-week prior and is being treated with anti-lymphocyte medication. What is the most likely diagnosis?**

Cytomegalovirus (CMV) pneumonitis and hepatitis is common after aggressive immunosuppression and usually occurs within the first month of transplantation. Those highest at risk are patients who are CMV-negative and receive a liver from a CMV-positive donor. Most centers now prophylaxis against infection with acyclovir.

❑❑ **What are the most common biliary complications following liver transplantation?**

Biliary strictures and leaks are the most common biliary complications. Eighty percent develop within the first 6 months. Biliary strictures at the anastomosis may be dilated or stented and rarely require surgical revision. Biliary leaks are managed with nasobiliary tubes, stents or sphincterotomy.

❑❑ **What vaccines are not safe after liver transplantation?**

Live or attenuated vaccines should be avoided (measles, mumps, rubella, oral polio, BCG). Hepatitis A, B and pneumococcal vaccines, if not given prior to transplantation, should be given.

❑❑ **T/F: Pregnancy is possible in patients following liver transplantation and pregnant transplant recipients should continue their immunosuppression medications.**

True. However, pregnancy after liver transplantation is complicated by a high rate of prematurity and low birth weight. Immunosuppressive agents should be continued throughout pregnancy.

❑❑ **What are the most common neoplasms that occur in recipients of liver transplants?**

Lymphomas (57%) followed by skin cancer (15%) and carcinomas of the colon were the top three neoplasms in a recent study of 329 patients surviving longer than 5 years.

❑❑ **What are the most likely causes of hyperlipidemia following liver transplantation?**

Long use of steroids, frequent use of bolus steroids for rejection, pretransplant hyperlipidemia and possibly the use of cyclosporine versus tacrolimus. Nearly 40% of patients develop hyperlipidemia and need some form of treatment.

❑❑ **A 50 year-old man presents with a painful and red swollen right first toe three years after receiving a liver transplant. What is your diagnosis and treatment?**

Gout is common after transplantation due to decreased excretion of uric acid caused by immunosuppressive medications. Treatment should not employ nonsteroidal anti-inflammatory medications due to the potential for precipitating renal failure. Initial management with colchicine usually relieves the acute attack.

ALCOHOLIC LIVER DISEASE AND NON-ALCOHOLIC STEATOHEPATITIS

Frank A. Anania, M.D., FACP

❑❑ **What are the primary risk factors for alcoholic liver disease?**

The amount and duration of alcohol consumption. Neither the pattern of drinking nor the beverage type are risk factors.

❑❑ **How are ounce-years calculated and what is its significance?**

Ounce-years are used to quantitate lifetime alcohol consumption. Grams of alcohol = volume (ml) x concentration (% alcohol) x 0.00798. Fluid ounces of alcohol = grams of alcohol/ 29.6. One mixed drink is equivalent in alcohol content (14 g of alcohol or 0.5 ounces of alcohol) to one glass of wine or one can of beer.

❑❑ **What percentage of alcoholics has antibody positivity to hepatitis C virus (HCV)?**

Forty percent of patients with alcoholic liver disease have antibodies to HCV.

❑❑ **What diseases are associated with non-alcoholic steatohepatitis?**

Hypertriglyceridemia, diabetes mellitus, obesity, hypothyroidism, hyperthyroidism, total parenteral nutrition, jejuno-ileal bypass and starvation.

❑❑ **What commonly prescribed medication can result in the histologic picture of non-alcoholic steatohepatitis?**

Amiodarone.

❑❑ **T/F: Cirrhosis caused by alcoholic liver disease can occur in the absence of necroinflammation, i.e. alcoholic hepatitis.**

True.

❑❑ **What is the current hypothesis for the development of alcoholic cirrhosis in the absence of inflammation?**

Aldehyde end-products, acetaldehyde, malondialdehyde, and other products of lipid peroxidation.

❑❑ **T/F: Patients with alcoholic hepatitis may have ascites and evidence of portal hypertension.**

True. Jaundice and stigmata of chronic liver disease may occur in patients with acute alcoholic hepatitis.

❑❑ **T/F: Alcoholic liver disease is the only liver disease that places patients at risk for acetaminophen toxicity.**

True. Alcoholic liver disease allows for increases in BPQIs or free radicals since glutathione stores are depleted and induction of cytochrome P450 2E1 occurs. This has not been demonstrated in other liver diseases. As little as 3 or 4 grams of acetaminophen can cause acute and occasionally fatal liver injury in this setting.

❑❑ In addition to abstinence, what is the most important therapy for patients with alcoholic hepatitis?

Good nutrition.

❑❑ Have corticosteroids been shown to benefit patients with acute alcoholic hepatitis?

Yes. A number of clinical trials and meta-analyses have shown benefit in a selected group of patients with acute alcoholic hepatitis.

❑❑ Which patients should be placed on corticosteroids for acute alcoholic hepatitis?

Patients with a discriminant function > 32 showed improved mortality at both 1 and 6 months after corticosteroid treatment compared to placebo-matched controls. Recall that the discriminant function is calculated as follows: 4.6 x (PT-control) + serum bilirubin (mg/dl).

❑❑ T/F: All patients with a discriminant function > 32 should receive corticosteroids.

False. Patients with gastrointestinal bleeding, renal failure or concomitant infection should not be treated with corticosteroids.

❑❑ What dose and what type of corticosteroid should be used?

Forty mg of prednisolone daily orally for 4 weeks. Methylprednisolone may also be used at a dose of 32 mg per day. Prednisone may be use instead of prednisolone.

❑❑ How long should a patient with end-stage alcoholic cirrhosis being considered for liver transplantation remain abstinent from alcohol?

While somewhat controversial, abstinence for at least six months is generally required.

❑❑ T/F: The short- and long-term outcomes of transplants done in patients with end-stage alcoholic liver disease are identical to the outcome in patients transplanted for non-alcoholic liver disease.

True.

❑❑ T/F: Generally, recidivism following liver transplantation for alcoholic liver disease is > 50%.

False. In fact, recidivism occurs uncommonly following liver transplantion for end-stage alcoholic liver disease. The longer a patient is abstinent from alcohol before transplant, the less likely they are to resume alcohol consumption following transplantation.

❑❑ Can acetaminophen be given to patients with alcoholic liver disease or should salicylates or nonsteroidal anti-inflammatory drugs (NSAIDs) be given?

Acetaminophen remains the drug of choice for pain in these patients; however, no more than 2 grams/day should be consumed. Aspirin and NSAIDs should be avoided for several reasons: increased risk of gastrointestinal bleeding and exacerbation of renal insufficiency in patients on diuretics.

❑❑ What other general classes of drugs should be avoided in patients with end-stage liver disease?

The most important group of drugs to avoid is aminoglycosides as they can precipitate renal failure.

❑❑ How does the recognition of alcohol withdrawal syndrome and delirium tremens differ?

Delirium tremens is a serious life-threatening end-stage condition related to the alcohol withdrawal syndrome and should be treated as a medical emergency. The defining symptom is delirium with delusions, agitation, disorientation, disorganized thinking, and vivid visual, auditory and tactile hallucinations. Autonomic hyperactivity is also present.

❑❑ **How is delirium tremens treated?**

Benzodiazepines are the drug of choice to treat this condition. Diazepam and chlordiazepoxide are the preferred drugs based on their pharmacokinetics. Careful monitoring reduces the likelihood of complications during treatment. Loading doses are given every 4 to 6 hours depending on the severity of the withdrawal symptoms.

❑❑ **What are the risk factors associated with delirium tremens?**

Male sex, age > 30, 5 to15 year drinking history, withdrawal seizures, previous history of delirium tremens and other comorbid illnesses such as pancreatitis, infections, trauma or gastritis.

❑❑ **What is the most important microsomal ethanol oxidizing enzyme related to the pathogenesis of both alcoholic liver disease and non-alcoholic steatohepatitis?**

Cytochrome P450 2E1.

❑❑ **What is the principal collagen-producing cell in the liver?**

Stellate cell.

❑❑ **T/F: Epidemiological data suggest that women are more sensitive than men to alcohol-induced liver injury.**

True. The mechanism(s) responsible remains unclear. In part, gastric alcohol dehydrogenase activity appears to be lower in women than men. This may result in less gastric detoxification of ethanol and a greater fraction reaching the liver.

❑❑ **T/F: The prevalence of antibody to hepatitis C (HCV) increases with the severity of underlying alcoholic liver disease.**

True. While there is a 20% prevalence of antibody to HCV in patients with alcoholic hepatitis and 40% in patients with cirrhosis, it is found in only 2% of alcoholic patients with normal liver biopsies.

❑❑ **In chronic alcoholics, which epidemiologic characteristics have been identified as independent risk factors for hepatocellular carcinoma?**

Cirrhosis, age greater than 50, male sex, Hepatitis B surface antigen positivity and anti-HCV positivity.

❑❑ **T/F: In aggregate, trials of parenteral and enteral nutritional support indicate that restricted intake of nutrients is associated with a poor prognosis in patients hospitalized with alcoholic liver disease.**

True. Feed the hospitalized alcoholic, especially those with acute alcoholic hepatitis.

❑❑ **What is the typical profile of a non-alcoholic steatohepatitis (NASH) patient?**

Middle-aged female with obesity, non-insulin-dependent diabetes mellitus, with or without hyperlipidemia.

❑❑ **What two pathophysiologic mechanisms are hypothesized to be responsible for the development of NASH?**

1) Tumor necrosis factor-α and interleukins 6 and 8 may be induced by 2) bacterial endotoxin.

❑❑ **What are the threshold levels of daily consumption of alcohol in males and females that may lead to significant liver disease?**

Twenty grams of ethanol per day in women and 80 grams of ethanol per day in men.

❑❑ **T/F: Currently available imaging modalities are relatively insensitive and nonspecific for NASH.**

True. Liver biopsy remains the gold standard for confirming a clinical suspicion of NASH.

❑❑ **T/F: NASH is histologically indistinguishable from alcohol-induced liver disease.**

True. NASH is, therefore, a diagnosis of exclusion.

❑❑ **What three variables independently increase the risk of progression of alcohol-related hepatic steatosis to cirrhosis?**

Continued alcohol consumption, severity of initial histologic injury and female gender.

❑❑ **What can be recommended to patients with NASH?**

Treatment consists of modifying the factors that are commonly associated with NASH - weight loss, reduction in serum lipids and glucose and cessation of responsible medications. Medical therapy, such as ursodeoxycholate, remains unproven.

❑❑ **What can be recommended to NASH patients about prognosis with steatosis? Steatohepatitis? Fibrosis?**

Steatosis often follows an indolent course. The probability of developing clinically significant complications of liver disease is increased in patients with steatohepatitis or fibrosis.

❑❑ **Define focal fatty liver, or fatty sparing.**

An important difference between NASH and the above named lesion is that NASH is diffuse. Focal fatty liver is incidentally found as a result of improved abdominal imaging techniques. This is not a pathologic diagnosis, needs no treatment and often regresses.

❑❑ **What is the most potent stimulus to alcoholic liver fibrosis?**

Transforming growth factor beta.

AUTOIMMUNE AND OVERLAP CONDITIONS

Howard J. Worman, M.D.

❏❏ **Antimitochondrial antibodies from individuals with primary biliary cirrhosis primarily recognize what family of proteins?**

The E2 subunits of oxoacid dehydrogenase complexes - most frequently, pyruvate dehydrogenase.

❏❏ **Primary sclerosing cholangitis is associated with what disease?**

Ulcerative colitis in 50% to 75%.

❏❏ **T/F: Cytoplasmic antineutrophil cytoplasmic antibodies (cANCA) are often present in individuals with primary sclerosing cholangitis.**

False. Atypical perinuclear ANCA (pANCA) have been reported in 30% to 80% of individuals with primary sclerosing cholangitis. cANCA are antibodies against proteinase 3 and are present, most commonly, in individuals with Wegener's granulomatosis.

❏❏ **What drug has been shown to increase the time to death or liver transplantation in primary biliary cirrhosis?**

Ursodeoxycholic acid.

❏❏ **What drugs form the cornerstone of treatment of autoimmune hepatitis?**

Prednisone and azathioprine.

❏❏ **What type of autoantibodies are present in individuals with type 2 autoimmune hepatitis?**

Antibodies to liver/kidney microsome antigen 1 (anti-LKM1). The antigen has been identified as cytochrome P450 2D6.

❏❏ **T/F: Antinuclear antibodies are almost never present in individuals with primary biliary cirrhosis.**

False. About 50% of individuals with primary biliary cirrhosis have antinuclear antibodies. The most commonly recognized nuclear antigens are nuclear pore membrane glycoprotein gp210 and "nuclear dot" protein Sp100.

❏❏ **T/F: Autoimmune hepatitis, primary sclerosing cholangitis and primary biliary cirrhosis are all more common in women than men?**

False. About 70% of cases of autoimmune hepatitis occur in women and 90% of cases of primary biliary cirrhosis occur in women but about 60% to 70% of cases of primary sclerosing cholangitis occur in men.

❏❏ **What are the typical cholangiographic findings in primary sclerosing cholangitis?**

Diffuse multifocal strictures of the biliary tract and multiple areas of ectasia, resulting in a "beading" pattern.

❑❑ **What bone diseases occur frequently in patients with primary biliary cirrhosis?**

Osteoporosis and osteomalacia.

❑❑ **T/F: Pruritus in primary biliary cirrhosis usually worsens with the degree of liver damage.**

False. There is no correlation between liver damage and pruritus in primary biliary cirrhosis.

❑❑ **T/F: Plasma cell infiltrates are more common in liver biopsies from patients with chronic viral hepatitis than chronic autoimmune hepatitis.**

False.

❑❑ **T/F: Liver biopsy is usually diagnostic in primary biliary cirrhosis.**

False. The florid bile duct lesion, which is essentially diagnostic for primary biliary cirrhosis, is only seen in a minority of cases. Usually, the liver biopsy is "consistent with" a diagnosis of primary biliary cirrhosis.

❑❑ **Ductular proliferation is seen in what histological stage of primary biliary cirrhosis?**

Stage 2. Stage 1 is the florid bile duct lesion while Stage 3 demonstrates fibrosis and Stage 4 displays cirrhosis.

❑❑ **In classical, or type 1, autoimmune hepatitis, what fraction is elevated in serum protein electrophoresis?**

Gamma-globulin concentration is elevated in most cases.

❑❑ **What autoimmune condition is most commonly associated with type 1 autoimmune hepatitis?**

Autoimmune thyroiditis. About 15% to 20% of patients with type 1 autoimmune hepatitis have a concomitant autoimmune disease and about 60% of them have thyroiditis.

❑❑ **T/F: Several studies have demonstrated an association between HLA haplotypes and a susceptibility to autoimmune hepatitis.**

True. Several studies have shown an association of autoimmune hepatitis with HLA A1, B8 and DR3.

❑❑ **T/F: Ursodeoxycholic acid has been shown to improve survival and slow the progression to cirrhosis in primary sclerosing cholangitis.**

False. No study has demonstrated that any medication is of benefit in altering the course of this condition.

❑❑ **Atypical antineutrophil cytoplasmic antibodies are most frequently present in which two liver diseases.**

Primary sclerosing cholangitis and autoimmune hepatitis.

❑❑ **Which immunoglobulin type concentration is elevated in the serum in most cases of primary biliary cirrhosis?**

IgM.

❑❑ **T/F: "Overlap syndrome" is a clearly defined entity with specific diagnostic findings on liver biopsy.**

False. "Overlap syndrome" is a poorly defined term often used for cases that have clinical, laboratory, immunological and histological features of two different autoimmune liver diseases, usually primary biliary cirrhosis and autoimmune hepatitis.

❑❑ **What drug has been associated with the development of autoimmune hepatitis in individuals with chronic hepatitis C.**

Interferon-alpha.

❑❑ **What malignancy occurs in 10% to 15% of subjects with long-standing primary sclerosing cholangitis?**

Cholangiocarcinoma.

❑❑ **Sjögren's syndrome is most commonly associated with what liver disease.**

Primary biliary cirrhosis. It has been reported to occur in 25% to 75% of these patients.

❑❑ **T/F: Elevated serum cholesterol concentrations in autoimmune hepatitis are caused by synthesis of an abnormal lipoprotein known as lipoprotein X.**

False. Elevated serum cholesterol concentrations are not associated with autoimmune hepatitis. Lipoprotein X is synthesized in association with increased serum cholesterol concentrations in long-standing bile duct obstruction. This is commonly seen in individuals with primary biliary cirrhosis.

❑❑ **Antimitochondrial antibodies are detectable in sera of about what percent of cases of primary biliary cirrhosis.**

Approximately 90%.

❑❑ **T/F: Primary biliary cirrhosis is inherited in an X-linked fashion.**

False. Primary biliary cirrhosis is not inherited in a Mendelian fashion.

❑❑ **T/F: There is a 25% chance that a sibling of an index patient with primary sclerosing cholangitis will have the same disease.**

False. Primary sclerosing cholangitis is not inherited in a Mendelian fashion. Although it may tend to run in families, it is still extremely unlikely that a family member of an index case will develop the disease.

❑❑ **Spontaneous remissions occur in approximately what percent of individuals with primary biliary cirrhosis.**

Zero percent. There are no carefully documented cases of spontaneous remission.

❑❑ **A 40 year-old woman presents with pruritus. Blood testing reveals an elevated serum alkaline phosphatase activity. Antimitochondrial antibodies are present in serum at a titer of 1:640. Which of the following tests would most likely provide the most useful information to make a solid diagnosis: liver ultrasound, endoscopic retrograde cholangiography (ERCP), liver biopsy or computed tomography (CT) of the liver.**

Liver biopsy. Based on the clinical presentation and laboratory test results, this patient very likely has primary biliary cirrhosis. Imaging studies such as ultrasound and CT would most likely be normal unless advanced cirrhosis was present. ERCP does not detect specific changes in primary biliary cirrhosis. A liver biopsy with consistent findings would confirm the diagnosis.

❑❑ **A 50 year-old man with a history of ulcerative colitis presents with jaundice. Routine laboratory testing demonstrates an elevated serum bilirubin concentration and elevated serum** alkaline phosphatase activity. An ultrasound examination of the liver, gallbladder and bile ducts is normal. What would you expect to find on ERCP?

Primary sclerosing cholangitis would be high on the differential diagnosis. On cholangiography, you would expect to find diffuse, multifocal strictures of the biliary tract and multiple areas of ectasia resulting in a "beading" pattern.

❑❑ T/F: Autoimmune hepatitis usually develops in individuals with systemic lupus erythematosis.

False. There is no association between autoimmune hepatitis, despite its old name "lupoid hepatitis," and systemic lupus erythematosis.

❑❑ T/F: Patients with cirrhosis as a result of primary biliary cirrhosis are generally poor candidates for orthotopic liver transplantation.

False. Since these patients are usually young to middle-aged women without other major organ disease, most transplant centers consider patients with primary biliary cirrhosis to be excellent candidates for liver transplantation.

❑❑ What is the most important test in which to diagnose primary sclerosing cholangitis?

Endoscopic retrograde cholangiography (ERCP). Diffuse, multifocal strictures of the biliary tract and multiple areas of ectasia, resulting in a "beading" pattern is most typically seen and virtually diagnostic. Liver biopsy is rarely diagnostic but may have consistent features. An "onion skin" lesion around bile ducts on biopsy is highly suggestive of the diagnosis. Liver biopsy is useful to establish if cirrhosis or fibrosis have developed. The histological staging system is similar to primary biliary cirrhosis.

❑❑ Infections of the biliary tree with what organisms can cause a condition similar to primary sclerosing cholangitis in individuals with acquire immune deficiency syndrome?

Cryptosporidium and cytomegalovirus.

❑❑ What is "autoimmune cholangitis?"

Autoimmune cholangitis has been considered by some to be an "overlap" syndrome between primary biliary cirrhosis and autoimmune hepatitis. There is bile duct damage or loss on liver biopsy often along with hepatocellular inflammation. These patients do not have detectable antimitochondrial antibodies against the E2 subunits of oxo-acid dehydrogenases.

❑❑ What drugs have been shown to be effective in the treatment of pruritus in individuals with primary biliary cirrhosis?

Ursodeoxycholic acid, cholesterol binding resins such a cholestyramine and colestipol, opioid antagonists such as naloxone and naltrexone, and rifampicin. Immunosuppressive agents such as steroids, cyclosporine A and methotrexate may also attenuate pruritus but are not generally used for this purpose.

❑❑ Approximately what percent of individuals with autoimmune hepatitis treated with corticosteroids develop cirrhosis within 10 years?

In a large study from the Mayo clinic, 40% of patients with autoimmune hepatitis treated with corticosteroids developed cirrhosis within 10 years.

❑❑ How are antimitochondrial antibodies, antinuclear antibodies and anti-smooth muscle antibodies most commonly detected in the routine clinical laboratory?

By indirect immunofluorescence microscopy.

❑❑ T/F: In about 60% of cases of autoimmune hepatitis, infection with the hepatitis C virus is thought to be a triggering factor.

False.

❏❏ Recurrent bacterial cholangitis is a common complication in which of the following liver diseases: primary biliary cirrhosis, primary sclerosing cholangitis, Wilson's disease or autoimmune hepatitis.

Primary sclerosing cholangitis.

❏❏ T/F: Epidemiological studies have shown a strong association between primary biliary cirrhosis and coronary artery disease.

False. Although serum cholesterol concentrations are elevated in many individuals with primary biliary cirrhosis, an association with coronary artery disease has not been demonstrated.

❏❏ In which liver disease might you order a Schirmer's test?

Primary biliary cirrhosis. A Schirmer's test is used to detect xerophthalmia which is a component of Sjögren's syndrome.

❏❏ T/F: Autoimmune hepatitis is the most common liver disease of pregnant women.

False. Viral hepatitis is the most common liver disease of pregnant women.

❏❏ The term "nonsuppurative cholangitis" best describes the histopathological lesion in what liver disease?

Primary biliary cirrhosis. The term means inflammation of the bile ducts without pus.

❏❏ T/F: Antinuclear antibodies are highly specific for the diagnosis of autoimmune hepatitis.

False. Antinuclear antibodies are present in individuals with many different conditions and even some healthy individuals, in low titers.

❏❏ T/F: The Gunn rat is an animal model for primary biliary cirrhosis.

False. The Gunn rat is an animal model for Crigler-Najjar Syndrome, Type I.

CIRRHOSIS AND ITS COMPLICATIONS

Bhupinderjit S. Anand, M.D.

❑❑ What is the World Health Organization definition of cirrhosis?

Cirrhosis is a diffuse process in which the architecture of the liver is replaced by abnormal nodules (pseudonodules, which lack the lobular arrangement of a normal liver) and which are separated by bands of fibrous tissue.

❑❑ What are common complications of cirrhosis?

Fluid collection (edema and ascites), portal hypertension (variceal bleeding), spontaneous bacterial peritonitis, hepatic encephalopathy, renal failure (hepatorenal syndrome) and hepatocellular carcinoma.

❑❑ What is the normal portal pressure and what is the definition of portal hypertension?

The normal portal pressure is 5 to 10 mmHg and pressures > 12 mmHg constitute portal hypertension. Since it is difficult to directly measure the portal pressure, an indirect method is to measure the hepatic vein pressure gradient which is the difference between wedged hepatic vein pressure and free hepatic vein pressure.

❑❑ At what pressure do esophageal varices form and when do they bleed?

A hepatic vein pressure gradient (HVPG) > 12 mmHg is required for the formation of esophageal varices. Similarly, variceal bleeding occurs only when HVPG is > 12 mmHg; however, there is no absolute level of HVPG that correlates with risk of bleeding. The higher the HVPG, the greater the risk of recurrent bleeding and worse survival.

❑❑ How frequently do esophageal varices occur in patients with cirrhosis?

Nearly 80% patients with alcoholic cirrhosis develop esophageal varices within 10 years of diagnosis. The risk is somewhat less in cirrhosis due to hepatitis C virus infection.

❑❑ What are the chances of bleeding in a patient with esophageal varices?

Nearly 30% cirrhotics with large varices experience variceal bleeding, usually within the first year of diagnosis.

❑❑ How common are recurrent episodes of variceal bleeding?

If left untreated, patients who have experienced an episode of bleeding have a 70% chance of recurrent bleeding within 6 months.

❑❑ What is the mortality rate of acute variceal bleeding?

Variceal hemorrhage is a serious medical emergency. Each episode of bleeding is associated with a 30% to 50% risk of death.

❑❑ What are the predictors of increased risk of variceal bleeding?

Factors associated with increased risk of bleeding include: large varices, presence of endoscopic signs such as cherry red spots and red wales over the varices, and advanced liver disease.

❑❑ What is the treatment of choice for acute variceal bleeding?

Endoscopic techniques - endoscopic sclerotherapy or endoscopic variceal ligation along with the use of vasoactive drugs which reduce the portal pressure. The drug used most commonly is somatostatin or its synthetic analogue, octreotide.

❑❑ T/F: There is no difference in the results obtained between endoscopic sclerotherapy (EST) and endoscopic variceal ligation (EVL).

False. EST (injection of sclerosing agent into varices) and EVL (placing a rubber band on the varices) are designed to obliterate varices. Both are equally effective; however, EVL is associated with fewer complications, lower rates of rebleeding and requires fewer sessions to achieve variceal obliteration.

❑❑ What drugs are effective in reducing portal pressure?

Portal pressure-reducing drugs are divided into two categories: 1) Vasoconstrictors (somatostatin, beta-blockers, vasopressin) cause splanchnic vasoconstriction and reduce portal blood flow; and, 2) Vasodilators (nitrates, prazosin) decrease the vascular resistance of the intrahepatic portal vessels.

❑❑ What is the treatment for patients with acute variceal bleeding who fail endoscopic/medical therapy?

About 15% patients continue to bleed despite all medical measures. The next line of treatment is the transjugular intrahepatic portosystemic shunt (TIPS) or a surgical shunt.

❑❑ What are the complications of the TIPS procedure?

The two most important complications are development of hepatic encephalopathy and shunt closure which may result in recurrent variceal rebleeding.

❑❑ Which patients should be referred for shunt surgery?

Patients with well-compensated cirrhosis (Child's class A). A popular procedure is the distal splenorenal shunt (splenic vein to renal vein) since it is associated with a lower risk of hepatic encephalopathy compared to a portocaval shunt.

❑❑ What is portal hypertensive gastropathy?

This refers to the development of vascular congestion of the gastric mucosa in patients with portal hypertension. Less frequently, other parts of the gastrointestinal tract may be involved (e.g., portal hypertensive colopathy). Portal hypertensive gastropathy may result in acute and chronic blood loss and anemia.

❑❑ What is the treatment of portal hypertensive gastropathy?

The treatment of choice is the use of vasoactive agents such as non-selective beta-blockers.

❑❑ T/F: Varices can form in areas of the gastrointestinal tract other than the esophagus.

True. Varices can develop anywhere in the gastrointestinal tract. After the esophagus, the next most common site is the stomach. Bleeding from extra-esophageal varices is difficult to control by endoscopic means. Initial treatment is with beta-blockers. If unsuccessful, the patients are considered for transjugular intrahepatic portosystemic shunt, surgical shunt or transplantation.

❑❑ How can we prevent the occurrence of the first episode of variceal hemorrhage?

Individuals with large varices are at an increased risk of bleeding. Such patients should be treated with non-selective beta-blockers (e.g., propranolol, nadolol) which reduce the risk of variceal bleeding by nearly 40%. The long-acting nitrate, isorsorbide mononitrate, has also been shown to be effective. Endoscopic techniques to obliterate the varices have not convincingly been shown to be effective in the primary prevention of variceal bleeding.

❑❑ What are the treatment options for patients with recurrent episodes of variceal bleeding?

Endoscopic variceal ligation (or sclerotherapy) until the varices are completely obliterated or use of non-selective beta-blockers. If bleeding recurs despite these measures, a surgical shunt, transjugular intrahepatic portosystemic shunt (TIPS) or transplantation should be considered.

❑❑ What are the characteristics of ascites in a cirrhotic patient?

The ascitic fluid has a low albumin content (often < 1 gram%) and the serum to ascitic fluid albumin gradient (SAAG) is ≥ 1.1. A SAAG ≥ 1.1 is characteristic of portal hypertension but may also be seen with congestive heart failure and myxedema. In contrast, a SAAG < 1.1 may be seen in tuberculous peritonitis, carcinomatosis, pancreatic ascites and nephrotic syndrome.

❑❑ Describe the treatment of cirrhotic ascites?

The most important step is to achieve negative sodium balance (i.e. > 88 mmol [2g]/day, the usual daily allowance of Na^+). In addition to sodium restriction, the diuretics, spironolactone and furosemide are very useful. The maximum doses are 400 mg and 160 mg, respectively.

❑❑ What is diuretic-refractory ascites? Diuretic-resistant ascites?

Diuretic-refractory ascites refers to persistent ascites despite sodium restriction and maximal diuretic therapy. Diuretic-resistant ascites refers to the development of diuretic-induced complications which prevent use of effective diuretic therapy.

❑❑ What are treatment options for diuretic-refractory and diuretic-resistant ascites?

The safest and most commonly used approach is periodic large-volume paracentesis. A less safe technique is the placement of a peritoneo-venous shunt (PVS) (e.g., Denver shunt) which drains ascitic fluid into the superior vena cava. The PVS is associated with complications such as infection, disseminated intravascular coagulation, congestive heart failure and shunt thrombosis. Transjugular intrahepatic portosystemic shunts and surgical shunts are also options.

❑❑ What is spontaneous bacterial peritonitis (SBP)?

Patients with cirrhosis are prone to develop peritonitis without a precipitating cause such as bowel perforation or inflammation, hence the term 'spontaneous'. The diagnosis is made by the finding of an ascitic fluid neutrophil count ≥ 250 /mm^3. A positive ascitic fluid culture is obtained in 90% patients and shows a single bacteria (usually *Escherichia coli*), unlike surgical peritonitis which is polymicrobial.

❑❑ What is the treatment of choice for spontaneous bacterial peritonitis?

The drug of choice is cefotaxime 2 g intravenously every 8 hours for 5 days.

❑❑ Why are aminoglycoside's not used in spontaneous bacterial peritonitis?

Aminoglycoside's are contraindicated in cirrhotic patients with ascites because they carry a high risk of nephrotoxicity.

❑❑ What is the risk of recurrence of spontaneous bacterial peritonitis?

Patients who have experienced an episode of spontaneous bacterial peritonitis have a 70% probability of a second episode within one year.

❑❑ Can recurrent episodes of spontaneous bacterial peritonitis be prevented?

Long-term administration of norfloxacin (400 mg daily), a poorly absorbed antibiotic reduces the risk of recurrent SBP to 20% from 70% compared to placebo. Trimethoprim-sulfamethoxazole has also been shown to be effective. Those with very low ascites albumin levels seem to benefit most. However, there are concerns regarding emergence of drug-resistant organisms with such long-term therapy.

❏❏ **What is the definition of hepatorenal syndrome?**

Progressive renal failure in patients with advanced liver disease and portal hypertension in the absence of a specific cause for renal failure. Typically, patients have oliguria (urine volume < 500 ml/24 hr) and low urinary sodium (< 10 mEq/L).

❏❏ **What is the pathogenesis of hepatorenal syndrome?**

The pathogenetic mechanism is reduction in renal blood flow. Structurally, the kidneys are normal and show complete recovery if the liver disease is reversed or after liver transplantation.

❏❏ **T/F: There are different types of hepatorenal syndrome.**

True. Type I is an acute process with a rapid increase in BUN and creatinine over 1 to 14 days; it is seen in fulminant hepatic failure and severe alcoholic hepatitis. Type II is associated with a more gradual renal failure over several weeks to months.

❏❏ **What is the prognosis of hepatorenal syndrome?**

Prognosis is extremely poor. The median survival for type I is less than 2 weeks. Survival is longer for patients with type II, but the overall prognosis is poor.

❏❏ **What is hepatic encephalopathy?**

Appearance of neuropsychiatric symptoms (mental confusion, personality change, sleep disturbance, unconscious state or coma) or signs (asterixis, hyperreflexia, muscular rigidity, extensor planters, decerebrate posturing) in patients with liver dysfunction in the absence of a specific etiology.

❏❏ **What is subclinical hepatic encephalopathy?**

Subnormal performance in psychometric tests in the presence of normal neurological examination. The most commonly performed test is the Reitan trail test in which the time taken by a patient to connect numbers is recorded. Subclinical hepatic encephalopathy is seen in nearly 70% patients with cirrhosis, but its significance is unclear.

❏❏ **What laboratory tests are specific for hepatic encephalopathy?**

Hepatic encephalopathy is a clinical diagnosis and is not based on any laboratory test. Blood ammonia levels are not diagnostic of hepatic encephalopathy.

❏❏ **What is the treatment of hepatic encephalopathy?**

The first step is to treat any precipitating factor (infection, fluid/electrolyte disturbance, drug overdose, renal failure, constipation, high protein diet). Specific treatment consists of a low protein diet and laxatives; lactulose, in a dose which results in 2 to 3 bowel movements per day, is the traditional agent of choice.

❏❏ **T/F: Diseases of the biliary tree can result in end-stage liver disease and cirrhosis.**

True. Chronic biliary obstruction of any etiology can cause progressive liver damage and cirrhosis. The most common causes are primary biliary cirrhosis and primary sclerosing cholangitis followed by persistent choledocholithiasis, biliary strictures and parasitic infestations.

❑❑ **What is the pathogenesis of primary biliary cirrhosis (PBC)?**

PBC is a chronic cholestatic disease of unknown etiology seen predominantly in middle-aged women. It is characterized by destruction of small bile ducts, presumably by activated cytotoxic T-cells.

❑❑ **How is primary biliary cirrhosis diagnosed?**

The diagnosis is made on the basis of elevated alkaline phosphatase, relatively normal aminotransferases and a positive anti-mitochondrial antibody test. Liver biopsy helps to confirm the diagnosis and provides the stage of the disease.

❑❑ **What is the treatment for primary biliary cirrhosis?**

Ursodeoxycholic acid (12 to 15 mg/kg body weight) reduces pruritus, improves liver tests and prolongs survival free of liver transplantation. Additional measures include cholestyramine for relief of pruritus, fat-soluble vitamins and use of medium-chain triglycerides in patients with steatorrhea.

❑❑ **What are the diagnostic features of primary sclerosing cholangitis (PSC)?**

PSC is a chronic cholestatic liver disease of unknown etiology occurring in middle-aged individuals. Over 75% patients have associated ulcerative colitis. The principal diagnostic study is endoscopic retrograde cholangiography which may show irregularity of the intra- and/or extrahepatic bile ducts.

❑❑ **T/F: Ursodeoxycholic acid is beneficial in primary sclerosing cholangitis.**

False. No drug therapy has been shown to be of benefit in primary sclerosing cholangitis. The only definitive treatment is liver transplantation

❑❑ **What is Budd-Chiari syndrome?**

Obstruction of the hepatic veins is termed Budd-Chiari syndrome. The blockage may be due to thrombosis or presence of an intraluminal membrane.

❑❑ **What is the clinical presentation of Budd-Chiari syndrome?**

Patients present with a triad of hepatomegaly, ascites and abdominal pain. Eventually, portal hypertension occurs and the cause of death is usually uncontrolled variceal bleeding.

❑❑ **What is veno-occlusive disease (VOD)?**

Obstruction of the terminal hepatic venules. The initial defect is subendothelial sclerosis followed by thrombosis of the vessels. Acute VOD may occur after bone marrow transplantation. Chronic VOD is seen after ingestion of toxic alkaloids (pyrrolizidine alkaloids) present in herbal teas.

❑❑ **What liver test abnormalities may be seen in congestive heart failure?**

The most common abnormality is an elevated serum bilirubin (usually < 4.5 mg/dl), nearly 50% of which is unconjugated due to mild hemolysis and reduced uptake and conjugation by the liver. Serum aminotransferases are increased less frequently. Aspartate aminotransferase (AST) is usually higher than alanine aminotransferase because cardiac myocytes are rich in AST. Elevation of alkaline phosphatase is uncommon.

CONGENITAL AND STRUCTURAL ABNORMALITIES AND PEDIATRIC DISEASES

Istvan Danko, M.D., Ph.D. and Glen R. Gourley, M.D.

❑❑ **What percentage of the total blood flow is received by the liver?**

About 28%. Seventy-five percent of this comes through the portal vein.

❑❑ **What are the major cell types in the liver?**

Hepatocytes comprise about 60% of the total cell population. Thirty-five percent is of mesenchymal origin (Kupffer, stellate and sinusoidal endothelial cells). The remaining 5% are bile ductular epithelial cells.

❑❑ **What is the physiological significance of the zonal division of the hepatic acinus?**

Cells are grouped into 3 zones based upon their distance from the portal triad. Cells of zone 1 (periportal area) are closest to nutrient-rich blood and least vulnerable to hypoxia. Zone 3 is the microcirculatory periphery, first to be damaged and last to regenerate after hypoxia. In zones 1 and 2, oxidative processes predominate. In zone 3 (perivenular area), glycolysis is more active.

❑❑ **Which part of the small bowel absorbs most of the bile acids?**

The terminal ileum. Small amounts are also absorbed from the proximal small bowel and colon.

❑❑ **Which of the commonly measured aminotransferases is more liver-specific?**

Aspartate aminotransferase (AST) is found in the cytosol and mitochondria of hepatocytes and in many extrahepatic tissues. Alanine aminotransferase (ALT) is found predominantly in the cytosol of hepatocytes. Usually both are elevated with liver cell damage. An increase in AST out of proportion to ALT elevation suggests an extrahepatic cause (e.g., hemolysis, muscle damage).

❑❑ **What enzymes are used to evaluate cholestasis?**

Alkaline phosphatase, gamma-glutamyl transpeptidase (GGT) and 5'-nucleotidase levels are elevated during cholestasis. The latter is the most specific but least available. Alkaline phosphatase levels may be high in pediatric patients due to active bone growth, rickets, or following intercurrent viral infection.

❑❑ **What coagulation factors are synthesized in the liver and what test is used to indirectly assess them?**

Factors I, II, V, VII, IX, X are synthesised in the liver. The prothrombin time (PT), a test that evaluates the extrinsic pathway, is prolonged when any of these factors are deficient, either alone or in combination.

❑❑ **In addition to liver synthetic failure what are other causes of a prolonged PT?**

Congenital coagulation factor deficiency, consumptive coagulopathy, disseminated intravascular coagulation, treatment with coumadin and vitamin K deficiency.

❑❑ **What are the vitamin K-dependent coagulation factors?**

Factors II, VII, IX and X.

❏❏ **T/F: The liver edge is normally palpable in children.**

True. The right lobe may be up to 3.5 cm below the costal margin during the first 6 months, 3 cm below before 4 years and 2 cm below before 12 years. The upper border is usually in the 5th intercostal space.

❏❏ **What is the major source of bilirubin?**

Hemoglobin metabolism.

❏❏ **What is the first enzyme in the pathway converting hemoglobin to bilirubin?**

Heme oxygenase.

❏❏ **How do metalloporphyrins prevent neonatal jaundice?**

They block heme oxygenase and prevent bilirubin formation.

❏❏ **What protects adults from absorbing bilirubin via the enterohepatic circulation?**

Bacterial conversion of bilirubin conjugates to urobilinoids.

❏❏ **Why are neonates different from adults in their susceptibility to the enterohepatic circulation of bilirubin?**

Infants lack bacterial flora in which to convert bilirubin conjugates to urobilinoids.

❏❏ **What constitutes physiological jaundice in the newborn?**

Probably due to greater erythrocyte mass and shorter life span, most otherwise normal neonates experience unconjugated bilirubin levels greater than 1.4 mg/dl in the first few days. Levels rise slowly and peak around 6 to 8 mg/dl on days 3 to 4.

❏❏ **What is breastfeeding jaundice and breastmilk jaundice?**

About 13% of breastfed babies experience unconjugated bilirubin levels > 12mg/dl within the first 10 days. The early onset (days 2 to 4) variant is called breastfeeding jaundice and probably develops as a consequence of suboptimal fluid and calorie intake and meconium output. Breastmilk jaundice develops after the first week of life and is thought to be caused by inhibition of bilirubin excretion by factors in breast milk. Prerequisite for the diagnosis is that the baby is otherwise healthy, full-term and with normal hemoglobin, reticulocyte count, peripheral blood smear, liver tests and coagulation studies. Blood group incompatibility, hemolysis and hypothyroidism also need to be excluded.

❏❏ **Hyperbilirubinemia should be presumed to be abnormal in an infant if what conditions are met?**

1)   Baby appears ill.
2)   Occurs before 36 hours of age.
3)   Persists after 10 days of age (2 weeks for preterm deliveries).
4)   Bilirubin level > 12 mg/dl at any time (15 mg/dl in preterm).
5)   Increase > 5 mg/dl/day, direct fraction > 2 mg/dl.

❏❏ **What hereditary hyperbilirubinemias are caused by defects of bilirubin conjugation?**

The autosomal recessive Crigler-Najjar syndrome type 1 in which bilirubin glucuronyl transferase is completely absent has the worst prognosis. In the autosomal dominant Crigler-Najjar syndrome type 2 (Arias), there is residual glucuronidase activity and the overall prognosis is good. Gilbert's syndrome is autosomal dominant and benign with hepatic bilirubin clearance reduced by approximately one-half due to impaired glucuronidation.

☐☐ At what age are familial unconjugated hyperbilirubinemias typically recognized?

Crigler-Najjar syndrome types 1and 2 are recognized in the newborn period while Gilbert's syndrome is usually discovered after puberty.

☐☐ How can Crigler-Najjar syndrome types 1 and 2 be differentiated from each other?

By the clinical response to phenobarbital, which induces residual enzyme activity in type 2 and causes a significant drop in total serum bilirubin level.

☐☐ What is the main risk of Crigler-Najjar syndrome type 1?

Kernicterus.

☐☐ What is the mainstay of daily treatment while awaiting transplantation for individuals with Crigler-Najjar syndrome type 1?

Phototherapy.

☐☐ T/F: Liver biopsy is indicated for the diagnosis of Gilbert's syndrome.

False. Unless other biochemical abnormalities are present, a modestly elevated serum unconjugated bilirubin without hemolysis or other laboratory indication of liver disease does not require any further studies.

☐☐ How does biliary bile composition differ in Gilbert's syndrome from normal?

In Gilbert's syndrome, there are more bilirubin monoglucuronides and less diglucuronides than in normal bile.

☐☐ What is the genetic marker for Gilbert's syndrome in caucasians?

Homozygous state for an extra TA in the TATA promoter region of the bilirubin glucuronosyltransferase gene.

☐☐ What liver function tests are abnormal in Gilbert's syndrome?

Only total serum bilirubin.

☐☐ What is the cause of Dubin-Johnson syndrome?

A genetic mutation causing deficient canalicular multispecific organic anion transport (cMOAT) protein in the apical canalicular membrane (cMOAT is also known as MRP2-multidrug resistance protein).

☐☐ How does hepatic pigmentation differentiate Dubin-Johnson syndrome from Rotor syndrome?

Dubin-Johnson syndrome has black pigment in hepatocytes while Rotor syndrome does not.

☐☐ What is the inheritance pattern, treatment and prognosis of Dubin-Johnson and Rotor syndromes?

Both are autosomal recessive, have good prognoses and do not require treatment.

☐☐ Measurement of what urinary component enables differentiation of Rotor syndrome and Dubin-Johnson syndrome?

Urinary coproporphyrins. Total coproporphyrin (I and III) is normal in Dubin-Johnson syndrome but over 80% is type I. Total coproporphyin (I and III) is 2- to 5-fold elevated in Rotor syndrome but less than 80% is type I.

❏❏ **What is the key test that helps to differentiate cholestasis from physiological or breast milk jaundice?**

Measurement of direct bilirubin: a direct fraction > 2mg/dl or > 20% of total indicate cholestasis.

❏❏ **What are the three most common causes of cholestasis in infants?**

Extrahepatic biliary atresia and idiopathic neonatal hepatitis are each responsible for about one-third of the cases. Alpha$_1$-antitrypsin deficiency is found in about 17% of the cases.

❏❏ **What is the best method to differentiate extrahepatic biliary atresia (EHBA) and idiopathic neonatal hepatitis?**

Liver biopsy. Histological features of EHBA include bile duct proliferation and bile duct plugs, portal fibrosis and edema, and preservation of normal lobular architecture. In neonatal hepatitis, typically there is inflammatory infiltration of the lobule, hepatocellular necrosis, lobular disarray and mild portal tract disarray. Multinucleated giant cells and pseudoglandular transformation (cells arranged around a dilated canaliculus) can be present in both.

❏❏ **T/F: There is good concordance for extrahepatic biliary atresia (EHBA) between siblings.**

False. The occurrence of EHBA in siblings is extremely rare.

❏❏ **T/F: Visualization of the gallbladder rules out extrahepatic biliary atresia.**

False. There still may be distal atresia

❏❏ **T/F: Pigmented stools exclude extrahepatic biliary atresia (EHBA).**

False. Usually pigment in the stool is proof of biliary patency; however, in some cases of severe hyperbilirubinemia, bilirubin can be excreted through the bowel wall and stools can be mildly pigmented even in the presence of EHBA.

❏❏ **T/F: Newborns with extrahepatic biliary atresia are ill-appearing at birth.**

False. Most are full-term and in good condition. Stools may be pale from the outset but may be initially pigmented in 15% to 20%.

❏❏ **What is the Kasai procedure?**

Surgical excision of the whole extrahepatic biliary system and anastomosis of an intestinal conduit to the denuded porta hepatis (portoenterostomy).

❏❏ **What are the major late complications of the Kasai procedure?**

Cholangitis develops in 40% to 60% of the patients during the first year. Portal hypertension leads to esophageal varices in 39% of patients.

❏❏ **What is the classical triad of symptoms characteristic of choledochal cysts?**

Abdominal pain, mass and jaundice. However, this occurs in only 38% of pediatric patients. Frequently, it presents as cholestasis indistinguishable from extrahepatic biliary atresia, recurrent abdominal pain, recurrent pancreatitis or acute abdomen resulting from cholangitis or perforation.

❑❑ **What is the preferred surgical treatment of choledochal cysts?**

Radical cyst excision if possible. If there is complicating hepatic disease, portal hypertension and cholangitis, an initial drainage procedure may be needed with later revision.

❑❑ **What is the histological criterion for the diagnosis of intrahepatic biliary atresia (paucity of interlobular bile ducts - PIBD)?**

The normal ratio between the numbers of interlobular bile ducts and portal tracts is 0.9 - 1.8. A ratio less than 0.6 suggests PIBD.

❑❑ **What is Alagille's syndrome?**

Alagille's syndrome is also referred to as arteriohepatic dysplasia or syndromic PIBD. In these patients, intrahepatic biliary atresia is associated with cardiac, facial, ocular and vertebral abnormalities.

❑❑ **What studies are necessary to diagnose Alagille's syndrome?**

Diagnosis rests upon careful evaluation of a liver biopsy specimen and non-hepatic phenotypic features in the patient and relatives. Keep in mind that the liver biopsy may be non-diagnostic during the first 3 months of life. Echocardiography, vertebral x-ray studies and ophthalmologic studies for posterior embryotoxon are helpful.

❑❑ **What is the typical cardiac defect in Alagille's syndrome?**

Peripheral pulmonary artery stenosis is most common. A cardiac murmur is present in almost all patients.

❑❑ **What eye abnormality is associated with Alagille's syndrome?**

Posterior embryotoxon.

❑❑ **What are treatment options for pruritus associated with cholestasis?**

Medical treatment includes cholestyramine and phenobarbital. A diet rich in polyunsaturated fatty acids may promote fecal excretion of bile acids.

❑❑ **What problems are associated with the administration of cholestyramine?**

Unpalatability, interference with absorption of fat soluble vitamins and constipation. It may also cause acidosis in Alagille's syndrome.

❑❑ **What are the criteria for diagnosing idiopathic neonatal hepatitis?**

Proof of biliary patency and exclusion of all known causes.

❑❑ **T/F: Giant cell transformation is pathognomonic of idiopathic neonatal hepatitis.**

False. Although more frequently observed in infancy, it can accompany various liver diseases in different ages. The histogenesis of the hepatic giant cell is not clear.

❑❑ **What does the acronym TORCH stand for?**

It was introduced as a reminder of the serologic testing for infectious agents that might cause neonatal hepatitis. T (Toxoplasma), O (Others: syphilis, etc.), R (rubella), C (CMV, coxsackie) H (Herpetoviridae: CMV, EBV, HSV). In practice, the most important infectious agents to evaluate for in suspected neonatal hepatitis are CMV, EBV and HSV.

❑❑ **What eye abnormality is commonly associated with infectious neonatal hepatitis?**

Chorioretinitis.

❑❑ Biliary atresia and intracranial calcifications suggest what diagnosis?

Cytomegalvirus or Toxoplasmosis.

❑❑ What is the most frequent metabolic cause of cholestasis in infancy?

Alpha$_1$-antitrypsin deficiency. It accounts for 17% of neonatal cholestasis cases.

❑❑ T/F: The quantitation of serum alpha$_1$-antitrypsin level is sufficient to make the diagnosis of alpha$_1$-antitrypsin deficiency.

False. One of the pitfalls of diagnosis is that levels of alpha$_1$-antitrypsin, an acute phase reactant, may rise to normal in hepatitis because of the inflammation. The phenotype (protease inhibitor (Pi) type) must always be obtained.

❑❑ Which electrophoretic alpha$_1$-antitrypsin phenotype is associated with the highest probability of liver disease?

The ZZ phenotype.

❑❑ Deficiency of which enzyme is responsible for tyrosinemia type I?

Fumaryl acetoacetate hydrolase - the last enzyme of tyrosine degradation.

❑❑ T/F: Dietary correction of tyrosinemia alters the course of the liver disease.

False. Tyrosine probably does not play a major role in the pathogenesis.

❑❑ What biochemical abnormality is diagnostic of tyrosinemia type I?

Urinary succinyl acetone. This compound can also be measured in amniotic fluid by 15 weeks of gestation.

❑❑ What role does succinyl acetone play in the development of symptoms in tyrosinemia type I?

This compound is hepatotoxic and an inhibitor of delta aminolevulinic acid dehydrogenase. The latter effect is responsible for the appearance of delta aminolevulinic acid in the urine and porphyria-like symptoms.

❑❑ T/F: Galactosuria is diagnostic of galactosemia.

False. Galactosuria may be seen in many severe liver diseases.

❑❑ What eye abnormality is associated with galactosemia?

Cataracts.

❑❑ What monosaccharides make up lactose?

Glucose and galactose.

❑❑ What assay is used for the diagnosis of galactosemia?

Measurement of erythrocyte galactose-1-uridyl-transferase. This assay must be done in any jaundiced, septic or bleeding neonate if there is history of siblings with cataracts or unexplained death.

❑❑ What is the significance of lactosuria in neonates?

Lactosuria may normally occur in healthy newborns.

❑❑ **What is the treatment of galactosemia?**

Galactose-free diet for life.

❑❑ **What enzyme deficiency causes benign fructosemia?**

Absence of fructokinase. This is asymptomatic.

❑❑ **Deficiency of which enzyme of fructose metabolism causes severe symptoms?**

Absence of fructose-1-phosphate-aldolase and fructose-1,6-diphosphatase both cause severe symptoms.

❑❑ **Deficiency of which enzyme of fructose metabolism causes hereditary fructose intolerance?**

Absence of fructose-1-phosphate-aldolase.

❑❑ **What are typical fructose-containing foods?**

Fruits and honey.

❑❑ **T/F: Patients with hereditary fructose intolerance are asymptomatic if they avoid fructose.**

True. In fact, older children develop an aversion to foods containing fructose.

❑❑ **What are the typical presenting symptoms of hereditary fructose intolerance in infancy?**

Vomiting, pallor, lethargy, sweating and/or convulsions following ingestion of fructose.

❑❑ **What is the most common physical finding in hereditary fructose intolerance?**

Hepatomegaly.

❑❑ **T/F: Patients with fructose-1,6-diphosphatase deficiency are asymptomatic if they avoid fructose.**

False. Fructose ingestion is not required in fructose-1,6-diphosphatase deficiency for symptoms to develop.

❑❑ **What is the toxic substance that accumulates in hereditary fructose inltolerance?**

Fructose-1-phosphate.

❑❑ **How does fructose-1-phosphate cause symptoms?**

It results in hypoglycemia by inhibiting glycogenolysis and gluconeogenesis. In addition, it is cytotoxic to the liver, kidneys and gut.

❑❑ **What renal manifestations may develop as a result of fructose-1-phosphate nephrotoxicity?**

Renal tubular acidosis, aminoaciduria, hyperuricemia, hypophosphatemia or hypocalcemia.

❑❑ **What methods are used in the diagnosis of hereditary fructose intolerance?**

Enzyme assays from intestinal or liver specimens.

❑❑ **Which glycogen storage disease is associated with the most severe liver manifestations?**

Glycogenosis Type IV (branching enzyme defect) regularly progresses to cirrhosis.

❑❑ **Which lysosomal storage disease is associated with parenchymal liver disease in children?**

Nieman-Pick type C.

❑❑ **What metabolites accumulate in the cells of Nieman-Pick disease patients?**

Sphingomyelin and cholesterol.

❑❑ **What is the most common cause of neonatal ascites?**

Obstructive uropathy.

DRUG-INDUCED, GRANULOMATOUS AND OTHER INFLAMMATORY DISEASES

David E. Johnston, M.D.

❏❏ How is idiosyncratic drug hepatotoxicity explained, in general?

One cause may be variations in cytochrome P450 or other enzymes of drug metabolism. Reactive P450 metabolites can react with proteins in the liver to create new antigens. Variations in the immune response may be another reason for idiosyncratic drug reactions.

❏❏ What are some of the important enzyme systems which detoxify reactive drug metabolites produced by cytochrome P450?

The most important protective system is glutathione and glutathione-S-transferase, which is very abundant in hepatocytes. Another important enzyme is epoxide hydrolase, which breaks down reactive epoxides produced from drugs such as phenytoin.

❏❏ Anti-LKM (liver-kidney-microsomal) antibodies are directed against what antigens?

Against forms of cytochrome P450. The naturally occurring anti-LKM antibodies, found in type 2 autoimmune hepatitis, are directed against P450 2D6 whereas the anti-LKM antibodies found in some forms of drug-induced hepatitis are directed against other forms of P450 involved in drug metabolism (e.g., P450 3A1 in patients with hepatotoxicity from aromatic anticonvulsants or P450 2C9 in patients with hepatotoxicity from tienilic acid).

❏❏ What drugs are commonly mentioned in association with fulminant liver failure?

Acetaminophen, phenytoin, isoniazid, niacin, valproic acid and troglitazone are a few examples.

❏❏ What are risk factors for overt liver injury from isoniazid (INH)?

Increasing age, female gender and heavy alcohol use. Concomitant use of drugs such as rifampicin may be a risk factor. Early studies suggested that rapid acetylators were at greater risk; however, this is now controversial.

❏❏ Describe the histology of the liver after an acute overdose of acetaminophen. What explains this pattern of liver injury?

The liver shows a nearly pure necrosis, most marked in zone 3, around the central vein. This probably results from the metabolism of acetaminophen by cytochrome P450, which is more abundant in zone 3.

❏❏ What is a safe dose of acetaminophen?

This is estimated to be up to 4 g/day for a healthy person, perhaps up to 2 g/day for a regular drinker, and probably less than this, or none, for a person with alcoholic hepatitis.

❏❏ List risk factors for acetaminophen hepatotoxicity.

Regular heavy use of alcohol, phenobarbital, isoniazid and other drugs which induce cytochrome P450. Obesity may increase the risk of toxicity because it is associated with increased cytochrome P450 2E1.

Fasting reduces glutathione levels. Gilbert's syndrome is associated with reduced UDP-glucuronosyl transferase, one of the enzymes involved in the conjugation and detoxification of acetaminophen.

❑❑ **Why does alcohol increase the risk of acetaminophen hepatotoxicity?**

Alcohol induces cytochrome P450 2E1 which metabolizes acetaminophen to a toxic, reactive quinoneimine compound. Alcohol also causes depletion of glutathione, which functions to detoxify such reactive substances in the liver.

❑❑ **What drugs or chemicals are inducers or substrates of P450 2E1?**

Isoniazid (INH) is the best inducer. Ethanol, acetaminophen, carbon tetrachloride, chloroform, halothane, cocaine, benzene, and nitrosamines are other substrates or inducers of P450 2E1. This explains some of the interactions among alcohol and a number of other toxins and carcinogens. Alcohol metabolism by P450 2E1 produces reactive oxygen species which are thought to contribute to the toxicity of alcohol.

❑❑ **In an alcoholic with recent ingestion of acetaminophen and suspected acetaminophen hepatotoxicity, how are acetaminophen blood levels used to guide treatment?**

In this situation, acetaminophen levels do not really guide treatment unless they are high. Treatment should not be withheld because the acetaminophen level is low, since acetaminophen toxicity can occur in an alcoholic without a high blood level of acetaminophen. Although treatment is most effective within 10 hours of ingestion, it may be beneficial for up to 36 hours.

❑❑ **How is prognosis estimated in patients with acute liver failure caused by acetaminophen?**

The O'Grady criteria are commonly used to predict a fatal outcome and the need for liver transplantation in patients with fulminant liver failure. For acute acetaminophen toxicity, these criteria include: pH < 7.3 or international normalization ratio (INR) > 6.5 and serum creatinine > 3.4 mg/dL.

❑❑ **Describe the acute phenytoin hypersensitivity syndrome.**

This is an acute allergic reaction that can occur during the first six weeks of therapy. It occurs more often in females and adults and is characterized by a flu-like syndrome with adenopathy, fever, rash and liver dysfunction. It may progress to acute liver failure.

❑❑ **What enzymatic defect is thought to explain why some individuals develop the acute phenytoin toxicity syndrome?**

Deficiency of epoxide hydrolase. This enzyme normally breaks down aromatic epoxides resulting from P450 metabolism of phenytoin. The resulting aryl epoxides presumably become attached to proteins and become antigenic.

❑❑ **What types of chronic liver injury can phenytoin cause?**

Phenytoin can result in chronic hepatitis or cholangitis centered around small bile ductules.

❑❑ **What is the difference between macrovesicular and microvesicular fatty liver, in terms of lipid composition and pathophysiology?**

Macrovesicular fat is mostly triglyceride accumulated due to increased influx and decreased efflux of lipid. Microvesicular fat is mostly unesterified fatty acid which accumulates in conditions in which mitochondrial oxidation of fatty acids is impaired.

❑❑ **What drugs or toxins often cause macrovesicular steatosis of the liver?**

Ethanol, glucococorticoids, methotrexate and chlorinated hydrocarbons (such as carbon tetrachloride) are good examples.

❑❑ What drugs or toxins result in severe microvesicular steatosis of the liver?

Aspirin in an overdose or in Reye's syndrome, tetracycline and valproic acid. Some nucleoside analogs used in treating HIV disease, such as zidovudine and lamivudine, can cause mitochondrial dysfunction with microvesicular steatosis. The nucleoside analog fialuridine, used in clinical trials for treatment of hepatitis B, caused severe mitochondrial dysfunction with microvesicular steatosis, lactic acidosis and liver failure.

❑❑ What drugs or toxins mimic histologic features of alcoholic hepatitis?

The best example is amiodarone. Nifedipine, diethylstilbesterol (DES) and tamoxifen can also cause Mallory's hyaline and steatosis.

❑❑ A liver biopsy shows extensive homogenous intracellular material in hepatocytes. Electron microscopy shows whorls of concentric intracellular membranes. What is this and what drugs or toxins can cause it?

This is phospholipidosis, caused by amiodarone, perhexiline maleate, chlorpheniramine and a few other drugs. A number of the drugs which cause this are lipophilic cations.

❑❑ What is peliosis hepatis?

Peliosis hepatis is a condition characterized by vascular pools in the liver, from a few millimeters to a centimeter in size, perhaps related to obstruction of the sinusoidal-central vein junction. Peliosis has been associated with hepatomegaly. Such livers are prone to bleeding after biopsy.

❑❑ What drugs or other conditions cause peliosis hepatis?

Peliosis is associated with use of anabolic steroids, estrogens, azathioprine, 6-thioguanine and Thorotrast. Peliosis is also seen in patients with tuberculosis or malignancy and in AIDS patients infected with *Rochalimea henselae*.

❑❑ What is nodular regenerative hyperplasia and what medications can cause this disorder?

Nodular regenerative hyperplasia is characterized by a diffusely nodular liver without fibrosis. Nodular regenerative hyperplasia is thought to result from diffuse obstruction of microscopic arterioles with regeneration of better perfused areas. It is associated with the use of oral contraceptives, anabolic steroids, azathioprine, busulfan and 6-thioguanine.

❑❑ List some drugs or toxins which cause hepatic veno-occlusive disease (VOD).

Bush tea from *Senecio*, *Crotalaria*, *Heliotropiu* and some comfrey tea contains pyrollizidine alkaloids. The metabolism of these substances by zone 3 (central-lobular) hepatocytes gives rise to reactive metabolites which damage the central veins resulting in fibrosis and obstruction. VOD often occurs in bone marrow transplant patients, perhaps due to the combined effects of radiation and alkylating agents or azathioprine.

❑❑ What is the best example of a drug which causes pure cholestasis?

The 17-alkylated steroids, such as those commonly used in oral contraceptives, can cause decreased bile flow without evidence of inflammation or other liver injury. Women with a history of cholestasis during pregnancy are predisposed to steroid-induced cholestasis.

❑❑ List some medications which cause elevated unconjugated bilirubin.

Rifampicin interferes with the uptake of unconjugated bilirubin by hepatocytes. Nicotinic acid can increase unconjugated bilirubin in patients with Gilbert's syndrome. Elevation of unconjugated bilirubin can also be a sign of hemolysis, which could be drug-induced.

❑❑ What drugs cause inflammation involving microscopic bile ducts?

Sulfa drugs often result in some combination of cholestasis and hepatocellular injury. Sulfonylurea use can lead to a syndrome histologically resembling primary biliary cirrhosis (PBC) but with negative anti-mitochondrial antibody (AMA). Diclofenac has caused a number of cases resembling PBC, sometimes with positive AMA. A large number of drugs cause chronic cholestasis. Carbamazepine may result in hepatic inflammation centered on bile ductules.

❑❑ Explain what is meant by "vanishing bile ducts" and list some drugs which can cause this.

This refers to the disappearance of microscopic bile ductules, which normally number one to two per portal triad on a liver biopsy. The syndrome of vanishing bile ducts occurs in advanced primary biliary cirrhosis or in chronic liver allograft rejection. Some drugs associated with this syndrome include carbamazepine, phenothiazines and thiabendazole. There is a report of vanishing bile ducts in a child with Stevens-Johnson syndrome following ibuprofen use.

❑❑ What drugs cause damage or inflammation to large bile ducts?

The best example is FUDR (5-fluoro-deoxyuridine) given by intra-arterial infusion. This results in a syndrome resembling sclerosing cholangitis and is probably due to vascular injury.

❑❑ What drugs can lead to a chronic hepatitis mimicking autoimmune hepatitis?

Sulfonamides, propylthiouracil, alpha-methyldopa, nitrofurantoin, minocycline and ecstasy (a drug of abuse, MDMA, methylene-3,4-dioxy-methamphetamine) are examples. Some of these drugs induce anti-nuclear antibodies and other autoantibodies. Halothane toxicity can be accompanied by features of autoimmune hepatitis, including antimitochondrial antibodies.

❑❑ List drugs which can cause cirrhosis with chronic use.

Cirrhosis, with only minimal abnormalities on liver enzymes, can occur following use of amiodarone, methotrexate and vitamin A. While valproic acid is best known for causing acute liver failure, long-term use has also been associated with the development of cirrhosis.

❑❑ List risk factors for methotrexate hepatotoxicity.

Obesity, alcohol consumption, pre-existing fatty liver or other liver disease.

❑❑ What dose of vitamin A is needed to cause hepatotoxicity?

Large doses, in the range of a million IU/day, cause acute toxicity. Chronic use of more than 40,000 IU/day for months can cause chronic hepatotoxicity. Lower doses may be toxic in heavy alcohol users and persons with hyperlipidemia and elevated chylomicrons.

❑❑ What is the appearance of vitamin A toxicity on liver biopsy?

The liver biopsy shows vitamin A droplets in sinusoidal fat storing cells, Kupffer cell activation, inflammation and fibrosis. This fibrosis can lead to portal hypertension without accompanying cirrhosis.

❑❑ What drugs or chemicals are associated with hepatocellular carcinoma?

The most recognized is aflatoxin, produced by the fungus *Aspergillus flavus*, which can contaminate peanuts. Estrogens and anabolic steroids have also been associated with hepatic adenomas, focal nodular hyperplasia and hepatocellular carcinoma (HCC). Thorotrast has been associated with HCC.

❑❑ What drugs or chemicals are associated with angiosarcoma?

Thorotrast (thorium dioxide) was used intravenously as an angiographic contrast agent from 1930 until 1953. It has been associated with angiosarcoma, cholangiocarcinoma and hepatocellular carcinoma in similar proportions. Arsenic and vinyl chloride are associated mainly with angiosarcoma. Diethylstilbesterol and anabolic steroids have also been associated with this tumor.

❑❑ What herbal medicines have been associated with hepatotoxicity?

Creosote bush (chaparral tea), germander, pennyroyal (containing pulegone), Jin Bu Huan and Ma-huang are some examples.

❑❑ What drugs cause granulomatous hepatitis?

Sulfa drugs, quinidine, allopurinol, nitrofurantoin, carbamazepine and phenytoin.

❑❑ What are clinical features of acute valproic acid hepatotoxicity and what is its treatment?

The anticonvulsant, valproic acid, can cause acute microvesicular steatosis and liver failure. Valproic acid is a branched-chain carboxylic acid and is converted to its coenzyme A thioester in mitochondria where it is further oxidized. Valproic acid metabolites interfere with mitochondrial fatty acid oxidation. Institutionalized patients with malnutrition and mental retardation are at increased risk of valproate-induced acute liver failure. Some persons with valproic acid hepatotoxicity may have mild inborn errors of mitochondrial metabolism. Retrospective studies suggest that high-dose carnitine can reduce the severity of acute liver failure; however, this is not a proven treatment.

❑❑ What is the significance of elevated blood ammonia in a patient taking valproic acid?

A significant fraction of persons taking valproic acid have mildly elevated blood ammonia levels. This does not necessarily indicate serious drug toxicity; however, ammonia levels can become elevated to such a degree as to cause mental status changes. Some studies suggest that administration of L-carnitine can reduce blood ammonia levels in those taking valproic acid.

❑❑ What are features of hepatotoxicity from nicotinic acid?

High dose nicotinic acid used to treat hypercholesterolemia can cause jaundice and severe hepatocyte necrosis, occasionally with fulminant liver failure. Hepatotoxicity seems to be more common with sustained-release formulations.

❑❑ Which nonsteroidal anti-inflammatory drugs (NSAIDs) are most prone to cause hepatotoxicity?

Significant hepatotoxicity is not common with the currently marketed NSAIDs. NSAIDs more commonly mentioned as a cause of hepatotoxicity are sulindac and diclofenac.

❑❑ What are features of sulindac hepatotoxicity?

Mild hepatitis with cholestasis.

❑❑ What are features of diclofenac hepatotoxicity?

This NSAID has caused rare cases of acute hepatitis with liver cell necrosis, often with associated anti-nuclear antibodies. Fulminant liver failure has occurred. Some patients have developed anti-mitochondrial antibodies with a histologic picture similar to primary biliary cirrhosis.

❑❑ What determines the relative hepatotoxicity of inhalational anesthetics?

For the halogenated alkanes, this generally is proportional to their rate of metabolism by cytochrome P450 (halothane > enflurane > isoflurane).

❑❑ Describe clinical and histologic features of carbamazepine hepatotoxicity.

Fever, rash, eosinophilia and other features of a systemic allergic reaction often occur. Histology can include hepatocellular necrosis, granuloma formation and injury to microscopic bile ductules.

❑❑ What types of hepatotoxicity do 6-mercaptopurine and azathioprine cause?

An acute allergic-type reaction can occur with hepatocyte necrosis and very elevated aminotransferases and cholestasis. Chronic use can cause nodular regenerative hyperplasia, peliosis hepatis and possibly contribute to veno-occlusive disease.

❑❑ **What are the features of tetracycline hepatotoxicity?**

Hepatotoxicity has occurred with high-dose intravenous use of tetracycline but can also occur with oral use. On liver biopsy, there is accumulation of microvesicular fat in hepatocytes. It appears to be a toxic effect on mitochondria.

❑❑ **In what setting do penicillins cause hepatotoxicity?**

In general, the penicillins rarely produce overt hepatotoxicity. A mild, non-specific hepatitis occurs with intravenous oxacillin. Semi-synthetic penicillins such as cloxacillin have caused cholestasis. Although cholestasis is very rare with amoxicillin, a number of cases have occurred with amoxicillin-clavulanic acid, suggesting that clavulanic acid is responsible.

❑❑ **What type of liver injury do tricyclic antidepressants cause?**

Cholestasis and hepatocyte necrosis. This is uncommon and not usually serious.

❑❑ **What type of hepatotoxicity is seen with tacrine?**

About half of patients will have elevation of the alanine aminotransferase (ALT) level but only 2% will have very high ALT. Overt liver injury is rare.

❑❑ **In what setting does cocaine hepatotoxicity occur?**

Hepatocyte necrosis usually occurs in the setting of an overdose, especially in a heavy alcohol drinker. Induction of cytochrome P450 2E1 by alcohol probably causes increased metabolism of cocaine to toxic products.

❑❑ **What toxins are found in toxic mushrooms?**

These are mainly the amatoxins and phallotoxins. The amatoxins include a variety of cyclic peptides which inhibit RNA polymerase type II and, thus, inhibit the synthesis of messenger RNA. The phallotoxins promote the polymerization of cellular actin.

❑❑ **What solvent used in manufacturing rubber products causes hepatotoxicity?**

Methyl formamide, used in manufacturing rubberized cloth, has caused a type of acute hepatitis when used without proper ventilation.

❑❑ **What type of food poisoning is associated with acute liver failure?**

Bacillus cereus is a sporulating bacterium that can cause diarrhea and vomiting when it grows in rice and other grain products that have been improperly cooked or reheated. *B. cereus* produces an emetic toxin which has lead to cases of acute liver failure by interfering with mitochondrial function.

❑❑ **What type of hepatotoxicity is associated with cyanobacteria?**

Some strains of cyanobacteria ("blue-green algae") produce microcystins. These interfere with the hepatocyte cytoskeleton and cause liver hemorrhage and necrosis. Such liver toxicity is best known to occur in cattle but multiple cases have also occurred in humans in a hemodialysis center due to contaminated water.

❑❑ **What are the two most common causes of hepatic epithelioid granulomas in the United States?**

Sarcoidosis and tuberculosis.

❑❑ **What is the most common symptom in patients with hepatic granulomas?**

Fever of unknown origin is the most common symptom; however, symptoms correlate with the underlying illness. Fever is present in most cases of sarcoidosis and tuberculosis.

❑❑ **What are the most common physical findings in patients with conditions that cause hepatic granulomas?**

Splenomegaly, hepatomegaly and moderate lymphadenopathy.

❑❑ **What is the most common pattern seen in biochemical tests that would suggest a granulomatous liver disease?**

A moderate to marked increase in serum alkaline phosphatase (3 to 10 times normal) and a slight increase in serum aminotransferases (2 to 6 times normal).

❑❑ **T/F: Granulomatous diseases of the liver usually result in a clinically significant alteration of hepatic function.**

False. Most diseases that cause granulomas of the liver do not cause significant alteration of hepatic function. Sarcoidosis and primary biliary cirrhosis are exceptions.

❑❑ **There is a histopathologic distinction between epithelioid granulomas and granulomatous necrosis. Which of these two categories do most granulomas associated with drugs fall into?**

Drug-associated granulomas are usually characterized by granulomatous necrosis; a term used to describe punched out clusters of histiocytes and/or lymphocytes.

❑❑ **Sarcoidosis is a disease characterized by epithelioid cell granulomas. What organs are affected by these granulomas?**

Granulomas occur in many organs in sarcoidosis, including the liver.

❑❑ **What percentage of individuals with sarcoidosis have granulomas in the liver?**

Approximately two-thirds will have liver granulomas. The majority of granulomas are located in the portal area, although they may appear anywhere within the hepatic nodule.

❑❑ **What is the major diagnostic test used to distinguish between primary biliary cirrhosis and sarcoidosis?**

The antimitochodrial antibody test. Results are positive in primary biliary cirrhosis and negative in sarcoidosis.

❑❑ **What is the most consistently abnormal lab value in sarcoidosis?**

Elevated serum alkaline phosphatase. Other commonly abnormal lab values include elevated serum angiotensin-converting enzyme (50% to 80% of cases), elevated serum calcium and a moderate normocytic anemia.

❑❑ **What disease is characterized by persistent hepatic granulomas, regardless of whether or not the patient has received corticosteroid therapy?**

Sarcoidosis.

❑❑ **What are the names of the two inclusion bodies found in approximately half of granulomas associated with sarcoidosis?**

Schaumann bodies and asteroid bodies. Schaumann bodies are basophilic structures with concentric proteinaceous calcified laminations. Asteroid bodies are star-like radiating structures found within a clear space.

❏❏ **What is the treatment for sarcoidosis?**

Corticosteroids are the mainstay of therapy. Small doses are usually rapidly effective; however, patients often relapse with fever after discontinuation of steroid therapy. Thus, many patients often receive long courses of steroids.

❏❏ **What liver condition may result in later stages of sarcoidosis?**

Portal fibrosis of the biliary type may occur and may result in portal hypertension.

❏❏ **What percent of patients with Hodgkin's disease have hepatic granulomas?**

Up to 12%. Up to 2% of patients with Non-Hodgkin's lymphoma have hepatic involvement.

❏❏ **What histologic characteristics are typical of Hodgkin's disease granulomas?**

These granulomas, which are seen in both portal tracts and parenchyma, are typically epithelioid without caseation and occasionally contain Langerhan's giant cells.

❏❏ **What type of surgery is associated with an unexplained increase in epithelioid noncaseating granulomas on liver biopsy?**

Intestinal bypass surgery.

❏❏ **What percentage of cases of primary biliary cirrhosis are associated with liver granulomas and/or granulomatous necrosis?**

Approximately 25%.

❏❏ **Name six drugs that have been associated with hepatic granuloma formation.**

Allopurinol, sulfonamides, quinidine, chlorpropamide, beryllium and phenylbutazone.

❏❏ **Name findings that might suggest that liver granulomas are from a drug reaction.**

Portal location of granulomas, peripheral eosinophilia and tissue eosinophilia. There is no pathognomonic characteristic of drug-related hepatic granulomas.

❏❏ **What is the typical sequela after the removal of the offending drug?**

None. The granulomas quickly resolve without fibrosis or calcification.

❏❏ **What disease of the colon can be associated with hepatic granuloma formation?**

Crohn's disease.

❏❏ **What is the most common cause of jaundice in AIDS patients?**

Drug-induced hepatitis.

❏❏ **What systemic vasculitis that usually manifests itself in the respiratory tract is also associated with granulomatous hepatitis, elevated alkaline phosphatase and/or aminotransferases and ascites in 15% to 30% of cases?**

Wegener's granulomatosis.

❑❑ **What percentage of patients with polymyalgia rheumatica, giant cell arteritis and temporal arteritis have liver test abnormalities?**

Approximately one-third.

❑❑ **T/F: Hypogammaglobinemia is associated with liver test abnormalities.**

True.

HEPATOBILIARY PATHOLOGY

Corey A. Roberts, M.D.

❑❑ **What is the function of the Ito cell (perisinusoidal lipocytes) in the liver?**

It functions as a storage vehicle, metabolizes vitamin A and aides in the production of collagen.

❑❑ **In ischemic liver injury, what general pattern of necrosis would be expected?**

Centrilobular necrosis. The pericentral region of the lobule or zone 3 of the acinus is farthest from the blood supply and most susceptible to ischemic injury.

❑❑ **A liver biopsy is performed on a patient with a drug-induced hepatitis and subsequently is examined using an electron microscope. What would be the most common ultrastructural finding in this case?**

Megamitochondria, including some gigantic mitochondria, are typical of a drug reaction.

❑❑ **What zone of the liver acinus is characteristically involved in acetaminophen toxicity?**

Zone 3.

❑❑ **What is the name of the complete hepatitis B virus virion which includes the surface antigen, core antigen, DNA polymerase and the e antigen.**

A Dane particle.

❑❑ **How does the pattern of necrosis in acute viral hepatitis B compare to that seen in acute viral hepatitis A infection?**

The necrosis in acute hepatitis B infection typically is centered in zone 3 while acute hepatitis A is characteristically a zone 1 pattern of necrosis.

❑❑ **In a case of mushroom poisoning, what zone of the acinus would you expect to see necrosis?**

Zone 1.

❑❑ **The presence of noncaseating granulomas that are characterized by a "fibrin ring" pattern in the center should raise the diagnostic possibility of what rare type of hepatitis?**

Q-fever hepatitis caused by *Coxiella burnetii*. Sometimes, this lesion is referred to as a "doughnut" granuloma.

❑❑ **What subtype of cirrhosis is classically associated with alcoholic liver disease?**

Micronodular.

❑❑ **What is the ultrastructural composition of a Mallory body?**

These are intermediate filament bundles. More specifically, there are three types of Mallory bodies identified ultrastructurally.
Type I - bundles of filaments arranged in a parallel fashion.
Type II - randomly arranged fibrils.
Type III - an amorphous substance with scattered fibrils in no certain arrangement.

❑❑ **What type of steatosis, microvesicular or macrovesicular, is associated with Reye's syndrome, valproic acid toxicity and acute fatty liver of pregnancy?**

Microvesicular steatosis.

❑❑ **What two items must be described in a liver biopsy pathology report when making the diagnosis of chronic hepatitis?**

Grade and stage. The degree of activity is referred to as the grade and the amount of fibrosis as the stage. Of course, the etiology is also included if known.

❑❑ **Of the various agents of viral hepatitis, which has the longest incubation period?**

Hepatitis B, a DNA virus, has an incubation period that ranges up to 180 days.

❑❑ **What is the most common etiology of peliosis hepatis?**

Peliosis hepatis refers to the presence of multiple large blood-filled spaces within the liver that lack an endothelial lining. Causes of peliosis hepatis include treatment with anabolic or androgenic steroids and tamoxifen, history of Thorotrast use, elevated levels of vitamin A and infection with *Bartonella henselae*.

❑❑ **What viral agent has been identified by ultrastructural analysis in some cases of so-called "giant cell" hepatitis?**

Paramyxovirus.

❑❑ **A young adult presents with acute liver failure. Tissues are obtained for electron microscopy. What would you expect to see on electron microscopy if the patient has Wilson's disease?**

Ultrastructurally, the mitochondria are pleomorphic and have widened intercristal spaces.

❑❑ **A 36 year-old woman presents with chronic hepatitis and is found to have an HLA B8 haplotype, liver/kidney microsome antibodies and elevated levels of serum IgG. What is the most likely diagnosis?**

Autoimmune hepatitis (type 2).

❑❑ **What specific mushroom is associated with liver toxicity and fulminant hepatic failure?**

Amanita phalloides.

❑❑ **Describe the typical histologic features of primary biliary cirrhosis?**

Destruction of small bile ducts with a portal lymphoplasmacytic infiltrate including lymphoid follicles and even granulomas. There may also be a loss of 50% or more of the original interlobular bile ducts.

❑❑ **The finding of periductal fibrosis or sclerosis resulting in an "onion skin" pattern in the portal areas is indicative of what disorder?**

Primary sclerosing cholangitis.

❑❑ **What specific antibody titer may be elevated in patients with primary sclerosing cholangitis?**

Perinuclear antineutrophil cytoplasmic antibody (p-ANCA).

❑❑ **How can you differentiate between Dubin-Johnson and Rotor's syndromes histologically? Grossly?**

Dubin-Johnson is characterized by a black discoloration of the parenchyma seen both grossly and histologically. Histologically, the pigment is contained within the hepatocytes in zones 2 and 3. In contrast, Rotor's syndrome is devoid of pigment and, histologically, the liver may be normal.

❑❑ **Dubin-Johnson syndrome and Rotor's syndrome share a common inheritance pattern. What is it?**

Autosomal recessive.

❑❑ **Glucuronyl transferase is deficient or abnormal in what rather innocuous condition?**

Gilbert's syndrome.

❑❑ **On what chromosome does the defect responsible for Wilson's disease lie?**

Chromosome 13.

❑❑ **What is the hepatic iron index and what value would you expect in a patient with hereditary hemochromatosis?**

The hepatic iron index is calculated by taking the hepatic iron concentration in mg/g dry weight, dividing it by 56 and dividing that total by the patient's age. In hemochromatosis, a value greater than 1.9 is characteristic.

❑❑ **T/F: A solitary, unilocular simple cyst of the liver is typically found in the right lobe.**

True. They are twice as common in the right lobe.

❑❑ **Discuss in general terms the histologic findings in the liver in a case of carbon tetrachloride toxicity.**

Steatosis and centrilobular necrosis.

❑❑ **What is the earliest and most common histologic finding in liver biopsies of alcoholic hepatitis?**

Steatosis, predominantly macrovesicular.

❑❑ **What is the inheritance pattern of genetic hemochromatosis?**

Autosomal recessive. The gene is on the short arm of chromosome 6.

❑❑ **T/F: The development of hepatocellular carcinoma in patients with hemochromatosis and cirrhosis is common.**

True. Up to 20% of patients will develop hepatocellular carcinoma in that scenario.

❑❑ **T/F: There an association between hereditary tyrosinemia and hepatocellular carcinoma.**

True. Over one-third of patients who live beyond the age of two will develop hepatocellular carcinoma, sometimes multifocally.

❑❑ **Foreign, polarizable material is seen in association with a foreign body giant cell reaction within expanded, fibrotic portal areas on a liver biopsy specimen taken from a patient on chronic renal dialysis. What is the foreign material?**

Silicon rubber from silastic tubing that is found in hemodialysis equipment. A similar reaction can also be seen from damaged prosthetic devices.

❑❑ **In a patient with Wolman's disease, what is the substance that is accumulated within cells of the reticuloendothelial system both in the liver (Kupffer cells) and in histiocytes throughout the body?**

Neutral lipid.

❑❑ **What are some causes of hepatic granulomas or granulomatous hepatitis?**

Sarcoidosis, primary biliary cirrhosis and drug injury are the most common causes. Other causes include polymyalgia rheumatica, berylliosis, Brucellosis, foreign body reaction, primary sclerosing cholangitis, systemic infection and extrahepatic malignancies.

❑❑ **What is the most common parasitic disease involving the liver that can produce a granulomatous response?**

Schistosomiasis.

❑❑ **In amyloidosis involving the liver, where is the amyloid deposited?**

It can either be found within the vessel walls or the parenchyma, specifically in the space of Disse with compression of the underlying hepatocytes.

❑❑ **What effect does Budd-Chiari syndrome have on the caudate lobe?**

The caudate lobe is not usually involved, owing to its unique, separate venous drainage and, in fact, may exhibit compensatory hypertrophy in an attempt to "make up" for the involved liver.

❑❑ **What is Banti's syndrome?**

Also referred to as idiopathic portal hypertension, it is characterized by splenomegaly, hypersplenism and portal hypertension.

❑❑ **What is Zieve's syndrome?**

This refers to the triad of hemolytic anemia occurring in a patient with alcoholic hepatitis who also has hypercholesterolemia. Hemolysis may also occur in Wilson's disease and the finding of hemolysis in a young patient with liver dysfunction is strongly suggestive of Wilson's disease.

❑❑ **What are some etiologic agents of veno-occlusive disease (VOD)?**

Ingestion of pyrrolizidine alkaloids, radiation, various cancer chemotherapies, urethane, azathioprine, dacarbazine and hypervitaminosis A.

❑❑ **T/F: The granulomas found in the liver in some cases of Brucellosis are found in the portal areas.**

False. The granulomas are typically rather ill-defined and found within the lobules. Associated hepatocellular necrosis may be present.

❑❑ **In general, what is included in the differential diagnosis of micronodular cirrhosis?**

Alcoholic liver disease (Laennec's cirrhosis), primary biliary cirrhosis, hemochromatosis, non-alcoholic steatohepatitis (NASH), Indian childhood cirrhosis, galactosemia and glycogenosis type IV.

❑❑ **What are some of the conditions that are associated with macronodular cirrhosis?**

Viral hepatitis, alpha$_1$-antitrypsin deficiency, hereditary tyrosinemia, Wilson's disease and some drug injury.

❏❏ **Compare Caroli's disease and Caroli's syndrome?**

Caroli's disease is a developmental condition of intrahepatic cystic dilatations of bile ducts. The lumens of the cystic dilatations can be filled with mucin, bile or pus if infected. Caroli's syndrome is Caroli's disease found in association with congenital hepatic fibrosis.

❏❏ **In what fashion is Caroli's disease inherited?**

Autosomal recessive.

❏❏ **What are some of the main clinical manifestations of congenital hepatic fibrosis?**

In general, patients present with hepatosplenomegaly or bleeding from esophageal varices due to portal hypertension. Cholangitis is a less common presenting condition.

❏❏ **What is Ivemark's syndrome?**

This syndrome consists of the histologic features of congenital hepatic fibrosis in addition to pancreatic cysts and dysplastic changes in the pancreas, liver, and kidneys.

❏❏ **What is Meckel's syndrome?**

It is characterized by features that are similar to congenital hepatic fibrosis with the addition of an association with encephalocele, polydactyly and cystic kidneys.

❏❏ **Name the two most common hepatic complications associated with autosomal dominant polycystic kidney disease.**

Infection of the liver cysts is the most frequent complication followed by cholangiocarcinoma.

❏❏ **What is a von Meyenburg's complex?**

This is a localized collection of abnormally dilated bile ducts in a fibrous stroma background.

❏❏ **Which lobe of the liver are most hydatid cysts located?**

Right lobe. Remember, in general, most things are more common in the right lobe of the liver.

❏❏ **Discuss the clinical and pathologic findings in mesenchymal hamartoma of the liver?**

It is a tumor that can be quite large, develops in children (average age less than 2, usually males) and is characterized by a loose, connective tissue stroma with admixed bile ducts and vascular structures. A chromosomal translocation involving the long arm of chromosome 19 (19q18.4) has been described.

❏❏ **Which of these two benign lesions carries a greater risk of hemorrhage or rupture - focal nodular hyperplasia or hepatocellular adenoma?**

Hepatocellular adenoma.

❏❏ **An otherwise normal liver contains a solitary mass 5 cm in diameter which is characterized by a central, stellate scar. What is your diagnosis?**

Focal nodular hyperplasia.

❏❏ **What are some of the associations with nodular regenerative hyperplasia of the liver?**

Nodular regenerative hyperplasia is associated with numerous conditions including rheumatoid arthritis, CREST syndrome and other autoimmune diseases. It typically occurs in adults and is sometimes confused with cirrhosis.

❑❑ **Name some inherent differences between bile duct adenomas and von Meyenburg's complexes?**

Von Meyenburg's complexes are frequently multiple and are often associated with cystic lesions of the liver. In contrast, bile duct adenomas are small, measuring less than 1 cm, and solitary.

❑❑ **Describe the typical patient and clinical presentation of someone with a bile duct cystadenoma.**

These more commonly occur in women in the fourth and fifth decades of life, are usually found in the right lobe of the liver and often cause abdominal pain owing to their large size. Serum levels of CA19-9 are often elevated.

❑❑ **What benign tumor of the liver has been shown to sometimes occur in patients with Fanconi's anemia who are taking anabolic steroids and in patients with familial diabetes mellitus and type I glycogen storage disease?**

Hepatocellular adenoma.

❑❑ **What special stain can be used to help differentiate histologically between hepatocellular adenoma and hepatocellular carcinoma?**

A reticulin stain. Adenomas are characterized by preservation of the reticulin framework which defines the one to two cell layer thick plates, while hepatocellular carcinoma has no such reticulin framework or it is markedly diminished.

❑❑ **What is the most common location of cholangiocarcinoma in the liver?**

The right lobe of the liver; although, 30% are multifocal.

❑❑ **What is the relationship of serum alpha-fetoprotein to cholangiocarcinoma?**

Usually none. The vast majority of cholangiocarcinomas have no increase in serum AFP.

❑❑ **Which histologic type of hepatocellular carcinoma is characterized histologically by PAS-positive cytoplasmic inclusions within the tumor cells and dense fibrous strips of stroma investing sheets of tumor cells?**

The fibrolamellar variant.

❑❑ **What is the most common variant of hepatocellular carcinoma?**

Trabecular.

❑❑ **In general, which is more suggestive of hepatocellular carcinoma, detection of serum alpha-fetoprotein or immunoperoxidase reactivity for alpha-fetoprotein in tissue sections?**

A markedly elevated serum AFP is much more suggestive. The reported sensitivity of AFP positivity in tissue sections varies widely and can be detected in adenocarcinomas of other origins.

❑❑ **What is the most common primary hepatic malignancy in children?**

Hepatoblastoma.

❑❑ **A tumor in an 18 month-old male infant is described histologically as consisting of an epithelial component comprising embryonal-type cells and fetal cells within a mesenchymal stroma and foci of extramedullary hematopoiesis. What tumor is this?**

Hepatoblastoma.

❑❑ **What is the gross appearance of an epithelioid hemangioendothelioma of the liver?**

They are typically multicentric, involve both lobes of the liver and are firm and white-tan in color. Although both epithelioid hemangioendothelioma and angiosarcoma can be multifocal, the firm, white-tan appearance of the former is quite different than the hemorrhagic appearance of the latter.

❑❑ **What are the typical demographics and presentation of a patient with epithelioid hemangioendothelioma?**

It is more common in females in the sixth decade of life. The presenting symptoms are nonspecific but include pain and jaundice. Although the tumor grows slowly, it has a five-year survival of around 30%. Liver transplantation has been used to prolong survival.

❑❑ **What liver tumor has been associated with exposure to Thorotrast and vinyl chloride monomer?**

Angiosarcoma.

❑❑ **What are the histologic features of acute graft-versus-host disease involving the liver?**

The most noteworthy finding is that of damage to the bile ducts. In addition, individual hepatocyte necrosis may occur and endotheliitis may be present. It is very similar to acute allograft rejection.

❑❑ **T/F: Chronic graft-versus-host disease can occur in the absence of previous acute graft-versus-host disease.**

True. This occurs in about a quarter of the cases.

❑❑ **In bone marrow transplant patients who develop chronic graft-versus-host disease, how frequently is the liver involved?**

About 90% of the time.

❑❑ **What are some of the classic histologic alterations of the hepatocytes in zone 1 of the acinus in patients with chronic cholestasis?**

They typically exhibit a so-called "feathery" degeneration (enlarged, often cleared out cytoplasm) and they often contain increased copper and even Mallory's hyaline.

❑❑ **What substance usually binds to and detoxifies acetaminophen within the liver and becomes overwhelmed in cases of acetaminophen toxicity?**

Glutathione.

❑❑ **What parasitic infection can result in the so-called "pipestem fibrosis" of portal areas and/or a granulomatous reaction in the liver?**

Schistosomiasis.

❑❑ **What area of the brain is classically involved and damaged in Wilson's disease?**

The basal ganglia, particularly the putamen of the lenticular nucleus. Hence, the alternative designation "hepatolenticular degeneration".

❑❑ **What would happen to the steatosis seen in a liver biopsy of an alcoholic if he or she were to quit drinking alcohol for an extended period of time?**

It resolves.

❑❑ **What is the most common cause of death in patients with long-standing hereditary hemochromatosis?**

Hepatocellular carcinoma.

❑❑ **What percentage of patients with alpha$_1$-antitrypsin deficiency characterized by a PiZZ (homozygote) phenotype have demonstrable liver disease?**

Less than 20%; however, 100% will have PAS-positive, diastase-resistant globules within the cytoplasm of hepatocytes.

❑❑ **T/F: It is uncommon for patients with primary sclerosing cholangitis (PSC) to have concomitant ulcerative colitis (UC).**

False. These two conditions coexist 70% of the time; however, patients with UC have concomitant PSC in less than 5% of cases.

❑❑ **What gallbladder lesion is characterized by histologically normal epithelial crypts which exist amidst a hyperplastic muscularis?**

Adenomyosis. When localized to the fundus, it is called an adenomyoma although that term is somewhat misleading as it is not a true neoplasm.

INFECTIOUS DISORDERS

Tariq Akbar, M.D. and Nicholas Ferrentino, M.D.

❑❑ **What percentage of patients with an amebic liver abscess has a history of dysentery or diarrhea?**

Only about 10% to 20%

❑❑ **T/F: All amebae are pathogenic.**

False. *Entamoeba histolytica* is pathogenic while *E. dispar* is nonpathogenic. Zymoden analysis and RNA/DNA probes can differentiate these two forms.

❑❑ **What are high risks groups for amebic liver abscess?**

Lower socioeconomic status in endemic areas, immigrants from endemic areas, male homosexuals, travelers and institutionalized individuals.

❑❑ **What are poor prognostic signs in cases of amebic liver disease?**

Jaundice, peritonitis, elevated transaminases and pericardial rub.

❑❑ **What are the sensitivities of serological tests in amebic liver disease?**

Indirect hemagglutination assay (IHA) has a sensitivity of 85% to 95%. A combination of the immunofluorescent antibody test (IFAT) and the cellulose acetaldehyde precipitin test (CAP) gives 100% correlation between positive results and invasive amebic liver disease. These tests are positive in all forms of invasive amebic disease, including dysentery. A positive IFAT may persist for more than six months after treatment and IHA titers may be raised for more than two years. The CAP may become negative within one week of treatment.

❑❑ **What factors predispose to complications of an amebic liver abscess?**

Age > 40, multiple abscesses, large abscess (> 10 cm in diameter), immunosuppression and corticosteroid use.

❑❑ **What is the drug of choice for treatment of an amebic liver abscess?**

Nitroimidazoles. Alternative therapies include dehydroemetine and choloroquine. Luminal amebicides (diloxanide furoate, diiodohydroxyquin, paramomycin) must always be used following the above regimens.

❑❑ **Which lobe of the liver is more commonly affected by a liver abscess?**

Right lobe. Abscesses of biliary origin are commonly bilateral.

❑❑ **What is the leading cause of pyogenic liver abscess?**

Malignant biliary obstruction.

❑❑ **What are the most common organisms isolated from pyogenic liver abscesses?**

Gram negatives.

❑❑ **How have the trends of pyogenic liver abscess changed during the past two decades?**

The incidence of pyogenic liver abscess has increased while the overall mortality has decreased. Due to increased use of indwelling biliary stents and use of broad-spectrum antibiotics, the prevalence of *pseudomonas*, *streptococcal* and fungal species has increased and the percentage of patients with abnormal liver functions has decreased.

❑❑ **T/F: The number of abscesses predicts mortality in pyogenic liver abscess.**

True. Mortality from pyogenic liver abscesses is directly related to the number of abscesses.

❑❑ **What is the most common presenting symptom of a pyogenic hepatic abscess?**

Fever, which is present in about 90% of patients. The next most common symptom is right upper quadrant abdominal pain.

❑❑ **What is the most common complication of pyogenic liver abscess?**

Bacteremia.

❑❑ **What factors are associated with increased mortality in pyogenic liver abscesses?**

Multiple abscesses, associated malignancy, septic shock, fungal infection, presence of jaundice, hypoalbuminemia, leukocytosis and presence of bacteremia. Advanced age, biliary etiology and elevated aspartate aminotransferase are no longer considered to be risk factors.

❑❑ **What is the most common infectious cause of hepatic cysts?**

Echinococcus granulosus.

❑❑ **What are the hosts of *Echinococcus*?**

Carnivorous animals, especially the dog. Other hosts include the fox, coyote and wolf.

❑❑ **What organs other than the liver are involved in echinococcal infections?**

Kidney, spleen, brain, heart, lungs and bones.

❑❑ **T/F: Most hydatid cysts are asymptomatic.**

True.

❑❑ **What is the sensitivity of serological tests for echinococcus in cases of hydatid cysts?**

ELISA or indirect hemagglutinations are positive in about 90%.

❑❑ **What stages of the malarial (*Plasmodium* spp.) life cycle involve the liver?**

Pre-erythrocytic phase and exo-erythrocytic phase.

❑❑ **What factors influence the extent of hepatic injury in cases of malaria?**

Severity of infection and malarial species.

❑❑ **Name the causative organism of visceral leishmaniasis or kala-azar?**

Leishmania donovani.

❑❑ **What characteristic findings on liver biopsy are seen in cases of visceral leishmaniasis?**

A "peculiar cirrhosis" or so-called Rogers' cirrhosis. This is characterized by severe intralobular fibrosis with normal architecture and no regenerative nodules. This intralobular fibrosis is completely reversible after treatment.

❑❑ **T/F: Visceral leishmaniasis in an HIV-infected person is an AIDS-defining illness.**

True.

❑❑ **What is the diagnostic procedure of choice in case of visceral leishmaniasis?**

Examination and culture of needle splenic aspirate. This has an accuracy of nearly 100%.

❑❑ **What is the drug of choice in the treatment of leishmaniasis?**

Pentavalent antimonial compounds (sodium stibogluconate).

❑❑ **Name the schistosomes that affect the liver.**

S. mansoni, S. japonicum, S. mekongi and S. intercalatum.

❑❑ **What factors affect the severity of hepatic schistosomiasis?**

Intensity of egg deposition in the affected organ and HLA type (HLA A1 and B5).

❑❑ **What are typical clinical findings of hepatic schistosomiasis?**

Normal liver architecture and cellular function in the presence of portal fibrosis and portal hypertension.

❑❑ **What is katayama fever?**

This is a serum sickness-like syndrome triggered by the onset of tissue egg deposition in heavy infection with schistosomiasis.

❑❑ **What malignancy is associated with hepatic schistosomiasis?**

Follicular lymphoma of the spleen.

❑❑ **What is the most useful diagnostic method in case of active infection with schistosomiasis?**

Stool examination for eggs. This becomes negative after successful treatment.

❑❑ **What is the drug of choice for schistosomiasis?**

Praziquantel.

❑❑ **What is the drug of choice for *Fasciola hepatica*?**

Bithionol.

❑❑ **Name the malignancy commonly associated with clonorchiasis and opisthorchiasis?**

Cholangiocarcinoma.

❑❑ **What characteristic abnormality in liver tests is seen in bacterial sepsis?**

A cholestatic picture is noted even when no organisms are isolated in cultures. Endotoxin-mediated injury of the hepatocyte bile canalicular membrane is regarded as the pathogenesis of the cholestasis.

❑❑ **How does *salmonella* hepatitis differ from viral hepatitis?**

Salmonella hepatitis can be indistinguishable from acute viral hepatitis; however, *salmonella* hepatitis is associated with lower peak alanine aminotransferase (ALT) levels and higher peak alkaline phosphatase levels. High fever, relative bradycardia and a left shift of the leukocyte count favors *salmonella* hepatitis. The best discriminator is the ratio of ALT to lactate dehydrogenase (LDH) on admission. This is significantly lower (< 4) in *salmonella* hepatitis and higher (> 5) in case of viral hepatitis.

❑❑ **What is Fitz-Hugh-Curtis syndrome?**

Perihepatitis occurring as a complication of gonorrhea. It is marked by fever, severe right upper quadrant pleuritic pain, lower abdominal tenderness and a hepatic friction rub.

❑❑ **What are the manifestations of primary hepatobiliary tuberculosis?**

Tuberculomas, ascites, porta-hepatis adenopathy, hepatic abscess and cholangitis.

❑❑ **What group of patients is at high risk of developing a complicated *Yersinia* infection?**

Yersinia is an iron-dependent bacterium that requires exogenous iron for growth. Therefore, patients with hemochromatosis or secondary hemosiderosis are prone to develop hepatic abscesses from *Yersinia* infection.

❑❑ **What stages of syphilis can involve the liver?**

Secondary syphilis (up to 50% of cases) and tertiary syphilis (usually asymptomatic).

❑❑ **What is Weil's disease?**

It is a severe icteric form of leptospirosis and is characterized by marked jaundice, azotemia, hemorrhagic phenomena and hypotension. Minimal elevation of aminotransferases differentiates leptospirosis from acute viral hepatitis.

❑❑ **What form of granuloma is seen in Q fever?**

'Doughnut' or lipogranuloma in which a ring of fibrinoid necrosis and lymphocytes surrounds a centrally located fat vacuole. While this lesion is highly suggestive of Q fever, it is not pathognomonic. Similar lesions can be seen in visceral leishmaniasis, lymphoma and allupurinol hypersensitivity.

❑❑ **Name the parasite that most commonly affects the biliary tract?**

Ascaris.

❑❑ **What is the most common infection of the liver in acquired immunodeficiency syndrome (AIDS)?**

Mycobacterium avium complex (MAC).

❑❑ **What is the name of the organism known to cause bacillary peliosis hepatitis?**

The Gram-negative bacillus, *Rochalimaea henselae.* Peliosis hepatis refers to blood filled cystic changes in hepatic parenchyma that may or may not have an endothelial lining.

METABOLIC DISORDERS

Frank A. Anania, M.D., FACP

❑❑ **What is the least likely liver disease to also cause hepatocellular carcinoma?**

Wilson's Disease.

❑❑ **T/F: Children less than age 3 should be screened for Wilson's Disease.**

False. Clinical manifestations are rarely, if ever, seen before age 5.

❑❑ **In addition to the liver, brain and joints, what other vital organ can be affected by Wilson's Disease?**

Although the heart, pancreas and eyes have been reported to be involved, the most important other vital organ involved is the kidney. Wilson's Disease can cause Fanconi's syndrome resulting in low serum phosphorus and uric acid, and failure to excrete acid in the urine.

❑❑ **What other gastrointestinal disease is associated with copper storage overload and what molecular mechanism is defective?**

Menke's disease affects the copper transporter in the proximal small intestine and results in hyperabsorption of copper.

❑❑ **T/F: Wilson's Disease is inherited in Mendelian fashion as an autosomal dominant allele.**

False. Although Wilson's Disease is inherited in a Mendelian fashion, it is inherited as an autosomal recessive allele. Except for adult polycystic disease, all inheritable liver disorders are autosomal recessive.

❑❑ **If the transferrin saturation is > 55% and the ferritin level is > 1000 mg/dl in a male patient, what is the next step in the evaluation of genetic hemochromatosis (HHC)?**

Perform a percutaneous liver biopsy. Currently, genetic testing for mutations is not the next step in establishing the diagnosis.

❑❑ **How do you calculate the hepatic iron index?**

The hepatic iron index (HII) is calculated by taking the hepatic iron concentration and dividing by the patient's age in years. Keep in mind that the hepatic iron concentration must be in μmol iron/gram of dry weight of liver. Remember that the molecular weight of iron is 56.0 because the hepatic iron concentration may be reported in μg iron/gm of dry weight of liver. A value > 1.9 is consistent with homozygous HHC. A value < 1.5 is not due to homozygous HHC.

❑❑ **What stain is used to examine liver tissue for iron?**

Perl's Prussian blue stain.

❑❑ **Where is iron stored in genetic hemochromatosis?**

Iron is almost entirely within hepatocytes in a periportal distribution. The cirrhosis resulting from genetic hemochromatosis is typically micronodular, and regenerative nodules may have less-intense staining.

❑❑ **T/F: The survival rate in patients with genetic hemochromatosis following orthotopic liver transplantation (OLT) is equal to that of patients who undergo OLT for primary biliary cirrhosis.**

False. The survival rate for patients with genetic hemochromatosis following OLT is significantly less - about 60% after 5 years - than patients with other causes of end-stage liver disease because of cardiac arrhythmias related to iron overload in the myocardium.

❑❑ **Which of the organ(s) involved in genetic hemochromatosis will not improve with phlebotomy?**

Patients with advanced cirrhosis, arthropathy and hypogonadism do not improve with therapy.

❑❑ **Which members of a family should be screened for genetic hemochromatosis when it has been diagnosed in one member?**

The sibship of the proband and all first-degree relatives.

❑❑ **What is the best screening test to identify relatives of individuals with genetic hemochromatosis?**

Genetic testing is now available. A specific point mutation in the hemochromatosis gene on the short arm of chromosome 6 is the cause of up to 83% of cases of genetic hemochromatosis. This is a point mutation - substitution of cysteine for tyrosine (Cys282Tyr) at position 282. There is a second point mutation (His63Asp), which does not seem to be responsible for clinical expression of the disease.

❑❑ **T/F: In patients with genetic hemochromatosis, excess iron deposition is found predominantly in parenchymal cells (hepatocytes) with very little iron in cells of the reticuloendothelial system.**

True. This differs from other, secondary, causes of iron overload.

❑❑ **Recall all the possible rheumatoid conditions associated with HHC.**

Arthropathies involving the second and third metacarpophalangeal joints, joint space narrowing, chondrocalcinosis, subchondral cyst formation, osteopenia and joint swelling.

❑❑ **What infections are more common in iron-loaded patients?**

Vibrio vulnificus, Listeria monocytogenes, and *Pasteurella pseudotuberculosis.*

❑❑ **How is the transferrin saturation calculated?**

Serum iron/total iron binding capacity x 100%.

❑❑ **When is the serum iron level falsely elevated?**

After meals and at night. A fasting serum iron level collected in the morning is most useful.

❑❑ **T/F: The serum ferritin level is both more sensitive and specific than transferrin saturation values.**

False. Ferritin is also an acute phase reactant.

❑❑ **What hepatic conditions may also cause an elevated ferritin level?**

Chronic viral hepatitis (including Hepatitis C), alcoholic liver disease and non-alcoholic steatohepatitis.

❑❑ **What is the typical hepatic iron index of a patient with alcoholic liver disease? What is a normal index value?**

1.1 to 1.6; < 0.7 to 1.1.

❑❑ **How much iron is typically needed to be removed by phlebotomy in a patient with HHC?**

10 to 20 g.

❑❑ **How many phlebotomies will this require?**

Each unit of whole blood removed = 250 mg of iron; therefore, at least 40 to 80 units will need to be removed.

❑❑ **How many units of blood should be removed per week to treat patients with HHC?**

Usually 1 or 2 units/week.

❑❑ **What are the goal values for transferrin saturation, serum iron and ferritin during maintenance phlebotomy (i.e., remove 1 unit every 2 to 3 months) in patients with HHC?**

Transferrin saturation < 50%, low serum iron level and ferritin < 50 ng/ml.

❑❑ **Patients with ineffective erythropoiesis who require transfusions will have iron deposition in which liver cell populations?**

In reticuloendothelial (RE) cells as well as parenchymal cells. Secondary iron overload predominately affects storage of iron in the RE cells.

❑❑ **T/F: A gene for Wilson's Disease has been determined.**

True. ATP7B localized to human chromosome 13.

❑❑ **T/F: The Wilson's Disease gene is expressed in the liver and kidney.**

True. It is also expressed in the brain, lungs and placenta.

❑❑ **T/F: The serum ceruloplasmin is always decreased (i.e., < 20 g/L) in patients with Wilson's Disease.**

False. Remember that up to 5% of Wilson's patients will have low-normal range of serum ceruloplasmin levels.

❑❑ **What two clinical laboratory tests may be low in patients with Wilson's Disease?**

Serum uric acid and phosphate concentrations may be low reflecting the renal tubular dysfunction that may occur in untreated Wilson's disease.

❑❑ **What is the hepatic copper content per gram of dry weight of liver considered diagnostic of Wilson's Disease?**

250 μg.

❑❑ **What foods are to be avoided in patients with Wilson's Disease?**

Organ meats, shellfish, nuts, chocolate and mushrooms.

❑❑ **Up to 30% of patients with Wilson's Disease develop a side effect of D-penicillamine that necessitates a change of treatment. What are the most common side effects that would necessitate stopping treatment?**

Dermatologic-rashes, pemphigus, nephrotic syndrome, Goodpasture syndrome, myasthenia syndrome, aplastic anemia (rare), leukopenia, thrombocytopenia, systemic lupus erythematosis-like syndrome. Gastrointestinal side effects are most common but usually mild.

❏❏ **What are alternative treatments to D-penicillamine for Wilson's Disease?**

Trientine, zinc, and ammonium tetrathiomolybdate.

❏❏ **What other drug must be administered with D-penicillamine?**

Pyridoxine (Vitamin B6, 25 mg/day).

❏❏ **T/F: D-penicillamine should be stopped during pregnancy.**

False. Therapy must be continued but at a lower dose. Stopping therapy can result in significant exacerbations.

❏❏ **T/F: D-penicillamine therapy should be continued for life.**

True. After initial high doses, lower maintenance doses (0.75 to 1 g/day) are instituted.

❏❏ **How is screening performed in the siblings of Wilson's Disease patients?**

Serum copper and ceruloplasmin measurements, 24-hr urinary copper measurement and a slit-lamp examination. Children younger than 5 or 6 are usually not affected and should be rechecked at intervals over the next 5 to 10 years. Genetic screening, while currently not commercially available, will eventually become the procedure of choice.

❏❏ **What is the normal phenotype for the alleles expressing the α_1-antitrypsin protease inhibitor (Pi)?**

PiMM is normal and PiZZ results in the lowest levels of α_1-antitrypsin.

❏❏ **How common is α_1-antitrypsin deficiency?**

α_1-antitrypsin deficiency occurs in approximately 1 in 2,000 individuals.

❏❏ **Where is the abnormal gene located?**

The gene, located on chromosome 14, results in the single amino acid substitution of glutamate by lysine at position 342 leading to a deficiency in sialic acid.

❏❏ **T/F: Cirrhosis occurs in less than 20% of patients with the PiZZ phenotype.**

True. The PiZZ phenotype, in several studies, caused cirrhosis in only 12% of patients. In contrast, chronic obstructive pulmonary disease occurs in roughly 75% of these patients.

❏❏ **Do other α_1-antitrypsin phenotypes, i.e. heterozygotes, result in chronic liver disease?**

It must be remembered that certain heterozygous states can result in chronic liver disease. For instance, patients with PiSZ and PiZZ can develop cirrhosis. MZ heterozygotes usually do not develop disease unless there is some other superimposed liver condition, such as alcoholic liver disease or chronic viral hepatitis. Liver disease due to other causes may progress more rapidly in individuals who have an MZ phenotype.

❏❏ **What is an effective treatment for patients with α_1-antitrypsin deficiency?**

The only treatment for α_1-antitrypsin-related liver disease is symptomatic management of complications and liver transplantation. With liver transplantation, the phenotype becomes that of the transplanted liver. Recall that the liver is the site of production of this protease inhibitor.

❏❏ **T/F: The α_1-antitrypsin level is the best test to detect deficiency states associated with cirrhosis.**

False. The best diagnostic test is obtaining the phenotype. The level may be low-normal even in states of homozygous deficiency.

❑❑ What is the frequency of genetic hemochromatosis? Of Wilson's disease?

Genetic hemochromatosis (1 in 250 individuals); Wilson's disease (1 in 30,000 individuals).

❑❑ What is the hepatic lesion associated with cystic fibrosis?

Focal biliary cirrhosis.

❑❑ What is the most common of the acute porphyrias?

Acute intermittent porphyria (AIP) occurs in 5 to 10 per 100,000 people. Its inheritance pattern is autosomal dominant with incomplete penetrance.

❑❑ What is the enzyme deficiency in AIP?

There is a 50% reduction in porphobilinogen (PBG) deaminase activity.

❑❑ What are the major manifestations of AIP?

Derangements in the autonomic nervous system.

❑❑ What are the predominant heme by-products in the urine of a patient with an acute attack of AIP?

Porphobilinogen (PBG) and 5-aminolevulinic acid (ALA). PBG quantities are higher than ALA. These levels may be normal in between attacks.

❑❑ T/F: AIP is the only porphyria that is not associated with cutaneous manifestations.

False. AIP is one of two acute porphyrias with only neurologic findings. The other is ALA dehydratase deficiency.

❑❑ What precipitates episodes of the acute porphyrias?

Prescription or recreational drugs, particularly corticosteroids and derivative hormones. This is why diagnosis is, oftentimes, first made at puberty. Alcohol ingestion, smoking, fasting, infection, stress and pregnancy are other risk factors.

❑❑ T/F: All of the heme synthetic enzymes are expressed only in the liver.

False. Three enzyme deficiencies among the cutaneous porphyrias are expressed in the bone marrow.

❑❑ What is the most common of the porphyrias?

Porphyria cutanea tarda (PCT) is the most common of the porphyrias, usually presenting after the age of 20 years.

❑❑ What do AIP and PCT have in common?

Enzyme expression occurs only in the liver, both have autosomal dominant patterns of inheritance (the former with incomplete penetrance while the latter can be acquired), and both are the most common (the former being acute while the latter being of the cutaneous porphyrias).

❑❑ What is the typical lesion associated with PCT?

Photosensitivity-induced vesicles and bullous lesions, or blisters.

❏❏ **PCT is strongly associated with what other disorders?**

Excess alcohol intake, estrogen therapy, systemic lupus erythematosus, diabetes mellitus, chronic renal failure, acquired immunodeficiency syndrome and chronic hepatitis C. Of note, most patients have iron overload.

❏❏ **T/F: Patients with acute porphyrias are at increased risk of developing hepatocellular carcinoma.**

True. Even though hepatic involvement is variable and mild.

❏❏ **What two porphyrias are most commonly associated with liver complications?**

PCT and hepatoerythropoietic porphyria (HEP).

❏❏ **What clinical clues should lead to consideration of the diagnosis of porphyria?**

Recurrent bouts of severe abdominal pain, constipation, neuropsychiatric disturbances and typical dermatologic findings.

❏❏ **What are the two bile acid transport disorders in which a genetic defect of primary bile acid secretion is believed responsible?**

Byler's syndrome and Alagille's syndrome.

❏❏ **T/F: No medical therapy been shown to benefit patients with cystic fibrosis-related liver disease.**

False. Controlled studies have demonstrated the beneficial effects of ursodeoxycholic acid in terms of improvement in cholestasis and nutritional status.

TUMORS AND CYSTS

Thomas Schiano, M.D.

□□ **What are some paraneoplastic syndromes associated with hepatocellular carcinoma?**

Secondary polycythemia, hypoglycemia, hypercholesterolemia and, rarely, hypercalcemia.

□□ **What is the differential diagnosis of an elevated alpha-fetoprotein (AFP) in a patient with known liver disease?**

AFP levels are elevated in a number of liver diseases including viral hepatitis and in some metastatic tumors to the liver (pancreas, stomach). Levels exceeding 1000 ng/ml may be seen in the presence of fulminant hepatitis, teratomas or in yolk sac tumors. An elevated AFP level is most commonly seen in hepatocellular carcinoma with a cut off level of 300 to 500 ng/ml being strongly suggestive.

□□ **T/F: The fibrolamellar variant of hepatocellular carcinoma manifests with an elevated alpha-fetoprotein (AFP).**

False. Patients with the fibrolamellar variant of hepatocellular carcinoma are almost always young and female and are always AFP-negative. They do, however, have increased serum concentrations of vitamin B12 binding proteins and neurotensin.

□□ **T/F: In a female patient with cirrhosis and ascites, the presence of an elevated CA-125 level strongly suggests the presence of an ovarian tumor.**

False. The CA-125 level is elevated in several benign and malignant neoplasms, most commonly ovarian carcinoma. In addition, it is also frequently elevated in the presence of ascites, from any cause, in the absence of malignancy.

□□ **What carcinogens have been linked to the development of angiosarcoma of the liver?**

Previous exposure to thorotrast, vinyl chloride, arsenic, radium and inorganic copper.

□□ **What are the most common modes of presentation of an hepatocellular adenoma?**

1) Intra-abdominal catastrophe due to hemorrhage.
2) Right upper quadrant abdominal pain.
3) Discovery of a palpable liver mass.
4) Incidental discovery of a mass on hepatic imaging performed for other reasons.

□□ **What are the different histologic patterns of hepatocellular carcinoma?**

Trabecular (plate-like), pesudoglandular (pseudoacinar), compact (solid), fibrolamellar, sclerosing and encapsulated.

□□ **What unique complications occur with hepatic arterial infusion of chemotherapy for colon cancer metastatic to the liver?**

Gastroduodenal ulceration and inflammation may occur in up to 50% of patients and appears to be related to exposure of the gastroduodenal mucosa to high concentrations of the chemotherapeutic agents. Rarely, patients may develop sclerosing cholangitis-like biliary stricturing. Actual surgical morbidity and mortality are limited.

❏❏ **What is the most common cause of hepatic cysts worldwide?**

Echinococcosis (hydatid disease).

❏❏ **In the setting of hepatocellular carcinoma (HCC), how often does ascitic fluid cytology reveal malignant cells?**

Involvement of the peritoneum by HCC occurs very infrequently; thus, ascitic fluid cytology is rarely positive.

❏❏ **Why does Mozambique have the world's highest incidence of hepatocellular carcinoma (HCC)?**

The population of Mozambique has a very high incidence of hepatitis B viral infection and its soil has one of the world's highest aflatoxin B1 contents. Hepatitis B-related cirrhosis and the aflatoxin exposure appear to cumulatively increase the predisposition for HCC.

❏❏ **In what patients is ultrasound-guided percutaneous ethanol injection (PEI) a viable treatment option for hepatocellular carcinoma?**

PEI is an acceptable mode of therapy for small tumors, especially those 3 cm in diameter or less, that occur in patients unable to undergo resection. Multiple injections may be required to eliminate the tumor but they are generally well tolerated and several lesions can be treated during the same session. Lesions involving the dome of the liver are often not accessible to these injections.

❏❏ **What is the importance of portal vein thrombosis in a liver transplant candidate with known hepatocellular carcinoma?**

Though portal vein thrombosis frequently occurs in the setting of cirrhosis, it may also be due to vascular invasion by the tumor. This would constitute extra-hepatic spread of tumor and, thus, preclude transplantation.

❏❏ **What are the characteristic histologic findings of focal nodular hyperplasia (FNH)?**

FNH is most often solitary and usually subcapsular. The presence of a central fibrous scar with thin fibrous septae and abnormal arteries radiating outward is most characteristic. Portal tracts are absent but there is often bile duct proliferation within the fibrous septae.

❏❏ **What are the most important variables associated with recurrence of hepatocellular carcinoma (HCC) following liver transplantation?**

Extra-hepatic spread of tumor, micro- or macrovascular invasion by tumor, size of a single HCC > 5 cm, cumulative size of three or more HCC > 10 cm and histologic grade.

❏❏ **What predisposing factors are associated with the development of cholangiocarcinoma?**

Primary sclerosing cholangitis, Caroli's disease, choledochal cysts, chronic hepatolithiasis and liver fluke infestation.

❏❏ **T/F: Orthotopic liver transplantation (OLT) is an accepted treatment for polycystic liver disease.**

True. Afflicted patients rarely, if ever, develop symptomatic liver disease and hepatic synthetic dysfunction. However, OLT is sometimes needed as definitive treatment because of massive hepatomegaly that causes refractory abdominal pain and distention, anorexia and malnutrition.

❏❏ **What are CT scan characteristics of an echinococcal cyst?**

Echinococcal cysts are parenchymal, sharply circumscribed defects with rim enhancement and usually have calcification within the cyst wall and daughter cysts within them.

❑❑ **Apart from kidney cysts, do patients with polycystic liver disease have other organ involvement?**

Approximately 5% of patients have cysts in other viscera including the pancreas, spleen, uterus, ovaries and seminal vesicles. There is also an increased incidence of berry aneurysms in the brain.

❑❑ **From what blood vessel does a hepatocellular carcinoma (HCC) receive its entire blood supply?**

The hepatic artery (the vessel used in therapeutic embolization and chemoembolization) serves as the main blood supply of HCC.

❑❑ **What is the best evidence of a causative role for aflatoxin in the pathogenesis of hepatocellular carcinoma (HCC) in humans?**

The high frequency of a unique mutation in codon 249 of the p53 suppressor gene in HCC of patients from geographic areas of high aflatoxin contamination and its absence in HCC occurring in regions of low aflatoxin exposure.

❑❑ **T/F: The presence of small peri-hilar lymphadenopathy in patients with primary sclerosing cholangitis increases the suspicion for a malignancy.**

False. Peri-hilar lymphadenopathy is commonly seen in patients with cirrhosis due to hepatitis C and in most forms of cholestatic liver disease in the absence of a liver neoplasm.

❑❑ **T/F: A patient with cirrhosis and a liver lesion noted on CT scan has a normal alpha-fetoprotein level (AFP). This excludes hepatocellular carcinoma (HCC).**

False. A normal AFP level never completely excludes the diagnosis of HCC.

❑❑ **What complications may occur following chemoembolization of a hepatocellular carcinoma?**

Virtually all patients experience marked right upper quadrant abdominal pain, nausea, vomiting and high fevers. Additionally, all patients develop transient elevations of liver tests and a minority may develop liver abscess and liver failure.

❑❑ **How does angiography differentiate between hepatocellular carcinoma (HCC) and a simple cyst?**

On angiography, a HCC is hypervascular with prominent neovascularity and arteriovenous shunting while a simple cyst is avascular with vessels seen stretching around the cyst.

❑❑ **How does a CT scan differentiate between hepatocellular carcinoma (HCC) and a hemangioma?**

HCC appears hyperdense on CT scan with preferential filling during the arterial phase of a dynamic scan while a hemangioma enhances from the periphery inward with additional and persistent enhancement on delayed scans.

❑❑ **What is Stouffer's syndrome?**

Stouffer's syndrome refers to the constellation of constitutional symptoms and non-specific elevation of liver tests in a patient with renal cell carcinoma, in the absence of metastatic disease to the liver.

❑❑ **What are the most common sites of metastatic spread in patients with hepatocellular carcinoma?**

In decreasing order of frequency, lung, portal vein, hepatic vein, regional lymph nodes, bone, bone marrow and peritoneum.

❏❏ **What is the drug of choice to treat an echinococcal infestation?**

Mebendazole, 40 mg/kg/day.

❏❏ **For what tumors has liver transplantation carried the greatest success rate for cure?**

Hepatocellular carcinoma found incidentally at the time of transplantation. The majority of these tumors are small and singular.

❏❏ **What are the most common tumors metastasizing to the liver?**

Carcinomas of the lung, breast, colon and pancreas account for the overwhelming majority of hepatic metastases in adults whereas neuroblastoma, Wilm's tumor and rhabdomyosarcoma are most common in the pediatric age group.

❏❏ **What is the chance for recurrence of cholangiocarcinoma after liver transplantation in a patient with sclerosing cholangitis?**

The recurrence rate is extremely high. Thus, a pre-operative diagnosis of cholangiocarcinoma generally precludes liver transplantation.

❏❏ **What is a Klatskin's tumor?**

Also termed hilar cholangiocarcinoma, Klatskin's tumor occurs at the section of the common bile duct between the cystic duct junction (common hepatic duct) and the confluence of the hepatic ducts at the hilum.

❏❏ **What other conditions mimic Klatskin's tumor by causing obstruction at the hilar confluence of the liver?**

Gallbladder carcinoma, primary sclerosing cholangitis, benign biliary stricture, biliary stones or sludge and metastatic carcinoma.

❏❏ **What is Caroli's disease?**

Caroli's disease (type 5 biliary cyst) is a congenital malformation characterized by multifocal intrahepatic bile duct dilation. It may be associated with congenital hepatic fibrosis, cirrhosis and portal hypertension.

❏❏ **What renal abnormality is associated with Caroli's disease?**

Medullary sponge kidney is present in 60% to 80% of cases.

❏❏ **Hepatocellular carcinoma (HCC) occurs seldomly in what etiologies of cirrhosis?**

HCC occurs rarely in patients with autoimmune hepatitis, alpha$_1$-antitripsin deficiency and in cholestatic conditions like PBC. In contrast, HCC occurs commonly in hemochromatosis.

❏❏ **In what liver condition do macroregenerative nodules occur and why are they important?**

They are typically seen in the setting of cirrhosis. Dysplasia arising within them often predisposes to the development of hepatocellular carcinoma.

❏❏ **What is Kasabach-Merritt syndrome?**

Thrombocytopenia related to a giant cavernous hemangioma.

❏❏ **What is the most common primary hepatic tumor?**

The cavernous hemangioma, usually an incidental findings, is detected in about 1% of all autopsies. These tumors are found in all ages and in both sexes, although they are most frequently seen in adults. Large cavernous hemangiomas (> 10 cm) are best managed by surgical resection given the risk of rupture.

❏❏ **What are complications of hepatic hydatid disease?**

Complications include biliary obstruction from compression of large intrahepatic ducts, cholangitis due to rupture into the biliary tract, secondary infection and anaphylaxis from peritoneal, pleural or pericardial rupture.

❏❏ **T/F: Patients with chronic active hepatitis B (HBV) infection without cirrhosis need to be screened for hepatocellular carcinoma (HCC).**

True. HBV-viral DNA appears to integrate into the host genome resulting in malignant transformation. HCC can arise in non-cirrhotic HBV patients but it usually does not develop in patients with HCV, unless they have cirrhosis. Thus, all patients with HBV infection should be screened for HCC. Screening is not recommended in those with HCV without cirrhosis.

❏❏ **T/F: Hepatocellular carcinoma (HCC) is among the world's most common malignancies.**

True. HCC is the most common visceral cancer in the world and may be the most common cancer overall. It represents 20% to 40% of all cancers in regions of high prevalence, where the incidence may reach 150/100,000 population per year.

❏❏ **In the absence of cirrhosis, how much liver parenchyma can be removed safely during the surgical extirpation of a liver tumor?**

60% to 80%. Many patients with liver tumors have cirrhosis, however, which precludes major resections.

❏❏ **T/F: Chemoembolization prolongs survival in hepatocellular carcinoma.**

False. Chemoembolization is utilized in patients for whom surgical resection of hepatocellular carcinoma is not possible. Gelfoam or other particles along with infusion of chemotherapy are injected into the hepatic arterial system feeding the tumor, producing a temporary reduction in blood flow and more direct exposure to the chemotherapy. Though studies have regularly shown significant reduction in the size of large tumors, there is no increase in patient survival with chemoembolization.

❏❏ **T/F: An elevated carcinoembryonic antigen (CEA) level in a patient with cirrhosis strongly suggests the possibility of a colonic neoplasm.**

False. Minor elevations of CEA are seen in many patients with hepatocellular carcinoma and in cirrhosis, in general.

❏❏ **How effective is chemotherapy in the treatment of hepatocellular carcinoma (HCC)?**

HCC is in a class of tumors that is highly resistant to chemotherapy. The vast majority of responses to chemotherapeutic agents are partial and very short-lived. The impact of chemotherapy on patient morbidity and mortality is negligible.

❏❏ **What are the imaging studies of choice in diagnosing a hemangioma of the liver?**

In most cases, a hyperdense, well-defined lesion is noted on ultrasound and a corresponding confirmatory lesion is seen on sequential dynamic bolus CT scan or MRI. Scintigraphy may also be used to confirm the diagnosis of hemangioma.

❏❏ **What is nodular regenerative hyperplasia (NRH)?**

NRH is characterized by diffuse nodularity of the liver in the absence of fibrosis. It's a rare condition that may, at times, be difficult to distinguish from focal nodular hyperplasia, hepatic adenoma and hepatocellular carcinoma. It is most often an incidental finding but may present with complications of portal hypertension. NRH may be idiopathic or found in association with hematologic disorders (multiple myeloma) or collagen vascular diseases (rheumatoid arthritis).

❏❏ T/F: Oral contraceptive use is linked with the the development of focal nodular hyperplasia (FNH).

False. While the development and growth of hepatic adenomas and cavernous hemangiomas have been linked to oral contraceptive use, the same cannot be said for FNH.

VASCULAR DISORDERS

Mohammed R. Annes, M.D. and Nicholas Ferrentino, M.D.

❑❑ **What is the average total blood flow to the liver in ml/min?**

Blood flow normally ranges between 800 and 1200 ml/min. The portal vein supplies the majority of the blood (approximately two-thirds) with the hepatic artery supplying the remainder.

❑❑ **What is the approximate amount of oxygen that the liver is able to extract from the blood and how does this compare to most other gastrointestinal organs?**

The liver is relatively unique in its ability to extract oxygen from the blood - up to 95% - making it much more efficient than most gastrointestinal organs.

❑❑ **What is the proposed mechanism of ischemic reperfusion injury?**

Formation of oxygen free radicals, predominately by the enzymes NADPH oxidase and xanthine oxidase.

❑❑ **T/F: Ischemic liver diseases are more common in the elderly.**

True. While ischemic liver disease may occur at any age, it most commonly occurs in the older population. This age group is more susceptible to severe cardiac and pulmonary diseases that predispose to ischemia.

❑❑ **What are common symptoms of ischemic liver disease?**

Common complaints include right upper quadrant (RUQ) abdominal pain, nausea, vomiting and anorexia. In its mild form, ischemic liver disease may be asymptomatic and abnormalities only detected by abnormal liver tests.

❑❑ **What physical findings are common in ischemic liver disease?**

Jaundice, in approximately 40%, and hepatomegaly, in up to 95% of patients. Laboratory findings almost invariable include a marked increase in serum aminotransferases and lactate dehydrogenase and often an increase in unconjugated bilirubin (25%).

❑❑ **What is the hallmark histopathologic finding in ischemic disorders of the liver?**

Centrilobular hepatocyte necrosis.

❑❑ **What are the most common causes of Budd-Chiari syndrome?**

Etiologies include thrombosis/occlusion of the major hepatic veins, mass lesions of the major hepatic veins or inferior vena cava and mass lesions/webs located between the liver and the right atrium.

❑❑ **How many major hepatic veins drain into the inferior vena cava?**

Three.

❑❑ **Name two diseases commonly associated with vascular thromboses.**

Polycythemia rubra vera and paroxysmal nocturnal hemoglobinuria.

❑❑ **What three symptoms characterize acute, rapidly progressive Budd-Chiari syndrome?**

Hepatomegaly, RUQ pain and ascites.

❑❑ **An enlarged spleen is often found in patients with Budd-Chiari syndrome. Name two possible causes of an enlarged spleen in this disorder.**

Portal hypertension and an underlying myeloproliferative disorder.

❑❑ **What is the prognosis for symptomatic, untreated patients with Budd-Chiari syndrome?**

Poor. The average life span is from three months to three years after initial diagnosis. The patients often develop renal failure, variceal bleeding, hepatic encephalopathy and jaundice.

❑❑ **What is the prognosis for asymptomatic individuals with Budd-Chiari syndrome?**

Excellent. This suggests thrombosis of only two or three hepatic veins or adequate collateral compensation.

❑❑ **Patients often do not present acutely with Budd-Chiari syndrome. If an obstruction is established in this case, what is the treatment of choice?**

Surgical decompression of the liver via shunt surgery. In those with advanced fibrosis or cirrhosis, liver transplantation may be considered.

❑❑ **How does hepatic veno-occlusive disease typically present clinically?**

Nonthrombotic, fibrous, obliterative endophlebitis of small intrahepatic veins, originally described by Chiari, is now referred to as hepatic veno-occlusive disease. Hepatic veno-occlusive disease typically presents with hepatomegaly, ascites and weight gain.

❑❑ **Name the classic etiology of hepatic veno-occlusive disease.**

Pyrrolizidine alkaloid ingestion typically from plants used to make some herbal teas. Other etiologies include: irradiation and high-dose chemotherapy prior to bone marrow transplantation; systemic lupus erythematosis and familial immunodeficiency; and, agents such as azathioprine, cytosine arabinoside, 6-mercaptopurine, urethane and possibly oral contraceptives.

❑❑ **T/F: Serum aminotransferases are typically elevated in hepatic veno-occlusive disease.**

True (80% to 85%). Other manifestations include hyperbilirubinemia (bilirubin 15 to 20 mg/dl) and elevated alkaline phosphatase (250 to 300 IU/L).

❑❑ **What percentage of bone marrow transplant patients are thought to acquire hepatic veno-occlusive disease?**

10% to 20%.

❑❑ **What is the reported mortality rate from hepatic veno-occlusive disease in bone marrow transplant patients?**

20% to 40%.

❑❑ **What is the classic order of manifestation of signs and symptoms in hepatic veno-occlusive disease in the bone marrow transplant setting?**

Weight gain occurring 8 or 9 days following the transplant, hyperbilirubinemia in 11 to 12 days, elevated aspartate aminotransferase and alkaline phosphatase in 13 to 15 days and hepatomegaly and ascites within one to two weeks of bone marrow transplantation.

❑❑ How is the diagnosis of hepatic veno-occlusive disease made?

If the patient is status post bone marrow transplant and the clinical syndrome typical, presumptive diagnosis can be made without further studies. In less clear cases, liver biopsy is warranted. Unfortunately, these patients are usually severely thrombocytopenic complicating the performance of any invasive procedure. The transjugular approach to liver biopsy may be a less risky alternative in this situation. Ultrasound with Doppler flow study, CT scan and MRI are all options to determine hepatic vein patency to rule out Budd-Chiari syndrome.

❑❑ What are the characteristics on liver biopsy that suggest hepatic veno-occlusive disease?

The hepatic venule is typically obliterated, hepatocyte dropout is noted and sinusoidal dilation is present.

❑❑ What is the mainstay of treatment for hepatic veno-occlusive disease secondary to pyrrolizidine alkaloid ingestion?

One-half of patients recover completely with fluid and sodium restriction.

❑❑ What etiology of hepatic veno-occlusive disease is associated with a higher incidence of severe, chronic and often fatal disease progression?

Up to 25% of patients following bone marrow transplantation suffer from severe disease. Treatment includes sodium restriction, diuretics and management of complications.

❑❑ What disease is associated with "atrophic infarcts of Zahn"?

Nodular regenerative hyperplasia.

❑❑ Name three processes associated with peliosis hepatis.

Tuberculosis, AIDS and drugs.

❑❑ What are common causes of Budd-Chiari syndrome in the western world?

Hypercoagulable states and neoplasms are common causes in the western world. Membranes or webs are important causes of outflow obstruction in Asia and South Africa.

❑❑ What are causes of occlusion of the hepatic veins and the inferior vena cava?

Myeloproliferative disorders, paroxysmal nocturnal hemoglobinuria, antithrombin III deficiency, protein C and S deficiencies, neoplasms, infections, collagen vascular diseases, Behcet's disease, sarcoidosis, oral contraceptives, pregnancy, inflammatory bowel disease, cirrhosis, polycystic liver disease and idiopathic.

❑❑ Name neoplasms associated with Budd-Chiari syndrome.

Primary hepatocellular, renal, adrenal, pulmonary, pancreatic and gastric carcinomas. Benign and malignant vascular neoplasms (leiomyomas, leiomyosarcomas and rhabdomyosarcomas) arising within the hepatic veins or vena cava have also been associated with Budd-Chiari syndrome and hepatic failure.

❑❑ Describe the histological appearance of the liver in Budd-Chiari syndrome.

Acute obstruction reveals significant centrilobular congestion and dilation of sinusoids. Atrophy, necrosis and drop out of centrizonal hepatocytes with extension to periportal regions is present with severe injury. With chronic disease, complete obliteration of central veins associated with midzonal and centrilobular fibrosis with or without cirrhosis is noted.

❑❑ What is the typical clinical presentation in Budd-Chiari syndrome?

A spectrum of disease is possible, ranging from an asymptomatic state to fulminant hepatic failure or cirrhosis with associated complications. Acute obstruction is associated with right upper quadrant pain, nausea and vomiting, hepatomegaly and ascites. Jaundice and splenomegaly may be noted but are usually mild. Most patients present with a subacute course of less than 6 months and complain of vague right upper quadrant discomfort, hepatomegaly, mild-to-moderate ascites and splenomegaly. Jaundice is either absent or mild. Symptomatic disease of more than 6 months presenting as fatigue, bleeding varices, encephalopathy, coagulopathy, hepatorenal syndrome and/or malnutrition suggests chronic obstruction. Massive hepatocellular necrosis with fulminant hepatic failure is a rare manifestation of Budd-Chiari syndrome and typically follows rapid and complete occlusion of all hepatic veins. Progressive encephalopathy, coagulopathy and death are inevitable within 8 weeks of occlusion if treatment is not provided.

❑❑ What laboratory abnormalities are usually present in Budd-Chiari syndrome?

Standard laboratory investigations are rarely helpful. Twenty-five to 50% of patients with venous outflow obstruction present with either normal or mildly abnormal aspartate and alanine aminotransferases. However, patients presenting with acute disease or fulminant hepatic failure may display values greater than 1,000 IU/L, especially if there is accompanying portal vein thrombosis. In addition, serum bilirubin, alkaline phosphatase and prothrombin time are usually normal or mildly elevated.

❑❑ How would you diagnose Budd-Chiari syndrome?

Radiologic imaging and liver biopsy.

❑❑ What is the sensitivity of ultrasound in the evaluation of Budd-Chiari syndrome?

85% to 95%. The addition of Doppler to conventional ultrasound is more sensitive than real-time investigation alone.

❑❑ What is the role of the CT scan in the evaluation of Budd-Chiari syndrome?

The CT scan is helpful in evaluating abnormalities of the hepatic veins and vena cava including membranes, the extent of hepatic parenchymal disease and the presence of ascites and spenomegaly.

❑❑ What is the gold standard in the diagnosis of Budd-Chiari syndrome?

Angiography. It not only provides information regarding cause and location of obstruction but is also helpful in obtaining pressure measurements which are important for surgeons before decompression. Ideally, all patients considered for surgery should undergo angiography in addition to liver biopsy.

❑❑ What medical options exist for the treatment of Budd-Chiari syndrome?

Medical therapies, while generally ineffective, include sodium restriction, diuretics and therapeutic paracenteses. In patients who present with acute incomplete thrombotic obstruction, anticoagulation and thrombolysis are alternatives.

❑❑ Discuss the role of interventional radiology in the treatment of Budd-Chiari syndrome.

Percutaneous transluminal balloon angioplasty is an exciting and emerging therapy for hepatic outflow obstruction secondary to caval webs or hepatic venous stenosis. Initial experience suggests excellent short term results but a 2-year patency rate of 50% and 50% failure rate in the first 6 months.

❑❑ What surgical shunts are useful in the treatment of Budd-Chiari syndrome?

Decompressive shunts should be considered the standard of care for patients with acute or subacute venous occlusion. Options include 1) side-to-side portocaval shunts, 2) mesocaval shunts (for patients with compression of the retrohepatic cava by caudate lobar hypertrophy) and 3) mesoatrial shunts (for patients with caval obstruction and a significant gradient between the cava and right atrium). After surgery, long-term anticoagulation is recommended to minimize the chance of recurrent thrombosis.

❑❑ **When should liver transplantation be considered in patients with Budd-Chiari syndrome?**

1) Fulminant liver failure, 2) End-stage liver disease, 3) Patients with significant liver disease who decompensate after receiving decompressive shunts, 4) Shunt failure, and 5) Venous thrombosis attributable to protein C, protein S or antithrombin III deficiency.

VIRAL HEPATITIS

Mark E. Mailliard, M.D.

❒❒ What are the antiviral actions of interferons?

Interferons are naturally-occurring glycoproteins produced by cells in response to a variety of stimuli including viral infection. Interferons have direct antiviral effects postulated to occur through induction of cellular enzymes that interfere with viral synthesis. Inhibition of viral RNA and DNA transcription and translation is likely but unproven. In addition, interferons have immunomodulatory properties and may exert antiviral actions through augmentation of cellular immune function.

❒❒ What percentage of patients treated with interferon-alfa for chronic hepatitis will develop autoimmune thyroid disease?

Two to three percent (equal incidence of autoimmune hyperthyroidism and hypothyroidism).

❒❒ What percentage of patients will develop neuropsychiatric side effects (primarily depression) during monotherapy of chronic hepatitis C with interferon-alfa?

20%.

❒❒ T/F: It can be challenging to differentiate autoimmune hepatitis from chronic hepatitis C (HCV).

True. Low titers of antinuclear antibodies (ANA) occur in 40% to 70% of patients with chronic HCV. ANA titers of over 1:160 can occur in 20% of patients with chronic HCV. Hypergammaglobulinemia is associated with a false positive ELISA test for HCV in 20% (predominantly young women). Steroid therapy of chronic HCV will decrease alanine aminotransferase levels but elevate HCV RNA levels. Severe hepatitis can occur when autoimmune hepatitis is treated with interferon. Unless the diagnosis of HCV infection is supported by the presence of HCV RNA, steroid therapy should be the primary initial treatment choice.

❒❒ A patient with chronic hepatitis B (HBV) develops a rise in aminotransferases four weeks after initiation of interferon alfa, 5 million units daily. What should be the response of the treating gastroenterologist?

During or immediately after interferon therapy for HBV, patient responders (those that lose HBeAg and HBV DNA) frequently will develop increased ALT levels. Continued interferon therapy with close monitoring of the patient and symptomatic treatment of side effects is indicated. Because of the cost, side effects and toxicity of interferon therapy for chronic HBV, patients selected for therapy should exhibit elevated ALT, low HBV DNA and have no evidence of decompensated liver disease.

❒❒ What is the mechanism of the antiviral action of lamivudine in the therapy of chronic hepatitis B (HBV)?

Lamivudine is a nucleoside analog that inhibits viral DNA synthesis by terminating the nascent proviral DNA chain through interference of the reverse-transcriptase activity of HBV (and HIV).

❒❒ What is the incidence of the appearance of YMDD mutants in HBV patients undergoing therapy with lamivudine?

Fiteen to 35% of patients treated with lamivudine (100 mg/d) for twelve months develop escape mutations in the active site of the HBV polymerase gene (YMDD locus). This molecular virologic event is associated with an increase in ALT and reappearance of HBV DNA.

❑❑ **Scleral icterus and jaundice occur frequently in adults with symptomatic hepatitis A (HAV) infection. How can jaundice secondary to HAV differ from other acute hepatitis infections?**

Jaundice can persist for weeks to months in adults with HAV. Rarely, a syndrome of prolonged cholestasis can persist for 3 to 4 months. Relapsing hepatitis can also occur in as many as 10% of HAV patients. Cholestatic and relapsing HAV infections do not have an increased mortality.

❑❑ **What are indications for Hepatitis A vaccination?**

The candidate pool for HAV vaccination is expanding. Foreign travelers, military personnel, male homosexuals, drug abusers, institutional workers and individuals in endemic areas should be targeted. Recent attention to the morbidity of HAV infection in chronic HCV patients has led to a call for vaccination of all HCV patients. Vaccine should be given three weeks before travel. Immediate protection may be accomplished by simultaneous administration of immune serum globulin and HAV vaccine.

❑❑ **What is the clinical utility of hepatitis B core antibody?**

In acute HBV infection, IgM anti-HBc appears one month after HBsAg appears and shortly before the ALT rises. IgM anti-HBc will usually indicate acute HBV infection and is the only marker of HBV infection during the window period (after HBsAg declines and before anti-HBs appears). IgG anti-HBc persists in patients with anti-HBs and patients that develop chronic HBV with HBsAg. The clinical significance of an isolated IgG anti-HBc is unknown; however, affected individuals are not allowed to donate blood and their organ donation may be associated with transmission of HBV infection.

❑❑ **What is the significance of an HBV mutant?**

Mutations of HBV DNA replication are not unusual. The pre-core mutation involving a G to A change at nucleotide 1896 is well described. This mutation prevents synthesis of HBeAg. The presence of the A1896 mutant should be suspected in patients with elevated ALT, presence of HBsAg, absence of HBeAg and positive anti-HBe. HBV DNA should be present.

❑❑ **What is the clinical significance of a "HBsAg carrier"?**

Classically, these patients have undetectable HBV DNA, negative HBeAg, normal ALT, and have no hepatic inflammation despite the presence of HBsAg. However, HBV DNA may persist at very low levels and reactivate with liver disease if these patients receive immunosuppression.

❑❑ **What percentage of patients with hepatocellular carcinoma have cirrhosis from HCV or HBV infection?**

The prevalence of HBsAg in patients with hepatocellular carcinoma varies from country to country and ranges from 7% (United States) to 87% (Korea). Over 80% of all hepatocellular carcinoma patients have cirrhosis. Cirrhosis is a risk factor for the development of hepatoma when patients have HCV or HBV. Cirrhotic patients with HCV have a 7% risk of hepatoma at five years and a 14% at 10 years after diagnosis.

❑❑ **How is chronic hepatitis D diagnosed?**

The presence of HDV-RNA by polymerase chain reaction assay is the "gold standard" for the diagnosis of HDV infection. The presence of IgM antibody to HDV may indicate hepatic injury from HDV.

❑❑ **What is the role of liver transplantation for end-stage liver disease associated with hepatitis D infection?**

Liver transplantation in HDV infected individuals coinfected with HBV carries a much lower risk of graft reinfection than does transplantation in patients infected with HBV alone. Overall patient survival matches that for other indications.

❑❑ **What subsets of patients with end-stage HBV infection would be expected to have improved survival after liver transplantation?**

Patients with acute fulminant hepatitis from HBV, HDV coinfection or undetectable HBV DNA would have a lower incidence of graft reinfection than patients that are HBeAg positive and have HBV DNA. Long-term immunoprophylaxis with hepatitis B immunoglobin decreases the incidence of HBV graft reinfection and enhances survival in patients with evidence of pre-transplant HBV DNA.

❑❑ **Describe the pathological grading and staging scoring system for chronic hepatitis.**

Grade (inflammation)	Stage (fibrosis)
1 – minimal activity	1 – mild expansion of portal tracts
2 – mild piecemeal necrosis	2 – periportal fibrosis
3 – moderate activity with spotty lobular necrosis	3 – bridging fibrosis
4 – severe activity with piecemeal and lobular necrosis	4 – cirrhosis

❑❑ **Describe the clinical manifestations of hepatitis E virus (HEV).**

HEV causes only an acute hepatitis. Fulminant hepatitis may occur in as many as 1% to 2% and there is a remarkable increase in mortality for infected pregnant women. Its route of transmission is similar to HAV.

❑❑ **What percentage of patients with infectious mononucleosis have liver involvement?**

Approximately 90% have ALT elevations while 11% become icteric.

❑❑ **Describe the clinical spectrum of cytomegalovirus (CMV) hepatitis.**

In general, 50% to 80% of individuals have serum antibodies to CMV by age 35. CMV hepatitis in normal children and adults is usually asymptomatic and subclinical. Neonates may develop jaundice and liver failure. Primary and secondary (reactivation) CMV infections may occur in immunosuppressed patients. The diagnosis of CMV hepatitis requires IgM antibody or a rise in IgG titer and a liver biopsy. Liver pathology classically shows giant cells with intranuclear inclusions. The virus may be identified from culture of liver tissue or body fluid.

❑❑ **Fulminant herpes simplex hepatitis typically occurs only in which individuals?**

Neonates, pregnant women in the third trimester and immunocompromised patients.

❑❑ **T/F: There is no conclusive evidence to suggest that hepatitis G virus (HGV) causes acute or chronic liver disease.**

True. HGV was originally identified in patients with abnormal liver enzymes secondary to HCV infection. There is no evidence that HGV, by itself, causes any liver disease and there is no conclusive evidence to suggest that it worsens HCV in any way.

❑❑ **What are possible extrahepatic manifestations of HCV infection?**

Most likely	Possible
Cryoglobulinemia	B-cell lymphoma
Vasculitis	Sjogren's syndrome
Glomerulonephritis	Idiopathic thrombocytopenic purpura
Porphyria cutanea tarda	Lichen planus
Thyroiditis	

❏❏ **What are the genotypes and the quasispecies of HCV?**

HCV has a high mutation rate during replication. The accumulation of mutations during the evolution of HCV worldwide has led to genetic heterogeneity among isolates and at least six major genotypes (1 to 6). Quasispecies refer to the heterogeneity within an infected individual and can number greater than 100 isolates.

❏❏ **What are the major etiologies of chronic liver disease in the United States?**

HCV	26%	Alcohol	24%
Cryptogenic	17%	HCV + Alcohol	14%
HBV	11%	Other	5%
HBV + Alcohol	3%		

❏❏ **How is hepatitis A transmitted and what is its prevalence in the United States?**

Although the primary route is fecal-oral, through contaminated food or water, transmission of HAV has been documented by parenteral and sexual means via blood transfusion and homosexual activity, respectively. The prevalence of IgG antibody to HAV is 10% in children and 37% in adults.

❏❏ **T/F: The standard therapy of hepatitis A is supportive/symptomatic.**

True. Other than supportive symptomatic therapy, there is no defined protocol. There is no evidence that corticosteroids are helpful. Postexposure prophylaxis is accomplished by serum immunoglobulin (0.02 mL/kg) administered by intramuscular injection. There is also evidence to suggest that immediate HAV vaccination, by itself, may be effective in the setting of postexposure prophylaxis.

❏❏ **What are the three phases of perinatally-acquired chronic HBV?**

Initial phase: Immune tolerance – HBeAg positive, high HBV DNA level, normal ALT.

Second phase: Immune clearance – between the ages of 15 and 35, HBeAg clearance, elevated ALT, mostly asymptomatic, rare hepatic failure or cirrhosis.

Third phase: Non-replicating – HBsAg negative, loss of or very low HBV DNA, normal ALT.

❏❏ **How is the diagnosis of acute HCV infection made?**

Because anti-HCV by ELISA is often undetectable for 5 or 6 weeks, testing for HCV RNA is necessary.

❏❏ **What is the major side effect of oral ribavirin therapy for HCV?**

A dose-dependent hemolytic anemia occurs within 2 to 6 weeks after beginning ribavirin with 15% of hemoglobin tested falling 4 grams when 1200 mg per day is administered.

❏❏ **What is the difference in the natural history of HDV infection between coinfection with HBV versus superinfection of HBV?**

Only 2% of coinfections become chronic compared to 90% of superinfected patients.

MISCELLANEOUS TOPICS

BIOSTATISTICS FOR THE GASTROENTEROLOGIST

Elizabeth Lyden, M.S., Jane Meza, M.S. and James A. Lynch, Ph.D.

❑❑ **Differentiate between Type I and Type II errors in hypothesis testing.**

Type I error (false-positive): rejecting the null hypothesis when it is true; alpha is the probability of a type I error.

Type II error (false-negative): failing to reject the null hypotheses when it is false; beta is the probability of a type II error. The power of a statistical test is 1-beta.

❑❑ **In tests used for screening purposes, differentiate between sensitivity and specificity.**

Sensitivity: indicates how good a screening test is at identifying the disease it is testing for. It refers to the proportion of patients with the disease who test positive. Sensitivity can be calculated as follows: True positive/True positive + False negative × 100%.

Specificity: indicates how good a screening test is at identifying the nondiseased group. It refers to the proportion of patients without the disease who test negative. Specificity can be calculated as follows: True negative/True negative + False positive × 100%.

❑❑ **What does the positive predictive value of a screening test indicate?**

This measure is the proportion of true positives among all patients with positive test results. The prevalence of the condition in the population being tested is an important consideration when determing predictive values. The higher the prevalence of the disease in the population being tested, the more likely a positive test is predictive of the disease.

❑❑ **Calculate the sensitivity, specificity, positive predictive value, negative predictive value and prevalence from the following 2 X 2 table which shows the results of screening for *Helicobacter pylori* in detecting peptic ulcer disease (PUD) in dyspeptic patients < 45 year of age (*Lancet 1991; 338:94-96*).**

	PUD	No PUD
H. pylori positive	90	287
H. pylori negative	2	423

Sensitivity: 90 / (90 + 2) = .978 or 97.8%
Specificity: 423 / (287 + 423) = .596 or 59.6%
Positive predictive value: 90 / (90 + 287) = .238 or 23.8%
Negative predictive value: 423 / (2 + 423) = .995 or 99.5%
Prevalence: (90 + 2) / (90 + 287 + 2 + 423) = .115 or 11.5%

❏❏ Journal articles commonly provide P-values as part of the results of statistical analyses. Explain the meaning of a P-value.

The P-value is the probability of obtaining the observed study results by chance if the null hypothesis is true.

❏❏ What does a 95% confidence interval imply?

It implies that if we repeatedly select random samples from the same population as our data and construct such interval estimates, 95 out of 100 of the intervals would be expected to contain the true parameter.

❏❏ Differentiate between a two-tailed and a one-tailed test.

Two-tailed (or nondirectional) test: occurs when researchers do not know *a priori* the direction of the value they expect to observe in the sample. For example, they want to know if the sample mean differs from the population mean.

One-tailed (or directional) test: occurs when researchers know *a priori* the direction of any true difference between the value observed in the sample and the population parameter. For example, they want to know if the sample mean is larger (or smaller) than the population mean.

❏❏ Define odds ratio.

The odds ratio is the odds that a patient is exposed to the risk factor divided by the odds that a control is exposed to the risk factor.

❏❏ What does an odds ratio of 1 indicate?

An odds ratio of 1 indicates no association between a potential risk factor and the disease of interest.

❏❏ The odds in favor of disease A are twice as high in vegetarians as in nonvegetarians (i.e., odds ratio = 2). The corresponding odds ratio for disease B is 0.5. Which disease is more strongly associated with eating habits?

They are the same, only the direction of the association differs.

❏❏ Distinguish between relative risk reduction (RRR) and absolute risk reduction (ARR).

Relative risk reduction (RRR): reduction of adverse outcomes achieved by a treatment expressed as a proportion of the adverse outcomes in the placebo group.

$$\frac{(\% \text{ of control patients with bad outcome}) - (\% \text{ of treatment patients with bad outcome})}{(\% \text{ of control patients with bad outcome})}$$

Absolute risk reduction (ARR): estimates the actual decrease in adverse outcomes among patients treated with the experimental therapy.

(% of control patients with bad outcome) - (% of treatment patients with bad outcome)

❏❏ Define what is meant by the number needed to treat (NNT).

NNT is the number of patients that need to be treated with a new therapy in order to prevent one additional adverse outcome.

1 / ARR = NNT

❑❑ How are the odds ratio and the relative risk reduction (RRR) related?

1 - odds ratio approximates the RRR assuming that the frequency of bad outcomes in the placebo group is low.

❑❑ In a study comparing endoscopic ulcers among patients (who were free of ulcers at the onset of the study) with osteoarthritis who received ibuprofen 800 mg three times daily or rofecoxib 25 mg daily, results at 12 weeks show 28.5% of the patients receiving ibuprofen to have endoscopic ulcers and 4.7% of the patients receiving rofecoxib to have endoscopic ulcers (*Laine, et al. Gastroenterology 1999; 116:A229, Abstract*). Calculate the ARR, RRR and NNT (with the ibuprofen group considered to be the control).

ARR = 28.5% - 4.7% = 24% or .24
RRR = (28.5% - 4.7%) / 28.5% = .84
NNT = 1 / .24 = 4.2

❑❑ Explain the meaning of the 95% confidence interval: $(23 < \mu < 35)$.

If a large number of such confidence intervals are constructed, about 95% of them will contain the true mean. It does not mean that the probability that μ is between 23 and 35 is 95%.

❑❑ Explain the difference between an observational study and an experimental study.

In an observational study, patients are observed (no intervention is applied) and the characteristics of interest are recorded. In an experimental study, an intervention is applied and the effect of the treatment on the subjects is analyzed.

❑❑ What is a double-blind trial and what is its purpose?

The experimenter and the subject do not know whether they are in the control group or the treatment group. The purpose is to prevent the researcher from interpreting the results in a manner which supports the researchers goals, especially in a trial with a subjective outcome.

❑❑ What does concealment of allocation mean with respect to clinical trials?

Concealment of allocation means that the researcher who enrolls patients into a trial (i.e., attempts to get informed consent from the patient) does not know if the next patient to enter the trial will get the experimental treatment or a placebo.

❑❑ Differentiate between an intention-to-treat analysis and per protocol analysis.

Intention-to-treat analysis: all patients who enrolled in a clinical trial are included in the final data analysis, regardless of whether or not the patient completed the trial.

Per protocol analysis: only patients who properly complete the clinical trial are included in the final data analysis.

❑❑ Describe how to calculate the mean and the median and explain the major difference between these two measures of central tendency.

To calculate the mean (average), add up all of the observations and divide by the number of observations. The median is the middle observation when all of the observations have been ordered. The mean can be influenced by extreme data values.

❑❑ For a skewed distribution, which is a better choice as a measure of central tendency, the mean or the median? Why?

The median, since the mean can be influenced by extreme values.

❑❑ **What is the most common measure of dispersion (spread)? Name another measure of dispersion.**

The most common measure of dispersion is the standard deviation. Other measures of dispersion are range, coefficient of variation and the interquartile range.

❑❑ **Name a distribution which has a bell shape and a distribution which is skewed.**

Normal distribution and Chi-Square distribution, respectively.

❑❑ **Define the coefficient of variation.**

The coefficient of variation is the standard deviation divided by the mean times 100%.

❑❑ **An investigator is interested in comparing two numerical distributions which are measured on different scales. Should the researcher use the standard deviation or the coefficient of variation? Why?**

The investigator should use the coefficient of variation since the coefficient of variation adjusts for the scales of the variables.

❑❑ **What statistic is most often used to describe the relationship between two numerical variables?**

Correlation coefficient.

❑❑ **For two variables X and Y, the correlation coefficient is $r = .89$. How does this describe the relation ship between X and Y?**

Since r is positive and close to 1, as the values of X increase, the values of Y tend to increase. In this case, we say that X and Y are positively correlated.

❑❑ **For two variables X and Y, the correlation coefficient is $r = .05$. Does this mean that X and Y are not correlated? Why or why not?**

No. The correlation coefficient r measures the *linear* relationship between X and Y. Since r is close to 0, we can only say that X and Y are not *linearly* correlated. They may, however, be correlated in some manner which is not linear.

❑❑ **The results from an experiment indicate that the probability that a person has blood type A is .45. What is the probability that a person does not have blood type A?**

$1 - .45 = .55$

❑❑ **Differentiate between the life-table method and the Kaplan-Meier method of calculating estimates of the survival distribution.**

Life-table method: the time axis showing the total observation period or follow-up time is divided into distinct intervals (not necessarily of equal length) and the number of deaths and withdrawals (censored patients) are shown for each interval. This method is useful when the exact times of death or withdrawal are unknown.

Kaplan-Meier method: exact times of death and withdrawal must be known as calculations are made at each time of death. Similar to the life-table method, the survival curve will resemble a step function; curves constructed by the Kaplan-Meier estimate will step down at each time of death.

❑❑ **Define median survival.**

Median survival is defined as the time at which 50% of the population under study has "failed" (died, progressed, relapsed, etc.).

❑❑ **The results from an experiment indicate that the probability a person has blood type A is .45 and blood type B is .11. What is the probability that a person has blood type A or blood type B?**

.45 + .11 = .56

❑❑ **T/F: The events described in the previous question are mutually exclusive.**

True. Mutually exclusive events are events that cannot occur simultaneously. These two events are mutually exclusive since a person cannot have both blood type A and blood type B.

❑❑ **Describe what it means for two events to be independent.**

Two events are independent if the outcome of the first event does not effect the outcome of the second event.

❑❑ **A study is designed so that every member of the population has an equal probability of being selected for the study. What sampling method is being used?**

Simple random sampling.

❑❑ **A researcher is interested in the following hypothesis test:**
$H_0: \mu \leq 0$
$H_1: \mu > 0$
Is this a one-tailed or a two-tailed test?

This is a one-tailed test. This can be determined by examining the alternative hypothesis. For this test, the null hypothesis is rejected if μ is sufficiently *greater* than zero. The hypothesis test $H_0: \mu = 0$ vs. $H_1: \mu \leq 0$ is an example of a two-tailed test since the null hypothesis is rejected if μ is sufficiently greater than zero *or* if μ is sufficiently less than zero.

❑❑ **A researcher is interested in the following hypothesis test with a .05 level of significance ($\alpha = .05$):**
$H_0: \mu \leq 0$
$H_1: \mu > 0$
The P-value is found to be .03. What is the conclusion of the test?

The P-value is the probability of obtaining a result as extreme or more extreme than the result obtained from the sample when the null hypothesis is assumed to be true. The P-value rule is to reject H_0 (Do not accept H_0) if the P-value is less than α and accept H_0 (Do not reject H_0) if the P-value is greater than or equal to α. Since the P-value is .03 and $\alpha = .05$, the conclusion is reject H_0 (Do not accept H_0).

❑❑ **How is the power of this type of test defined?**

The power of a test is the probability of rejecting the null hypothesis when in fact the null hypothesis is false.

❑❑ **A researcher is interested in the following hypothesis test with significance level .05 ($\alpha = .05$):**
$H_0: \mu = 0$
$H_1: \mu \neq 0$
The 95% confidence interval for μ is: ($-2.3 \leq \mu \leq 1.5$). What is the conclusion of the hypothesis test?

Since zero is included in the above confidence interval, zero is one of the likely values for μ. In other words, it is possible that in fact $\mu=0$. Therefore, the conclusion is accept H_0 (or Do Not Reject H_0).

❑❑ **What is meant by a nonparametric test?**

Nonparametric tests do not specify the distribution of the data. In other words, they are distribution-free tests.

❑❑ **The equation of the regression line for two variables X and Y is:**
Y = 12 - .9X
Are X and Y positively or negatively correlated. How do you know?

X and Y are negatively correlated. You can tell by examining the regression equation to see that as X increases, Y decreases.

GASTROINTESTINAL AND HEPATOBILIARY MANIFESTATIONS OF HIV AND AIDS

Themistodes Dasopoulos, M.D. and Eli D. Ehrenpreis, M.D.

❑❑ **What portions of the gastrointestinal tract may be involved in HIV-infected patients?**

The human immunodeficiency virus can affect any area of the gastrointestinal tract from the mouth to the anus. In addition, the liver, pancreas and biliary tree may be involved. In the intestines, HIV viral proteins and organisms can be seen in lymphocytes and macrophages of the lamina propria.

❑❑ **What is the most common presenting gastrointestinal symptom in HIV-infected patients?**

Diarrhea. Prevalence rates of 50% to 90% have been recorded. There are multiple etiologies of the diarrhea that occurs in HIV-infected patients including infections, neoplasms and direct viral effects.

❑❑ **According to the Centers for Disease Control and Prevention, what are the six gastrointestinal disorders that, along with HIV seropositivity, constitute an AIDS-defining illness?**

1) Esophageal candidiasis.
2) Cryptosporidosis.
3) Cytomegalovirus colitis, enteritis or hepatitis.
4) Herpes simplex virus ulcers or esophagitis (all for greater than one month).
5) Kaposi's Sarcoma (KS) in a patient younger than 60.
6) Disseminated *Mycobacterium avium* (MAI) or *Mycobacterium kansaii*.

❑❑ **What causes oral hairy leukoplakia?**

Epstein Barr virus (EBV). Oral hairy leukoplakia appears as white plaques that coat the lateral aspects of the tongue.

❑❑ **What is the most common infection of the small bowel in patients with AIDS?**

Cryptosporidiosis. This protozoa causes a self-limited diarrheal illness in normal hosts. However, in patients with AIDS, this infection can cause severe diarrhea (up to 17 liters of stool/day), malabsorption and weight loss. The disease course is worse with increasing degrees of immunodeficiency. While paromomycin may decrease protozoal load, there is no cure and treatment is aimed at controlling symptoms and immunologic improvement.

❑❑ **What measure can patients with CD_4 counts < 200 take to decrease infection with *Cryptosporidium*?**

Boil water. This eliminates oocytes.

❑❑ **In HIV-infected patients, name a treatable protozoal infection of the small bowel.**

Isospora belli. This infection is endemic in the Caribbean and South America. It can be treated with sulfonamides or pyrimethamine. Some patients develop recurrent infections.

❑❑ **An HIV-positive patient with chronic diarrhea undergoes small bowel biopsy. On electron microscopy, a "cat's eye" appearance of the enterocyte nucleus with a supranuclear indentation is noted. What is the cause of the diarrhea?**

The appearance of the nucleus is caused by a merozite indicating infection with microsporidium, probably the species *Enterocytozoon biensui*. This species accounts for about 80% of all microsporidial infections and is often refractory to treatment. *Encephalitozoon intestinalis* makes up the other 20% of microsporidial infections. It is responsive to albendazole but may become disseminated.

❑❑ **What is the most common viral infection that causes diarrhea in AIDS?**

Cytomegalovirus (CMV). The infection may be limited to the right side of the colon in up to 30% of patients.

❑❑ **What are unique complications of CMV enteritis and colitis?**

Mucosal ischemic ulceration and perforation. Patients may present with an acute abdomen. CMV enteritis or colitis should be suspected in this clinical setting in a patient with AIDS.

❑❑ **What is the initial treatment of choice for intestinal CMV infection?**

Ganciclovir. Patients may need central line placement for daily treatment which usually lasts for three to four weeks. This approach is effective in approximately 75% of treated patients. If relapse occurs, the patient may need long-term maintenance treatment. Prior to treatment, the patient should undergo ophthalmologic examination because CMV retinitis is an indication for lifelong therapy.

❑❑ **What is the most significant side effect of treatment with ganciclovir?**

Bone marrow suppression. AZT has potentiating effects on drug-induced neutropenia. Foscarnet is an alternative choice to ganciclovir and is less expensive and similar in efficacy. It causes renal toxicity and electrolyte disturbances (hypocalcemia, hypomagnesemia, hypophosphatemia). Use Foscarnet with caution in those being treated with pentamidine.

❑❑ **What enteric bacteria is AIDS-defining when recurrent infection occur in a patient with HIV?**

Salmonella. Infection with this organism is known for complications such as bacteremia and arthritis.

❑❑ **What is an unusual feature of bacterial enteridites in patients with AIDS?**

Relapse with discontinuation of treatment. This may occur as a consequence of the antibiotics being unable to reach intracellular organisms or ineffective killing of organisms by the host. Some antibiotics like ciprofloxacin exhibit good intracellular penetration.

❑❑ **What antibiotic should be considered first-line therapy when used as empiric treatment in an ill-appearing HIV patient with acute diarrhea?**

Ciprofloxacin. Use this initially pending culture results.

❑❑ **T/F: *Clostridium difficile* is an important pathogen in HIV-infected patients.**

True. The incidence of *C. difficile* in this population is increased due to the frequent use of antibiotics and increased amount of time spent hospitalized. The clinical course of *C. difficile* infection is more severe in immunocompromised patients.

❑❑ **How do the presentations of gastrointestinal *Mycobacterium tuberculosis* (MTB) and *Mycobacterium avium intracellulare* (MAC) in HIV-infected patients differ?**

MAC is the most common mycobacterial infection in patients with AIDS. MTB usually causes symptomatic illness and generally affects the ileocecal region. MAC usually presents as an asymptomatic infection, most commonly in the duodenum. Alternatively, massive small intestinal infiltration with MAC may cause diarrhea and malabsorption. MTB has been associated with the formation of fistulae, perforation and occasionally intussusception.

❑❑ **T/F: Octreotide plays a major role in the management of chronic diarrhea in patients with AIDS.**

False. Octreotide is a somatostatin analogue that acts as an antisecretory and anti-motility agent. Some research suggests that HIV shares amino acid sequences with vasoactive intestinal peptide (VIP), thus, upregulating the VIP receptors and contributing to chronic HIV-associated diarrhea. Octreotide has been postulated to interfere with this mechanism. Nevertheless, a recent randomized, placebo-controlled trial failed to show any benefit of octreotide as treatment of HIV-infected patients with chronic diarrhea.

❑❑ **What malabsorptive disease can *Mycobacterium avium*-complex (MAC) infection of the gastrointestinal tract mimic?**

Whipple's disease. After the atypical mycobacterium are ingested from contaminated water, they are phagocytosed by macrophages but are not killed. They invade tissues causing lymphadenopathy and organomegaly. In the gut, they invade the wall impairing lymph flow and causing fat malabsorption and exudative enteropathy. Histologically, foamy macrophages are seen in the small intestinal lamina propria. These are indistinguishable from Whipple's disease; however, an acid fast stain will show numerous acid fast organisms in the case of MAC.

❑❑ **How does *Mycobacterium avium*-complex cause peritonitis?**

Liquefaction necrosis. An abdominal lymph node may necrose and result in peritonitis.

❑❑ **What is the difference in presentation between diarrhea of small bowel origin and of colonic origin?**

Small bowel diarrhea is usually high volume and associated with nausea, cramps and flatulence. It is typically worsened by food ingestion. Increased frequency, small volume stools, lower abdominal pain and urgency are more suggestive of a colonic origin.

❑❑ **What initial single stool test strongly suggests the presence of a colonic source of diarrhea?**

Fecal leukocytes.

❑❑ **What are important limitations of barium-contrast radiography in HIV-infected patients?**

Findings are often nonspecific and nondiagnostic. Additionally, barium studies must be done after stool studies have been collected because barium may interfere with microscopic stool examinations.

❑❑ **Describe a rational step-wise approach to the evaluation of chronic diarrhea in patients with AIDS.**

The optimal approach remains controversial. Initially, multiple stool samples should be obtained. If non-diagnostic, consider sigmoidoscopy (or colonoscopy with biopsies of the terminal ileum) and/or upper endoscopy with small bowel biopsy. These tests may provide a diagnosis in an additional 50% of cases. A serum D-xylose test may be helpful in distinguishing between small intestinal and colonic sources of diarrhea; however, it is seldom necessary.

❑❑ **What is the AIDS wasting syndrome?**

The loss of greater than 10% of body weight in 6 months with no identifiable infectious or neoplastic cause.

❑❑ **What is the most significant cause of weight loss in AIDS patients without gastrointestinal symptoms?**

Decreased caloric intake. Stable weights are often punctuated by episodic short-term weight loss when patients develop opportunistic infections. In addition, altered energy expenditure and adrenal insufficiency may contribute.

❑❑ How do you perform a D-xylose test? How do you interpret the results?

Twenty-five grams of D-xylose is administered orally and a serum level drawn 1 hour later. A one-hour serum D-xylose value of less than or equal to 20 mg/dl indicates the presence of small intestinal malabsorption. Studies indicate that a value of less than 13 mg/dl has a positive predictive value of 83% for the AIDS wasting syndrome and a positive predictive value of 92% for death within one year. This may indicate patients in need of early aggressive nutritional supplementation.

❑❑ What cytokine has been associated with the AIDS wasting syndrome?

Tumor necrosis factor. This cytokine may cause anorexia, weight loss, fat metabolism and an increase in triglycerides.

❑❑ All patients with HIV disease should have what vitamin level checked because of a high prevalence of deficiency?

Vitamin B12. In a landmark paper on the subject, Harriman *et al.* found a 15% prevalence of vitamin B12 deficiency in an unselected group of patients with AIDS and a 7% prevalence in asymptomatic HIV infection. In AIDS patients with chronic diarrhea, the prevalence of B12 deficiency may be as high as 39%.

❑❑ What mechanisms are responsible for the development of vitamin B12 deficiency in HIV-infected patients?

The most important mechanism is ileal absorptive dysfunction. Additional factors include achlorhydria (causing decreased liberation of food-bound cobalmin), decreased intrinsic factor secretion, bacterial or parasitic overgrowth in the small bowel and pancreatic insufficiency.

❑❑ What percentage of HIV-infected patients have esophageal complaints?

About 33%.

❑❑ What is the most frequent esophageal infection in patients with AIDS?

Candida albicans esophagitis. Cytomegalovirus and herpes simplex virus esophagitis are second followed by idiopathic esophageal ulceration.

❑❑ What area of an ulcer would you biopsy to detect herpes simplex virus (HSV)? Cytomegalovirus (CMV)?

Biopsy the edge (area of viral replication) of the ulcer to detect HSV and the ulcer base (CMV does not invade squamous epithelium) to detect CMV.

❑❑ What name is given to an ulcer seen on endoscopy in an HIV-infected patient with histopathology showing no viral cytopathic effect and no clinical or endoscopic evidence of reflux or pill-induced ulceration?

Idiopathic esophageal ulcer. These ulcers often present with odynophagia and substernal chest pain and may be deep and multiple in number. Ninety percent respond to oral or intralesional steroids. They also appear to be responsive to thalidomide.

❑❑ What is a "double-barrel esophagus?"

Idiopathic esophageal ulcerations may result in the formation of fistulous tracts. When the fistula is esophageal-esophageal, it is referred to as a "double-barrel esophagus." Other fistulae may include mediastinal or broncho-esophageal fistulae.

❑❑ **What is the empiric treatment for a patient with HIV who is complaining of dysphagia without odynophagia and who has oral thrush on exam?**

Fluconazole. The presumptive diagnosis is esophageal candidiasis. Up to two-thirds of patients with candidal esophagitis have oral thrush.

❑❑ **Why is ketoconazole less effective than fluconazole in the treatment of candidiasis?**

The absorption of ketoconazole and itraconazole is pH-dependent – requiring an acid pH for absorption. Achlorhydria has been well described in HIV infection. Concomitant use of H2 blockers or proton pump inhibitors is common in HIV-infected patients and also decreases absorption. Absorption of fluconazole is not pH-dependent.

❑❑ **What is the most common cause of pancreatitis in patients with HIV/AIDS?**

Drug-induced. Common offending agents include pentamidine, didanosine and occasionally trimethoprim-sulfamethoxazole. Less common causes include infections, alcohol and, rarely, lymphoma or Kaposi's Sarcoma.

❑❑ **T/F: Pancreatic toxicity from pentamidine causes hypo- and hyperglycemia.**

True. Direct toxicity to the pancreatic islet cells causes insulin release and low blood sugar levels. Hyperglycemia occurs later as insulin deficiency worsens.

❑❑ **T/F: An increase in amylase always indicates pancreatitis in patients with AIDS.**

False. Patients with increased amylase levels may have macroamylasemia, a condition which has been reported in HIV infection. Macroamylasemia occurs when amylase complexes with immunoglobulins or other serum proteins. This complex is cleared poorly by the kidneys. Diagnosis is confirmed by low urine amylase levels. Serum amylase values greater than three times the upper limit of normal increase the specificity for acute pancreatitis, particularly in the setting of clinical symptoms suggestive of pancreatitis.

❑❑ **Anorectal carcinomas are associated with what infections in homosexual patients with HIV infection?**

Human papillomavirus types 16 and 18. A CD_4 count less than 500 is an independent risk factor.

❑❑ **What is the most common cause of drug-induced hepatomegaly in HIV-infected patients?**

Sulfonamides. AZT and didanosine have also been reported to cause hepatomegaly. These drugs are thought to act as mitochondrial toxins. Most patients with AIDS have an incidental finding of steatosis on liver biopsy.

❑❑ **What percentage of AIDS patients have drug-induced liver disease?**

8%.

❑❑ **What is the most common hepatic pathogen in AIDS?**

Mycobacterium avium-complex. The hallmark of this infection is poorly formed granulomas with acid fast staining organisms located within foamy macrophages.

❑❑ **What tumor seen in HIV infection is made up of spindle cells and originates from lymphatic endothelial cells?**

Kaposi's Sarcoma. This submucosal tumor may be found in up to 10% to 15% of HIV-infected individuals. In the alimentary tract, Kaposi's Sarcoma typically occurs as bulky gingival or palatal lesions, or gastrointestinal lesions resulting in difficulty with chewing, swallowing and obstruction to flow, respectively. Rarely, it is a cause of gastrointestinal bleeding.

❑❑ **What percentage of patients with cutaneous Kaposi's Sarcoma have gastrointestinal or hepatic involvement?**

33%. These are usually asymptomatic.

❑❑ **A 43 year-old HIV-infected man complains of abdominal pain. He has a fever, lymphadenopathy, skin angiomas, hepatomegaly and lytic bone lesions. What is the most likely diagnosis?**

Bacillary peliosis hepatis. Caused by *Bartonella henselae*, this infection causes dilated vascular lakes and blood filled spaces within the liver. It is the fourth-leading cause of abnormal liver tests and hepatomegaly in AIDS patients. It is treated with erythromycin or doxycycline.

❑❑ **What are the five most common causes of abnormal liver tests and hepatomegaly in patients with AIDS?**

Mycobacterial infection, drug-induced, cytomegalovirus, bacillary peliosis hepatis and lymphoma

❑❑ **What is AIDS cholangiopathy?**

This syndrome resembles sclerosing cholangitis and papillary stenosis. Patients present with upper abdominal pain and increased serum alkaline phosphatase levels. Occasionally, transaminase elevations are also seen. This syndrome usually results from infection with *Cryptosporidium*. Other potential causative organisms include cytomegalovirus and microsporidiosis.

❑❑ **How does the pattern of liver enzyme elevation assist in the diagnosis of HIV/AIDS-related disease?**

The elevation of aminotransferases is nonspecific and common. The pattern and extent is not useful to correlate with a specific diagnosis. An impressive rise in the alkaline phosphatase without extra- or intrahepatic obstruction is strongly suggestive of infection with *Mycobacterium avium*-complex.

❑❑ **T/F: HIV increases the risk of sexual transmission of Hepatitis C virus.**

True. HIV also increases the vertical transmission of HCV from mother to child.

❑❑ **How does HIV effect Hepatitis B infection?**

HIV-infected patients have a decreased response to hepatitis B vaccination and a decreased response to interferon-alfa. They also have an increased risk of reactivation and increased development of chronic disease after acute infection. Liver damage with chronic disease is less severe in these patients.

❑❑ **What is the most common cause of ascites in patients with AIDS?**

Lymphoma. Other common causes include tuberculosis, atypical mycobacterial infections, disseminated fungal infections, disseminated *Pneumocystis* and non-AIDS-related causes.

❑❑ **T/F: Primary gastrointestinal fungal diseases are common in patients with HIV/AIDS.**

False. Fungal infections typically occur as part of a disseminated infection causing chronic fever, anorexia, nausea, vomiting, hepatomegaly and abnormal liver tests. Histoplasmosis and coccidiomycosis are among the more common infections seen.

❑❑ **What is the most common cause of nausea and vomiting in HIV/AIDS patients?**

Medications.

❑❑ **What is the most common cause of odynophagia in HIV/AIDS patients?**

Esophageal ulcers – usually viral.

❑❑ **A 37 year-old man with AIDS presents with severe anorectal pain associated with defecation? What is the most likely cause?**

Ulceration of the anal canal - usually associated with herpes simplex virus or cytomegalovirus infection.

❑❑ **What is the relationship between inflammatory bowel disease and AIDS?**

An idiopathic colitis resembling ulcerative colitis that responds to steroid therapy has been described in patients with AIDS. Cytomegalovirus enterocolitis may develop in patients with ulcerative colitis or Crohn's disease. Remission in patients with Crohn's disease has been reported to occur after infection with HIV.

GASTROINTESTINAL AND HEPATOBILIARY DISORDERS IN PREGNANCY

Carolyn McIvor, M.B.B.S.

❑❑ **What is the risk of relapse of ulcerative colitis in a patient with inactive disease during pregnancy and the puerperium?**

The same as it is in the non-pregnant state. The most likely times for relapse of inflammatory bowel disease during pregnancy are the first trimester and the post-partum period.

❑❑ **What medications should be stopped when a female patient with inflammatory bowel disease is contemplating or has become pregnant?**

Sulfasalazine and other 5-ASA drugs are considered safe to use during pregnancy (pregnancy category B). Metronidazole has potential risk to the fetus, especially if used in the first trimester (pregnancy category B except in first trimester when it is not approved). Corticosteroids carry a slight risk of fetal malformations. Ciprofloxacin (pregnancy category C) and cyclosporine (pregnancy category C) also carry risk, although the absolute magnitude is not known. Cyclosporine should be avoided when breast feeding. Recent reports have suggested that azathioprine and 6-mercaptopurine may be safe to use during pregnancy; however, they are pregnancy category D. Methotrexate (pregnancy category X) and cyclophosphamide (pregnancy category D) should not be used. Of course, the ultimate decision to use any of these medications during pregnancy depends upon the severity of the patient's disease and their clear understanding of the potential risks, benefits and alternatives of these therapies. The risk of using these agents must be weighed against the benefits of preventing a flare during pregnancy. Often the greatest risk to the fetus and the mother is inappropriate and precipitous withdrawal of maintenance medications which may then result in a flare of disease that is difficult to control.

❑❑ **What dietary micronutrients are needed in much greater amounts during pregnancy?**

Nutrient	Recommended Daily Intake	Add This in Pregnancy/Lactation
Riboflavin	0.6mg/1000kcal	0.3-0.5mg
Niacin	6.6mg niacin equivalents/1000 kcal	2 to 5 niacin equivalents
Pyridoxine	1.6 to 2.0 mg	1mg
Folic acid	3µg/kg	400µg
Vitamin B_{12}	2µg	0.2-0.6µg
Ascorbic Acid	60mg	10mg (pregnancy), 35mg(lactation)
Iron	15mg	15mg
Zinc	0.6mg/1000kcal	0.3-0.5mg

❑❑ **What is the most frequent cause of an acute abdomen in pregnancy?**

Acute appendicitis (1 in 2000) occurs most frequently followed by ovarian cysts with torsion, rupture or hemorrhage, intestinal obstruction and acute cholecystitis.

❑❑ **Why should a normal appendix found at laparotomy during pregnancy not be removed?**

Removal of a normal appendix has been associated with a tripling of the risk of fetal loss.

❏❏ **T/F: Nausea and vomiting occurring without an underlying infectious or surgical cause is a serious risk to the fetus.**

False. Even in hyperemesis gravidarum, with appropriate treatment, there is no increase in toxemia, spontaneous abortion, low birth weight or deformity. In fact, the incidence of fetal death is lower than normal in mothers with nausea and vomiting during pregnancy.

❏❏ **What features distinguish hyperemesis gravidarum from the more common nausea and vomiting that occurs during early pregnancy?**

Fluid and electrolyte disturbance and/or nutritional deficiency (reduction of 5% or more in body weight) in addition to intractable vomiting.

❏❏ **What important conditions are associated with an increased incidence of hyperemesis gravidarum?**

Multiple pregnancies and hydatidiform mole.

❏❏ **What is the significance of new onset nausea and vomiting occurring in the third trimester of pregnancy?**

Serious pathology is more likely to be occurring. Disorders to consider include acute fatty liver of pregnancy, hyperthyroidism, acute abdomen, gallbladder/biliary disease, acute viral hepatitis and serious gastrointestinal and urinary tract infections.

❏❏ **What are the indications for liver biopsy in suspected acute fatty liver of pregnancy?**

Elevated aminotransferases, usually 200 to 500 IU/L, with no other obvious cause.

❏❏ **What is the most common cause of upper gastrointestinal hemorrhage during pregnancy?**

Mallory-Weiss tear, followed by erosive esophagitis.

❏❏ **What gastrointestinal motility disturbances may occur during pregnancy?**

1) Abnormal esophageal motility with increased nonpropulsive motor activity and decreased contraction wave amplitude and velocity.
2) Decreased lower esophageal sphincter pressure.
3) Prolonged transit through the stomach and small bowel.
4) Prolonged intervals between interdigestive small bowel myoelectric complexes.
5) Gastric dysrhythmias.
6) Slower colonic transit.
7) Slower gallbladder emptying.

❏❏ **What antisecretory medications are safe for use during pregnancy?**

H_2 receptor antagonist are probably safe and are pregnancy category B. Proton pump inhibitors have been used in pregnancy but safety has not been clearly established. They should only be used if the benefit outweighs the potential fetal risk. Lansoprazole is pregnancy category B while omeprazole is pregnancy category C. While not really antisecretory medications, antacids and sucralfate are safe to use during pregnancy.

❏❏ **When is cholecystectomy safe during pregnancy?**

Open cholecystectomy carries a definite but small risk to the fetus but less so in the first and second trimesters. Laparoscopic cholecystectomy is promising but should, in general, not be performed after mid-pregnancy.

❑❑ **What features are associated with a higher risk of nausea and vomiting of early pregnancy?**

Primigravid status, younger age, nonsmokers, obesity, less than 12 years of education, previous nausea with oral contraceptive use and corpus luteum primarily on the right side of the uterus.

❑❑ **What are abdominal causes of acute volume loss (with or without abdominal pain) during pregnancy?**

1) Ruptured ectopic pregnancy.
2) Placental abruptio placenta.
3) Ruptured liver.
4) Ruptured splenic artery aneurysm.

❑❑ **What causes of pancreatitis may be exacerbated during pregnancy?**

Gallstones are increased in incidence during pregnancy although pancreatitis is rare.
Pregnancy may worsen underlying hypertriglyceridemia and precipitate pancreatitis.
Hyperparathyroidism may first become manifest during pregnancy and cause pancreatitis.

❑❑ **What is the cause of acute granulomatous peritonitis in pregnancy or the puerperium?**

Rupture of fetal contents into the peritoneum or meconium spillage during cesarean delivery.

❑❑ **What are the excess energy requirements during pregnancy (kcal/day)?**

Pregnancy increases energy requirements by 300 kcal/day during the second and third trimesters. Lactation increases energy requirements by 500 kcal/day.

❑❑ **List the cholestatic disorders of pregnancy.**

Hyperemesis gravidarum, intrahepatic cholestasis of pregnancy, acute fatty liver of pregnancy, pre-eclampsia and HELLP (hemolysis, elevated liver tests, low platelets) syndrome.

❑❑ **What is the cause of the increased rate of spontaneous abortion after exploratory laparotomy in pregnancy?**

Twenty-five percent of exploratory laparotomies in pregnancy result in spontaneous abortion. The risk of spontaneous abortion is related to the extent of the underlying process.

❑❑ **Why is acute appendicitis more hazardous to the mother during pregnancy than in the non-pregnant state?**

Local perforation may be contained by the uterine wall on one side and result in premature delivery with free perforation and generalized peritonitis after the uterus empties and pulls away from the appendiceal abscess.

❑❑ **T/F: An ileostomy precludes a vaginal delivery.**

False. However, active perianal disease at the time of delivery in a patient with Crohn's disease is an indication for cesarean section.

❑❑ **What are the risks to the pregnancy when Crohn's disease is active at the time of conception?**

Increased rates of spontaneous abortion and premature delivery.

❑❑ **T/F: Active Crohn's disease is a relative contraindication to pregnancy.**

True. Only one-third of women with active disease at the time of conception achieve remission during pregnancy.

❑❑ **What presentations of gallstone disease are common during pregnancy? Which are rare?**

Biliary colic and acute cholecystitis are common; jaundice and acute pancreatitis are rare.

❑❑ **At what stage of pregnancy is pancreatitis most likely to occur?**

During the third trimester and the postpartum period.

❑❑ **What effect does Crohn's disease have on fertility?**

Current evidence supports the view that subfertility occurs in both males and females with Crohn's disease. The etiology of this subfertility is not entirely clear. There are obvious organic factors such as sulfasalazine and oligospermia and anatomical problems such as occluded fallopian tubes. There is also a 'voluntary' component independent of these factors that may relate to advice to avoid pregnancy or fears of pregnancy or sexual intercourse. Fertility appears to be normal in patients with ulcerative colitis.

❑❑ **T/F: The use of enemas is contraindicated during pregnancy.**

False. There is no evidence that therapeutic enemas for ulcerative colitis or Crohn's disease causes premature labor or other harm during pregnancy.

❑❑ **What is the most morbid form of acute viral hepatitis in pregnancy?**

Acute Hepatitis E is associated with up to 20% mortality in women during the third trimester of pregnancy. Fulminant hepatic failure in the third trimester has multiple causes including Hepatitis E, acute fatty liver of pregnancy and herpes simplex hepatitis.

❑❑ **What are typical features of fulminant hepatic failure due to herpes simplex occurring during the third trimester of pregnancy?**

Normal or near normal bilirubin at presentation, fever and upper respiratory symptoms.

❑❑ **T/F: A history of Budd-Chiari syndrome precludes a subsequent normal pregnancy.**

False.

❑❑ **T/F: Hepatomegaly is normal during pregnancy.**

False.

❑❑ **What risks are associated with pregnancy in women with chronic liver disease?**

Exposure of the infant to the disease-inducing agent can be a problem. Alcohol is teratogenic and causes fetal alcohol syndrome. Hepatitis B may be transmitted to the infant and active and passive immunization of the infant at birth is indicated. There is a small risk of transmission of Hepatitis C to infants of infected mothers. The risk of Hepatitis C transmission rises dramatically when there is coinfection with HIV. Other than direct teratogen exposure, there is no increased risk of congenital anomalies in infants of mothers with chronic liver disease. There is, however, an increase in maternal problems and increased risk of prematurity or stillbirth.

❑❑ **T/F: Cesarean section should be performed in all pregnant women with chronic hepatitis B.**

False. Appropriate immunoprophylaxis of the infant after delivery is sufficient.

❑❑ **T/F: Immunoprophylaxis of hepatitis B is necessary for the infants of e antigen negative, hepatitis B surface antigen positive mothers.**

True. While on average the risk of transmission is lower in this group, it is still significant.

❑❑ What treatments of chronic liver diseases may be continued during pregnancy?

The effects of interferon-alfa on pregnancy are unclear. Successful pregnancies during interferon monotherapy have been reported. Ribavirin is teratogenic and should not be used during pregnancy. Low-dose azathioprine to maintain remission in autoimmune chronic active hepatitis is recommended as flare-ups of disease are likely if therapy is stopped. Ursodiol for primary biliary cirrhosis is probably safe for continued use during pregnancy. Therapy for Wilson's disease with penicillamine should be continued during pregnancy because of the major risks to the mother if it is withdrawn and the relatively minor risks to the fetus.

❑❑ T/F: Pregnancy is contraindicated in patients with chronic cholestatic liver diseases.

False. Cholestasis may worsen but can be managed and usually returns to baseline after delivery in primary biliary cirrhosis, Dubin-Johnson syndrome and the familial intrahepatic cholestatic syndromes such as Alagille's syndrome.

TRAVEL MATTERS IN GASTROENTEROLOGY

Martin E. Gordon, M.D., FACP, FAAAS

☐☐ **An Ivy League swim team traveled to Key West, Florida to practice for the regional meets. Workouts were intense and fatiguing but worth the fun of seeing the sights, eating at the local street restaurants and enjoying the night life. Following ingestion of a tropical seafood dish, the team captain was seized with chest pain, nausea, vomiting, abdominal pain and dizziness and nearly collapsed. Upon arrival to the Emergency Department, the attending physician asked two astute questions: "Did the hot fish dish taste cold" and "Did he feel flushed?" Which of the following is most likely: the chef forgot to cook the food, ciguatera fish poisoning or scromboid poisoning?**

Ciguatera poisoning. The reversal of taste sensation is diagnostic of ciguatera poisoning. Large carnivorous tropical fish such as grouper, amberjack, red snapper, barracuda and sea bass commonly harbor the toxin which cannot be detected by odor, taste or color. As more scuba divers and oil riggers stir the coral reefs, toxic dinoflagellates such as *Gambierdiscus taxicus* enter the food chain. The enterotoxin activity seems to be mediated by intracellular calcium, not by cyclic AMP or cyclic GMP, and stimulates intestinal fluid secretion without causing mucosal damage. The neurotoxic sequelae of paresthesias and motor weakness can be prolonged for months to years. Priapism and painful erections have been reported by the Royal Navy Medical Unit. Orthostatic hypotension appears to be related to both parasympathetic excess and sympathetic failure. Travelers are especially at risk in such popular destinations as the Caribbean and Pacific Islands.

Scromboid poisoning results from bacterial decomposition of a fish surface, when there has been inadequate cold storage and spoilage, resulting in conversion of histidine to histamine. The histamine sensitivity reaction, characterized by flushing and anaphylactoid symptoms, is well-known. A peppery taste to the fish is frequently noted.

☐☐ **The Port of Miami hosts over three million cruise ship passengers annually, each vulnerable to other passengers carrier states and the chef's indescretions. On the sixth day of one particular cruise, 200 passengers became ill with nausea and vomiting. Match the most likely causative organism with the iced buffet choice:**

1. Sea-food mix salade
2. Choice of international cheeses
3. Chicken salad supreme
4. Chef Edward's custard delight
5. Sunshine stir-fries on a bed of rice

a. *Vibrio parahemolyticus*
b. *Listeria monocytogenes*
c. *Campylobacter* species
d. *Staphylococcus aureus* enterotoxin
e. *Bacillus cereus* preformed toxin spores

1=a, 2=b, 3=c, 4=d, 5=e.

☐☐ **A ship surgeon, moonlighting on a luxurious ship featuring only first class accommodations, recognized that an ongoing food-related gastroenteritis outbreak would make some passengers seriously ill. Which of the following passengers is vulnerable: a day trader who spends most of the trip at the bar insisting that his associations with both Alcoholics Anonymous and Gamblers Anonymous were totally worthless; a wealthy passenger who boasts that he donates a pint of blood to the Red Cross monthly; a woman, five months pregnant, with a history of hepatitis B and drug abuse; or, a gourmon who exhausted the supply of Tabasco sauce on his daily Oyster's Rockefeller appetizer?**

All are vulnerable. The excessive oyster eater is especially vulnerable to Hepatitis A, *Vibrio vulnificus* and *Cryptosporidium parvum*. A single oyster or mollusk can filter > 14 liters of estuary water which is subjected to adjacent sewage outlets. The oocysts of the latter remain on the gills and may be found in commercial harvesting sites.

Excessive iron in specific tissues and cells promotes the development of infection, neoplasia, cardiomyopathy, arthropathy and various endocrine and possibly neurodegenerative disorders. To contain and detoxify the metal, hosts have evolved an iron-withholding defense system; however, the system can be compromised by numerous factors. Iron can contribute to disease development in several ways. Excessive amounts of the metal in specific tissues and cells can hinder the ability of proteins, such as transferrin and ferritin, to prevent accretion of free iron. Moreover, in infectious diseases, inflammatory diseases and illnesses that involve ischemia and reperfusion, iron causes reactions that produce superoxide radicals. Iron can also increase disease risk by functioning as a readily available essential nutrient for invading microbial and neoplastic cells. Highly virulent strains possess exceptionally powerful mechanisms for obtaining host iron. Markedly invasive neoplastic cell strains can glean host iron more easily than less malignant strains or normal host cells.

❏❏ **A venture capital executive has spent the last year traveling internationally. He returns to your city complaining of girth distention and you detect ascites. What potential viruses, parasites, fungi, bacteria and ingestants may be responsible for the ascites?**

Hepatitis B, C; Clonorchiasis, Opisthorciasis, Filariasis, Echinococcosis, Fasciolopsis Buski, Schistosomiasis; Anthrax, Tuberculosis; and, Gordo-lobo-yerba tea toxicity.

❏❏ **As a consultant in gastroenterology, you are frequently asked to assist in the diagnosis and treatment of constipation, ileus or intestinal obstruction. Exposure to various organisms may alter your approach. What two protozoal conditions are often overlooked causes of the above-mentioned conditions?**

Amebiasis due to *Entamoeba histolytica* and Chagas Disease due to *Trypanosoma cruzi*.

❏❏ **A forestry graduate student, who went canoeing in the canadian northwest territory during the summer semester break, was evacuated by helicopter because of fever reaching 105 degrees and rigors. A prominent leukemoid reaction was noted as was a normal erythrocyte sedimentation rate. Which of the following reservoir wild-game hosts most likely resulted in this student's illness: brown bear served at the campfire dinner; carnivorous mammals, such as native dogs and wild boar, which made ideal rifle practice targets; or, huge rats that were feeding from the camp garbage?**

All the animals mentioned are potential vectors for *Trichinella spiralis*. A leukemoid reaction with a normal sedimentation rate is unique to trichinosis. The first manifestations of trichinosis are gastrointestinal, heralded by diarrhea and abdominal cramps, in over 58% of cases. In this patient, medium-rare bear steak, cooked over a campfire, had been ingested. The ingested third-stage larvae are released in the acid-pepsin gastric environment, pass into the small bowel crypts and eventually migrate to the striated muscles where they stimulate the host DNA to build a muscle cell membrane - encysting within striated muscle fiber bundles. Large amounts of glycogen are stored in the larvae and permit long term survival. The liver contributes nutritional substances for the early stage larvae and mild liver enzyme changes may occur transiently.

❏❏ **A scuba diver on NPH insulin was so intrigued with St. Thomas' coral reef fauna that he missed the tour group's final banquet. He barely made the departure of their return flight two hours later. During the flight, he experiences the sudden onset of abdominal pain and dyspnea followed by collapse and seizures. What happened and should the aircraft's crew perform an emergency landing?**

At least 24 hours are strongly recommended after scuba diving before undertaking air travel. Nitrogen gas expansion, related to Boyle's law and often be overlooked by clinicians, may result in an insufficiency of mesenteric and cerebral blood flow. In this case, the occurrence of the seizure would compel rapid descent of the aircraft.

❏❏ **During an eco-tour trip to Australia's aborigine tribes, refreshments were taken at a native stand at the base of Ayer's Red Rock. One month later, while back in the United States, a group** member developed fever, myalgias and unrelenting back pain. He was noted to have hepatosplenomegaly and mild liver function abnormalities did not resolve for weeks. A third-year clinical clerk, who noticed a persistent leukopenia, carefully questioned whether a specific canned beverage was taken at the Red Rock, thereupon solving the diagnostic dilemma. Which of the following beverages may have caused this patient's disease: Boomerang Cola; Wallabee Beer; Ayer's Refreshing Milk; or, Grandmother's Green Tea-For-Two?

Brucellosis is an often overlooked condition when consumption of raw milk or cheeses is not assessed. In this case, the goat's milk was not pasteurized and was the vehicle for the disease. A granulomatous reaction within the liver parenchema may persist for months. Diagnostic liver and/or bone marrow biopsies may be helpful. Treatment with doxycycline and/or rifampin or gentamicin is often curative provided therapy is continued for at least 6 weeks in order to prevent relapse.

❑❑ A 78 year-old man with peptic ulcer disease decided to spend his discretionary funds on a worldwide trip lasting 8 months. His gastroenterologist stopped his proton pump inhibitor, recognizing that his patient would have been vulnerable to which of the following diseases: shigellosis, giardiasis, cholera, salmonellosis, tuberculosis, or enterotoxigenic *E.coli*?

All are correct except shigellosis.

❑❑ A university-sponsored trip to the Galapagos Islands featured an overnight stay in a three-star Ecuadorian pension "for shopping and eating unique native dishes". Several trip members developed diarrhea but responded to treatment with Pepto Bismol and ciprofloxacin. Two months later, one member became aware of "noodles in my underwear." Name the likely cause and your treatment.

Ninety-eight percent of travelers commit dietary indiscretions within the first three days of a foreign trip and diarrheal occurrences are proportional to the mistakes. Cestodiosis is rampant in this area of South America and *Taenia saginata* is most likely. Roadside treats are frequently sold by natives who have a greater than 60% infection carrier rate. A party dish, steak tartare, not infrequently enjoyed in the United States, has been responsible for many embarassing and distressing episodes. The treatment for beef tapeworm (*Taenia saginata*) is niclosamide - chew 2 grams (4 tablets) then 2 tablets per day for six more days. Pork tapeworm (*Taenia solium*) may produce neurocysticercosis and seizures 20 years after the initial infection. The treatment is praziquantel 50 mg/kg. t.i.d. for 14 days. An alternative treatment is albendazole – 15 mg/kg for 30 days.

❑❑ Several travelers returning from sightseeing in the Andes complain to you, their trusted gastroenterologist, of fatigue, anorexia and nausea and liver enzymes are elevated. Before you invoke "jet-lag," you recall that both Hepatitis A and B vaccines were administered before the trip. However, you learn that ceviche, a native dish made from snails and raw seafood and overflowing with limes was "tried" by the group. You also learn that diarrhea during the trip was treated with an "herbal diarrhea medicine" that is also used by the natives for cough. What do you suspect?

Had you not given the prophylactic immunizations for hepatitis, the native dish would be a common source of viral hepatitis. The liver dysfunction may be due to "Gordo-lobo yerba tea," which, like germander and comfrey teas, contains pyrrolizidine alkaloids. Veno-occlusive liver disease may follow.

❑❑ An affluent Egyptian exporter is referred to you by his personal physician for treatment of a sigmoid polyp. An unresolved right middle lobe lung lesion does not deter you from proceeding with a polypectomy since you are confident that they may be related. After treatment, eight Egyptian relatives of the exporter request your knowledgeable advice and expertise. Why?

Schistosomal inflammatory colonic polyps appear grossly similar to hypertrophic and even adenomatous lesions. Suspecting the associated pulmonary lesion was part of a *S. mansoni* infection, treatment with praziquantel 20 to 30 mg/kg x 1 probably precluded the ordering of many unneeded studies.

❑❑ Your colleague, a pediatrician, refers a 10 year-old Vietnam refugee for treatment of intermittent diarrhea, anemia and lethargy. Your careful examination did not disclose a coin lesion. His growth was retarded but neither pallor nor rectal prolapse were found. You order a stool culture and stool concentrates for ova and parasites and perform a flexible sigmoidocopy. What mixed infection is likely?

Growth retardation is common when hookworm and *trichuris trichuria* coexist. Suspect trichuriasis or shigellosis when rectal prolapse is found. Purpuric coin-like skin lesions are often seen after treatment by natives.

❑❑ A 58 year-old phyto-pharmacologist had all necessary immunizations before embarking on an assigned 12 month expedition to the central Brazilian Amazon river area, seeking exotic plant candidates for his biotechnical company. He returned feeling fatigued, with occasional ill-defined chest discomfort and an awareness that a good steak "didn't sit well." On your examination, sentinel cervical adenopathy was absent and an occasional ectopic beat was noted on cardiac examination. Stool and chest x-ray exams were normal. Which of the following is most likely: esophageal carcinoma; functional esophageal spasm related to his company's downsizing; or, Chagas Disease with esophageal motor dysfunction and early apical myocardial infiltration by *Trypanosoma cruzi*?

Over 90 million individuals are at risk for Chagas Disease. Increasing travel to the Andes and, especially Brazil and Peru, enhance the risk. Co-infection with HIV can increase the blood parasitemia. Transmission of *Trypanosoma cruzi* in blood transfusions add to the risk. Verapamil has had a variable response in the treatment of the chronic esophageal neurodysfunction but is beneficial in increasing myocardial blood flow.

❑❑ A student entemologist presented complaining of fevers, an acute onset of a retrobulbar headache, nausea, vomiting, intense back pain and a transient blanching rash. The fever was intermittent and diphasic. She had been collecting arthropod species in the hills of Jamaica for her graduate thesis. Upon return, a Student Health physician at a well-known Texas university commented that he was seeing other students with a similar syndrome. What did he have in mind?

Dengue Fever, now transmitted by the Asian Tiger mosquito (*Aedes albopictus*), has been found in old discarded tires, styrofoam cups and stagnant waters. Approximately 40% of the world's population live in disease-endemic areas and dengue outbreaks have occurred in more than 100 countries. Its spreading presence in Texas and the southwestern United States may become a serious threat. Infected persons usually have high fever, chills, frontal headache, characteristic blanching rash, severe myalgias and malaise. A diphasic temperature is seen in the alpha-virus infections of the Bunyavirus group, as in dengue. Lysis of the fever may occur after the second bout of continuous fever.

❑❑ A 7 year-old boy you had previously treated successfully for malabsorption due to giardiasis was brought to the emergency department because of the acute onset of nausea and vomiting followed by lethargy. A confusional state, fever and mild neck stiffness were noted. Your questions to the apprehensive parents regarding potential exposures revealed a local swimming area where wooden ladders are immersed. Immediate initiation of a life-saving treatment demonstrates your skills as a clinician. What is the diagnosis?

Primary amebic meningoencephalitis is caused by the free-living amebae of the genera Naegleria species - *fowleri, gruben* or *acanthamebae*. The organism is found in shallow ditches, in water-saturated pool mats and near rotting boards because the high carbon dioxide environment is ideal for its growth. The organisms are thermophilic and thrive adjacent to power dams and quarries where hot water discharges from generators are attractive to both swimmers and the organisms. Death ensues rapidly if treatment is not given with 24 hours. Amphotericin B 1 mg/kg/day administered intravenously must be given for an uncertain time period.

❑❑ You are caring for a young computer software developer with inflammatory bowel disease who has required a prolonged course of corticosteroids. She is planning a trip to China. You agree that she can bike in a limited area of southwest China with her companions but suggest that she use permethrin-treated bednets to reduce the chance of developing malaria. During the trip, unusual fatigue followed by persistent vomiting and fever followed by a grand mal seizure suddenly abort her trip and necessitate an air evacuation to you, her trusted physician. Name the measures that could have prevented this outcome?

Japanese encephalitis vaccine prophylaxis and use of permethrin-saturated clothing to repel the Culex and Anopheles mosquitoes. Japanese encephalitis is the leading cause of viral encephalitis in Asia and is a potential threat to the 2 to 3 million United States citizens who travel or live in south and east Asia. The Biken monovalent Japanese encephalitis vaccine is seldom given unless outbreaks are reported; however, the 25% mortality and neurological deficits that accompany this disease warrant these preventitive measures, especially before prolonged rural trips to Myanmar (Burma), Malaysia and Lao People's Democratic Republic.

❑❑ **A 36 year-old Language Professor decided to finish her scholarly text in a Chinese province where her fluent Mandarin would be helpful. Her cultural interactions during her stay at the lakeside home of her host were most welcomed, especially eating their very prevalent water-borne vegetable delights. Upon return, her annual gynecologic exam detected ascites and weight gain. Referral to which of the following specialists would be most efficient in establishing the diagnosis: radiologist, oncologist, gastroenterologist or hepatologist?**

Gastroenterologist. *Fasciola hepaticus*, like most liver flukes such as *Clonorchis senensis* and *Opisthorchis viverrini* infect and reside in the biliary tract. The brown leaf-like fasciola fluke may be visualized on cholangiography. Fascioliasis, contracted from water vegetation, often produces a right upper quadrant "hot sensation," hepatomegaly and ascending cholangitis. Raw fish ingestion may lead to clonorchiasis that presents as pancreatitis. Cholangiography may detect the characteristic sacculated and dilated biliary tree of opisthorchiasis. Cholangiocarcinoma has been found in 30% of areas in Thailand where raw fish dishes are frequently consumed.

❑❑ **A couple, both retired physicians, take two cruises a year as rewards for their labors. Seasickness on a prior trip to the Aegean and Adriatic Seas prompted them to carry seasickness patches and antihistamines in their medicine kits. An unexpected storm in the Bermuda triangle was threatening. Four hours after a black tie dinner that same evening, his wife was found on the deck with a 4 cm forehead laceration. She had vomited copiously, was flushed and confused. The left pupil was dilated and fixed but she had no other abnormal neurological signs. Her lungs were clear to auscultation and percussion. Her husband insisted to the captain that the trip could be completed after a special maneuver. What was done?**

A transdermal scopolamine patch can be very effective for the prevention of seasickness but striking anticholinergic reactions are occasionally seen. Removal of the patch resulted in the return of a normal pupillary size within 12 hours. The journey was uninterrupted.

❑❑ **Profuse diarrhea and weight loss have not responded to medications previously prescribed for a 36 year-old "green card-carrying" Guatemalan employed as a housemaid. Because of the high prevalence of a particular water contaminant in her country, you suspect the correct diagnosis and, thus, prevent excessive loss of her meager salary by avoiding extensive testing. Which of the following is most likely?**

1) *Helicobacter pylori* **infection contracted during a recent trip to her Peruvian relatives.**
2) *Necator americanis* **contracted from walking barefoot in the muddy soil near her previous home.**
3) *Leptospira canicolaris* **associated with the domestic presence of dogs and the heavy mountainous rainfall.**
4) *Cryptosporidium parvum* **from drinking the well-water dispensed by a rubber hose.**
5) *Cyclospora cayetanensis.*

Cyclospora cayetanensis in Guatemala is very prevalent. Outbreaks have occurred following the North American importation and eating of Guatemalan raspberries. The source of contamination of the implicated raspberries has not been established. Fecal contamination of water used for spraying fungicides and other substances directly on the fruit seems most likely. In North America, patients have been infected with cyclospora by eating fresh raspberries, pesto dishes and mesclun lettuce. In Guatemala, the main vehicle of infection appears to be untreated water.

❑❑ **A hospital medical aid is seen in the Emergency Department two hours after a Christmas party because of an acute onset of excruciating abdominal pain associated with sweating and collapse. She intermittently used antacids and H$_2$ receptor blockers for heartburn. Narcotics were withheld despite the pleading of the patient. Other staff members recalled the many meat, poultry and fish**

stations at the party and the patient's obvious preference for the fish station. What is the most likely diagnosis?

Evaluating adventurous eating events or assessing intimate contact with pets, vectors and environmental exposures need not be confined to the vulnerable "World Traveler". Today's popular sushi and sashimi bars are attracting a variety of raw fish choices as well as patrons. The gustatory culprit in this case was the *Anisakis simplex* larvae imbedded in the Japanese sushi containing Skip Jack Tuna, sea eel and squid. The nematode larvae was first recognized in Netherland herring and global reports have increased exponentially. Deceptive clinical manifestations include granulomatous strictures mimicking Crohn's ileitis, transmural eosinophilic gastroenteritis and gastric tumors. In one recent report, United States west coast market fish lots averaged eight nematodes per fish while east coast market fish averaged less than one. Blast freezing of fish to -35 degrees Celcius for 15 hours is a safeguard for those that do not cook their fish thoroughly. Extraction by endoscopic forceps, as in this case, gives immediate relief. Eschewing the ingestion of raw fish is the best prophylactic measure!

❐❐ **You are seeing a 49 year-old pediatric dentist who had previously been seen by four different psychiatrists because of intractable "gaseous bloating" that had precluded sleep for many months. This distress had aborted his usual quarterly skiing trips in Colorado. He denied any appreciable diarrhea. A subtotal gastrectomy scar was evident. While he vented his anger and frustrations, you decide what the diagnosis might be and schedule a single diagnostic test to be performed on his day off. What is the definitive test that subsequently led to a cured patient and earned many other patient referrals?**

While repeated stool examinations for cysts or trophozoites of giardia may be unrevealing, direct duodenal sampling or slide examination of the mucous adherent to the extracted string of an enterocapsule may be immediately diagnostic. An enterocapsule "string test," seldom utilized nowadays, may conveniently assess for the presence of motile microorganisms such as nematodes or protozoa that reside in the duodenum (96% success rate). His exposure to daycare children, his gastrectomy status and the frequent ski trips each made him especially vulnerable to giardiasis. The pathogenesis of gut injury remains incompletely understood, however a cascade of abnormalities, including immunologically-mediated functional and structural enterocyte injury that impair absorption, occur.

❐❐ **Five weeks after spending a hectic month in Brazil arranging a major bank loan while also dining in the finest restaurants, a 56 year-old chief executive officer became aware of malaise, low-grade fever, mild mucoid diarrhea with flatulence and right lower quadrant aching. A 10-pound weight loss was attributed to resuming his morning workouts. After your evaluation, laboratory testing revealed fecal "green-tinted crystals" and a hypochromic microcytic anemia. Which of the following are correct?**

a) **A colonoscopy would aid in the diagnosis.**
b) **The persistent mucoid discharge suggests a right sided colonic lesion.**
c) **Ameboma, chronic appendiceal abscess, Crohn's ileitis and tubercular or yersinea infections are all diagnostic considerations.**
d) **A limited trial of medical therapy, while avoiding alcohol, is justified before surgical intervention.**

All are correct. A constricting cecal ameboma associated with colonic ulcerations was visualized on colonoscopy. These regressed on metronidazole and paromomycin therapy with negative biopsies two months later. Pineapple crystals display a greenish tinge with long acicular forms and are often mistaken for Charcot-Leyden and fatty acid crystals. The simple use of a flurochrome, calcoflor compound as a wet mount will enhance the detection of not only amebic cysts but filamentous fungi, microsporidia and *Pneumocystis carini*. During invasive amebiasis, the host's mucosal surface produces anti-amebic IgA and cytotoxic T-lymphocytes and lymphokine-activated macrophages are mobilized. The subsequent undermining of the submucosa leads to the familiar flask-shaped ulcer characteristic of amebic colitis.

PICTURE GALLERY

James L. Achord, M.D. MACG, FACP, Michelle O. DiBaise, PA-C, MPAS and Cory A. Roberts, M.D.

❑❑ **A 60 year-old man presents with moderate hematemesis but is hemodynamically stable. An endoscopic view just below the cardioesophageal junction is shown below What is your diagnosis?**

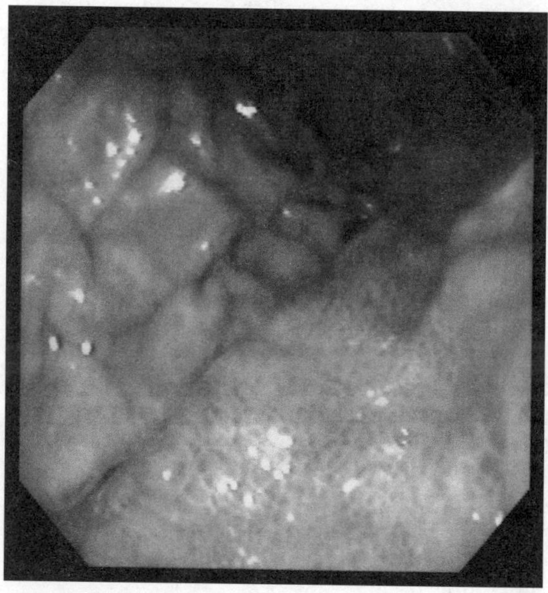

Adenocarcinoma of the stomach.

❑❑ **A 45 year-old woman presents with massive hematemesis. Shown below is the endoscopic view. What is your diagnosis and, given the findings, what is the likelihood that she will bleed again within the next few days?**

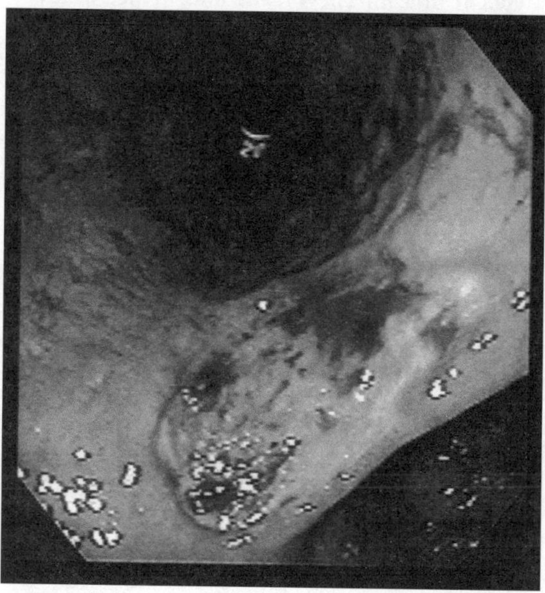

Gastric ulcer in an NSAID user. With a visible vessel, the likelihood of rebleeding within three days is 40% to 60%.

❑❑ **A 35 year-old man presents with massive hematemesis and anemia but active hemorrhage seems to have stopped promptly. What does the figure show?**

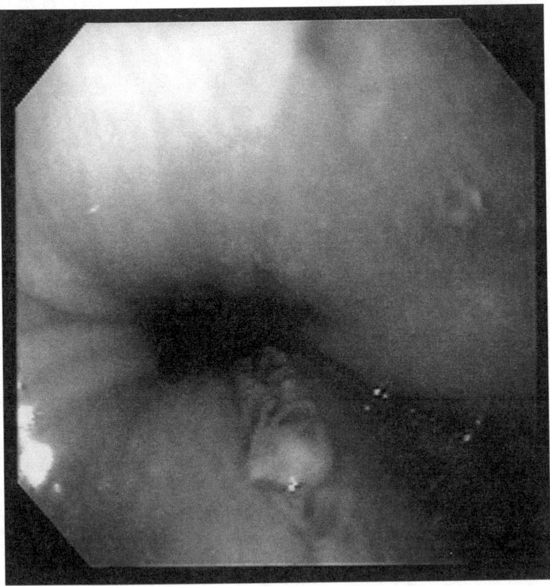

Mallory-Weiss tear.

❑❑ **A woman with melena was treated for 12 hours with nasogastric suction, blood transfusions and an intravenous histamine-2 receptor antagonist. When hemodynamically stable, upper endoscopy was performed and showed the lesions below What is your diagnosis?**

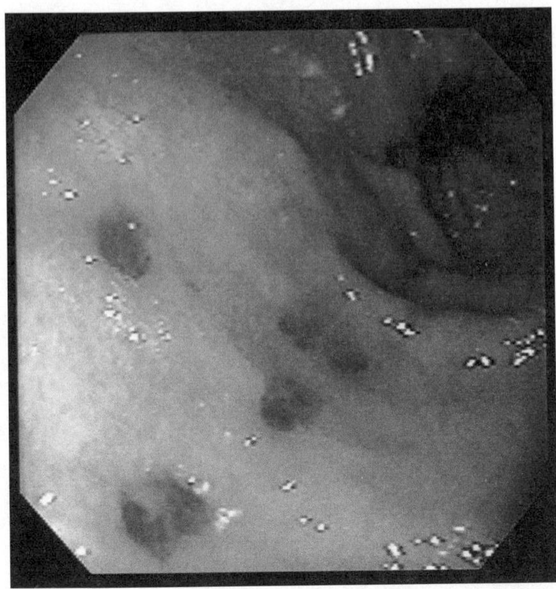

Suction injuries due to constant nasogastric suction. Obviously, this was not the cause of the melena.

❏❏ **T/F: Below is an endoscopic photograph from a patient who presented with hematemesis. This patient is an appropriate candidate for early discharge (from the ER or hospital).**

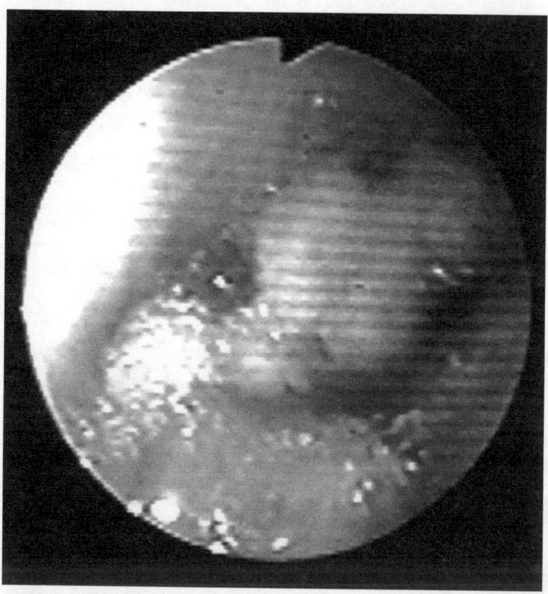

False. A visible vessel is present and predicts rebleeding in about 40% to 60% of patients, usually within 48 to 72 hours.

❏❏ **A 35 year-old woman presents with hematemesis. On upper endoscopy, a duodenal ulcer was found. What is the lesion in the esophagus?**

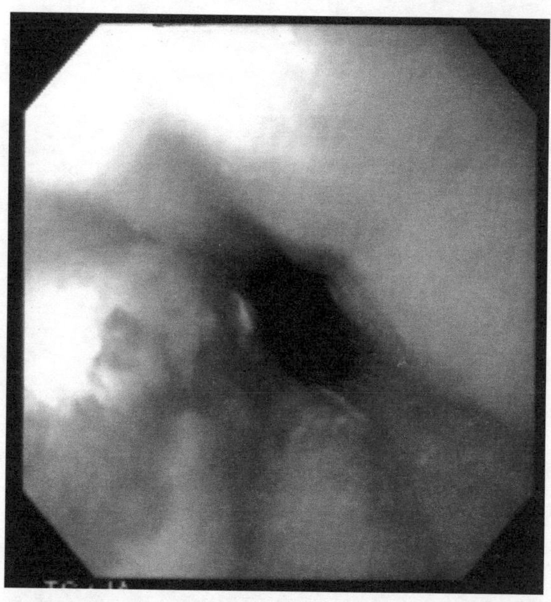

Barrett's epithelium. A biopsy would be necessary to confirm our endoscopic impression.

❑❑ **A 40 year-old man who receives hemodialysis for renal failure bleeds intermittently but significantly. On colonoscopy, the following lesion is seen in several areas. What is it? How is it treated?**

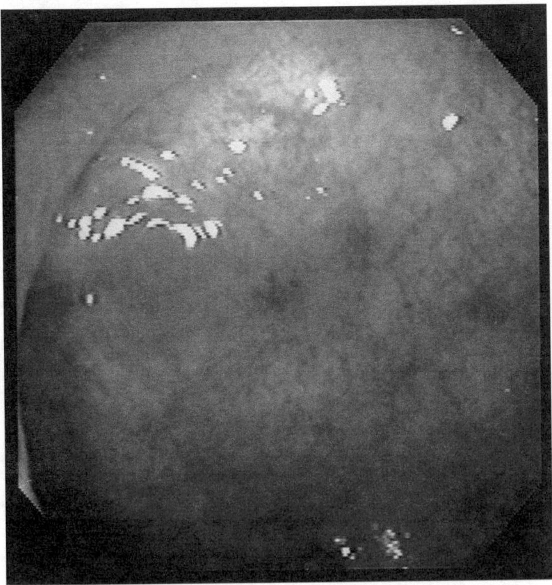

Angiodysplasia of the colon, commonly called arteriovenous malformation (AVM). Several endoscopic, angiographic and surgical methods are available to obliterate these lesions. Electrocautery, in the form of heater probe, seems to be the most popular method currently.

❑❑ **A patient presents with iron deficiency anemia and a 15 pound weight loss. He abuses nonsteroidal anti-inflammatory drugs. What is the gastric lesion shown below?**

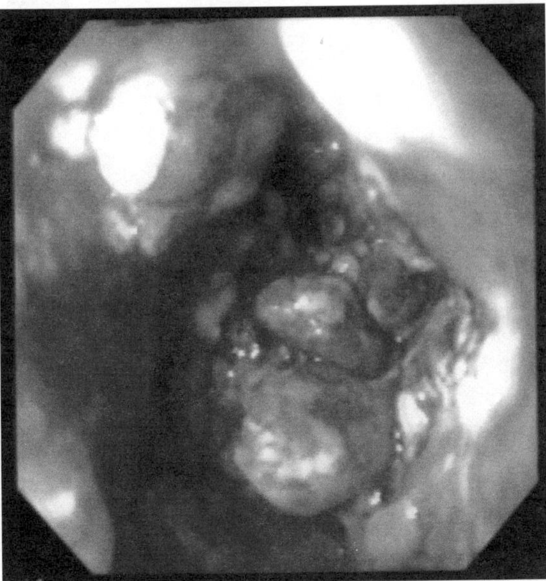

Carcinoma of the stomach.

❑❑ A patient appears in the emergency room stating that he passed "a lot" of gross blood the day before without any other symptoms. His hematocrit is 22%. What is the lesion seen below? Is it the source of his bleeding?

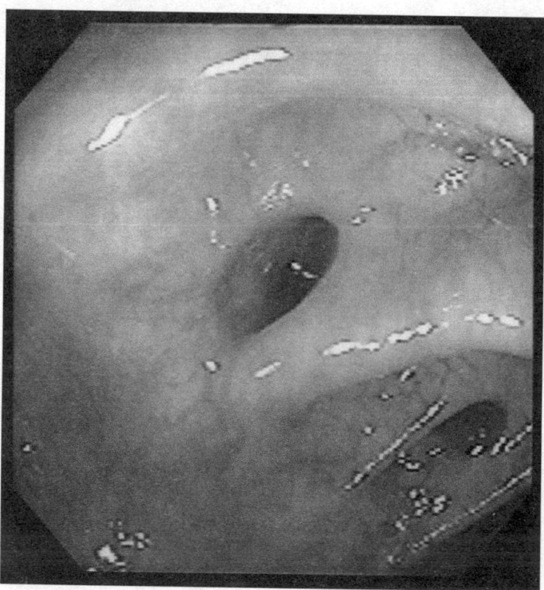

Diverticulosis. In the absence of any other demonstrable lesions, diverticulosis must be assumed to be the cause of the hemorrhage.

❑❑ A patient gives a history of intermittent painless hematochezia, always following defecation of a normal colored stool, and often with several drops of blood dripping into the commode. There is usually blood on the toilet tissue after defecation. What is the lesion shown below?

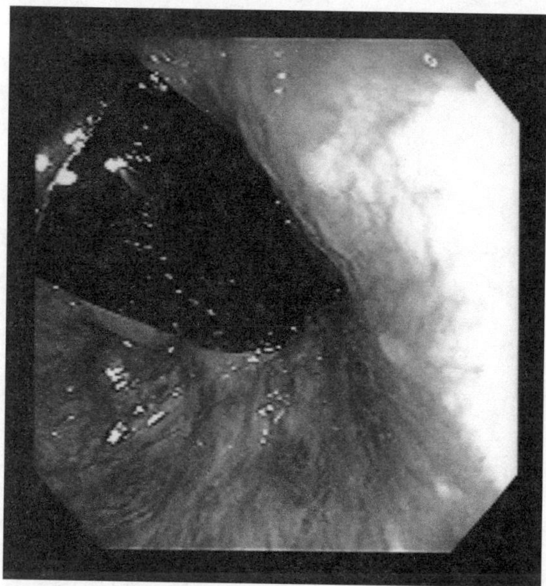

Internal hemorrhoids. An anal fissure should be considered in those who present with hematochezia and painful defecation.

❑❑ **What is the lesion shown below?**

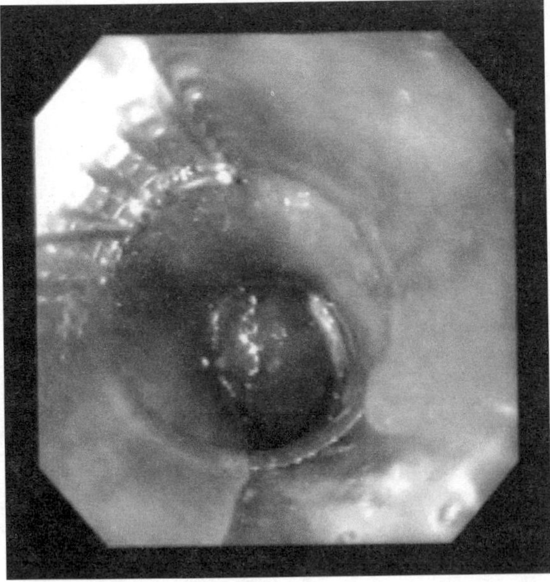

An esophageal varix that has just been banded. Note the rubber band at the base of the banded varix.

❑❑ **With a history of hematemesis the evening before, the following picture of the stomach was obtained on upper endoscopy. What is being demonstrated?**

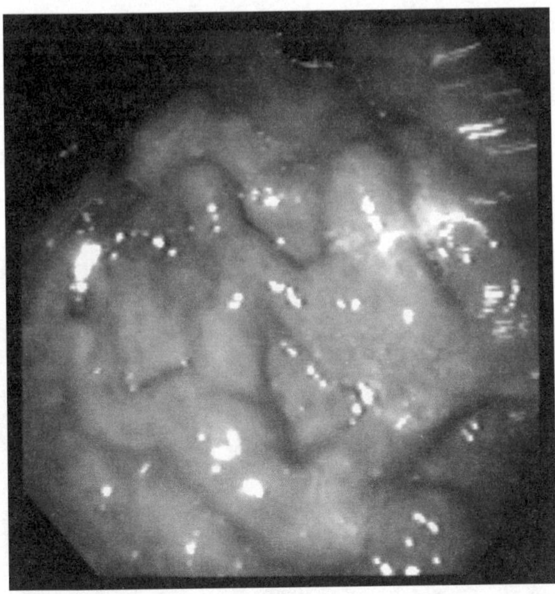

Gastric varices.

❏❏ **In a patient with melena but a normal hematocrit, the lesion below was found on upper endoscopy. Because of its appearance, what is the most likely contributing factor to this ulcer?**

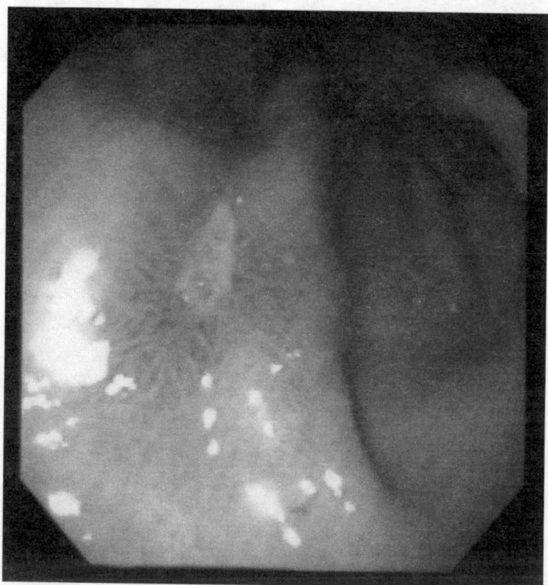

Nonsteroidal anti-inflammatory drug use.

❏❏ **A patient is transferred to your hospital with a history of hematemesis and melena the day before. What is the lesion?**

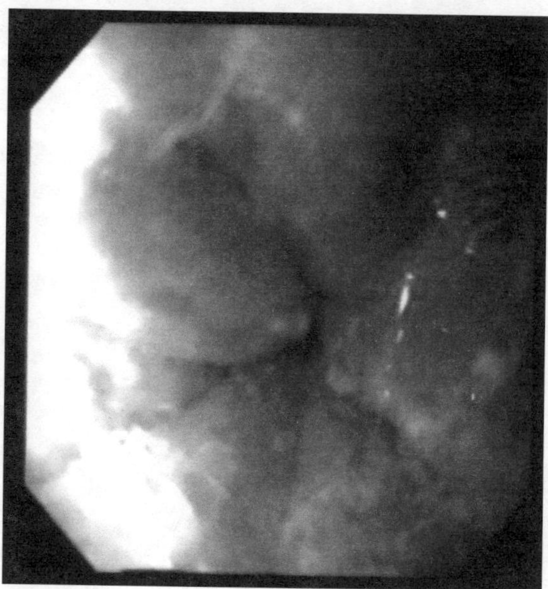

Esophageal varices at the cardioesophageal junction.

❏❏ **What percent of patients with the type of neurocutaneous porphyria shown in the figure will develop hepatic cirrhosis?**

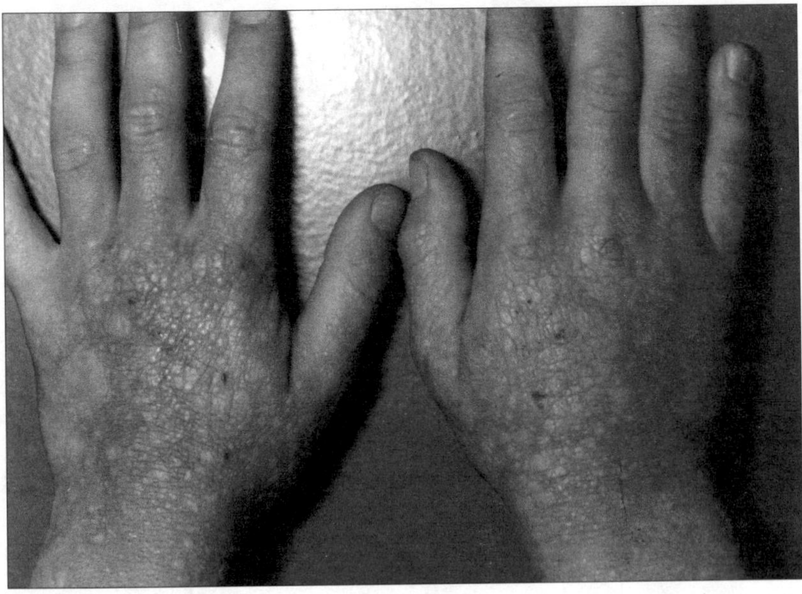

Five percent of patients with erythropoeitic protoporphyria (EPP) will develop cirrhosis. The enzyme defect responsible for EPP is ferrochelatase.

❏❏ **What skin reactions are found in porphyria cutanea tarda (PCT)?**

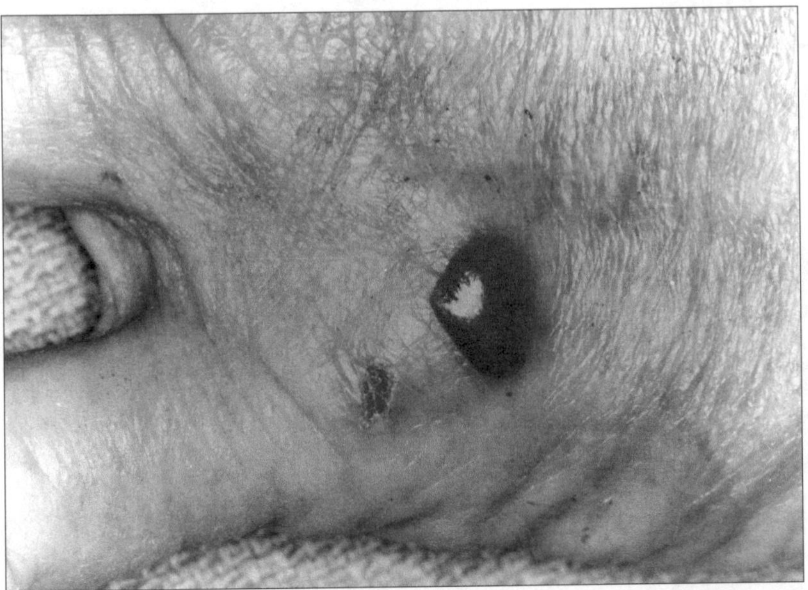

Vesicles/bullae on dorsa of hands/feet, skin fragility/scarring, hyperpigmentation and sclerodermoid plaques, milia on fingers/hands, and hypertrichosis. The enzyme defect responsible for PCT includes uroporphyrinogen decarboxylase in liver (Type I) and erythrocyte (Type II).

❑❑ **A 39 year-old man with a long history of recurrent epistaxis presents with melena. The oro-labial lesions demonstrated in the figure are noted. What is the most likely diagnosis?**

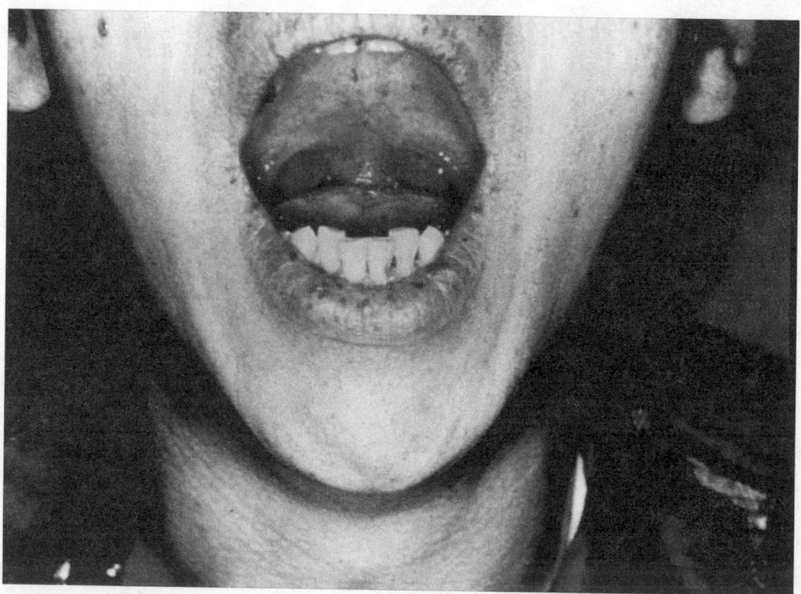

Hereditary hemorrhagic telangiectasia (Osler-Weber-Rendu syndrome).

❑❑ **Treatment for the condition illustrated in the figure includes what modalities?**

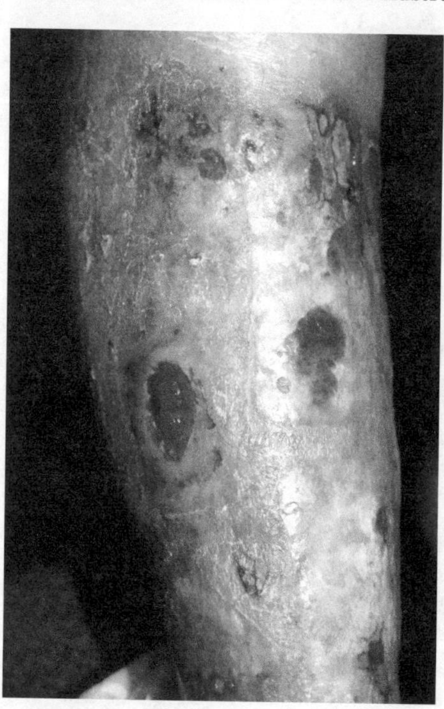

The figure demonstrates typical lesions of pyoderma gangrenosa. Treat the underlying disorder if one exists (40% to 50% of cases are idiopathic). Surgical debridement should be avoided as it can stimulate the development of new lesions. Systemic glucocorticoids, dapsone, sulfapyridine, sulfasalazine, cyclosporine, tacrolimus, 6-mercaptopurine, azathioprine, methotrexate, cyclophosphamide, chlorambucil, clofazimine, minocycline, colchicine, plasmapheresis and thalidomide have all been reported to cause significant improvement or resolution of these lesions.

❑❑ **A 59 year-old woman with diabetes presents with bilateral, symmetrical, pruritic vesicles on the elbows, knees, buttocks and lower back. A skin biopsy reveals granular dermal papillary deposits of IgA. What is the diagnosis?**

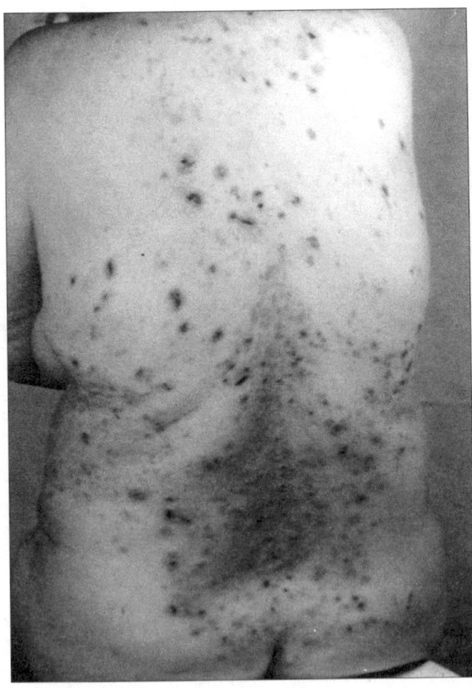

Dermatitis herpetiformis.

❑❑ **A 27 year-old man presented for sigmoidoscopy because of intermittent hematochezia. Numerous polyps were seen. A peculiar freckling pattern on his lips was also noted. What is the most likely diagnosis?**

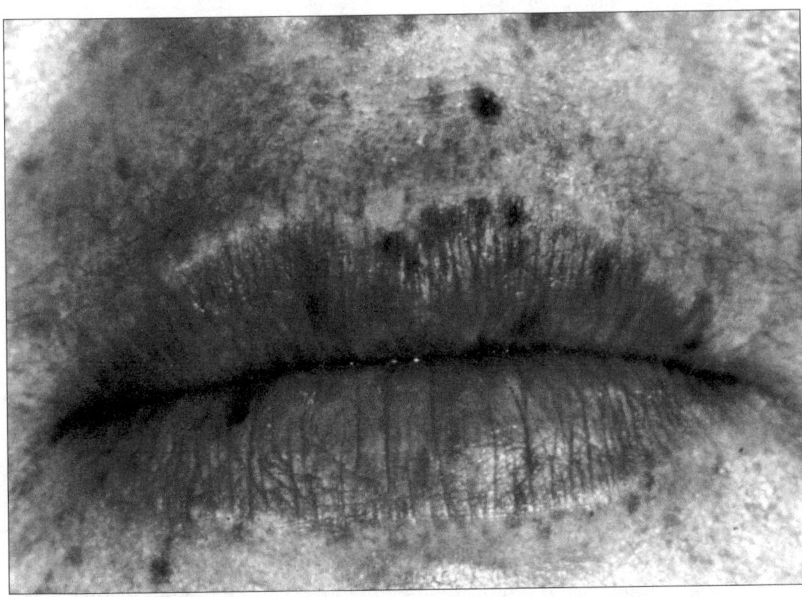
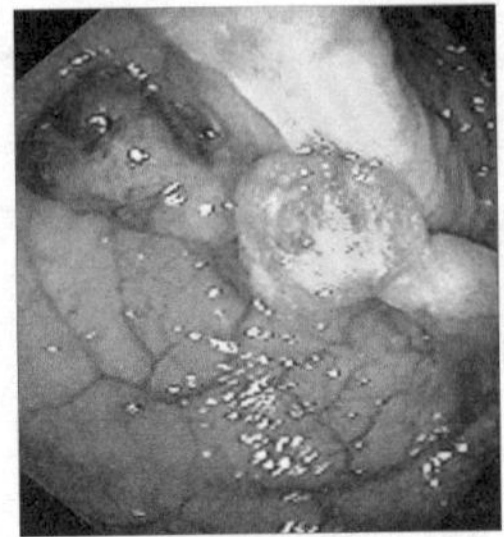

Peutz-Jeghers syndrome.

❑❑　A 72 year-old woman presents with periorofacial, intertriginous and perigenital circinate lesions with vesicles, crusting and postinflammatory pigmentation in association with glossitis, weight loss, diarrhea and diabetes. The rash is shown below. What is the diagnosis?

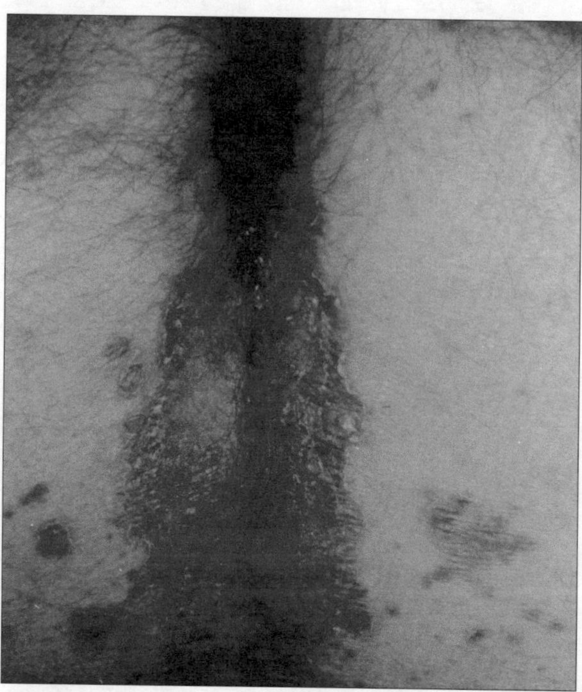

Glucagonoma. Arising in the islet cells of the pancreas, glucagonoma is associated with a distinctive dermatitis referred to as necrolytic migratory erythema (NME).

❑❑　What condition is associated with the nail changes illustrated in the figure?

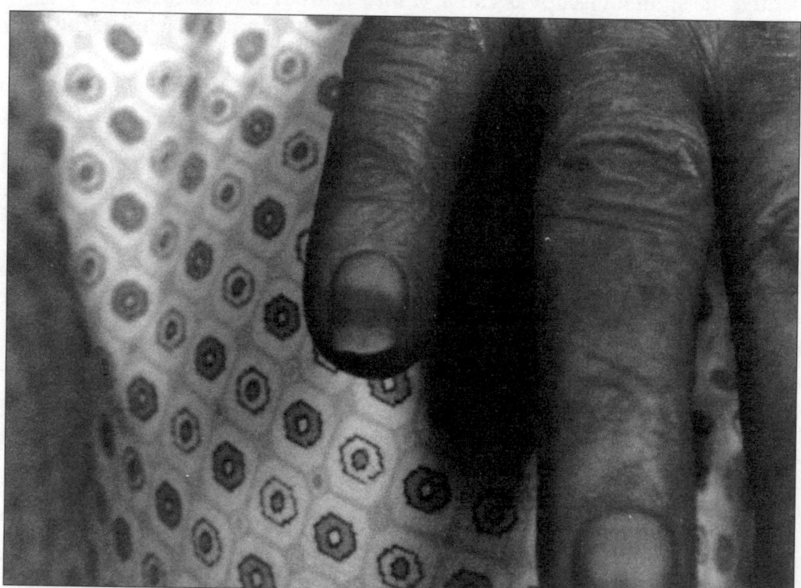

Cirrhosis. Skin and nail finding associated with cirrhosis include white nails referred to as Terry's nails; spider nevi; a diffuse muddy gray color of the skin or a blotchy brown pigmentation; linear pigmentation in skin creases; perioral and periorbital hyperpigmentation (chloasma hepaticum); guttate hypomelanosis; palmar erythema; portal-systemic collaterals over the abdomen; purpura; and, a decrease in facial and body hair growth.

❑❑ **A 32 year-old man with AIDS presents with melena. The skin lesions illustrated in the figure are noted. What is the cause of the skin lesions? Could these lesions be responsible for the gastrointestinal bleeding?**

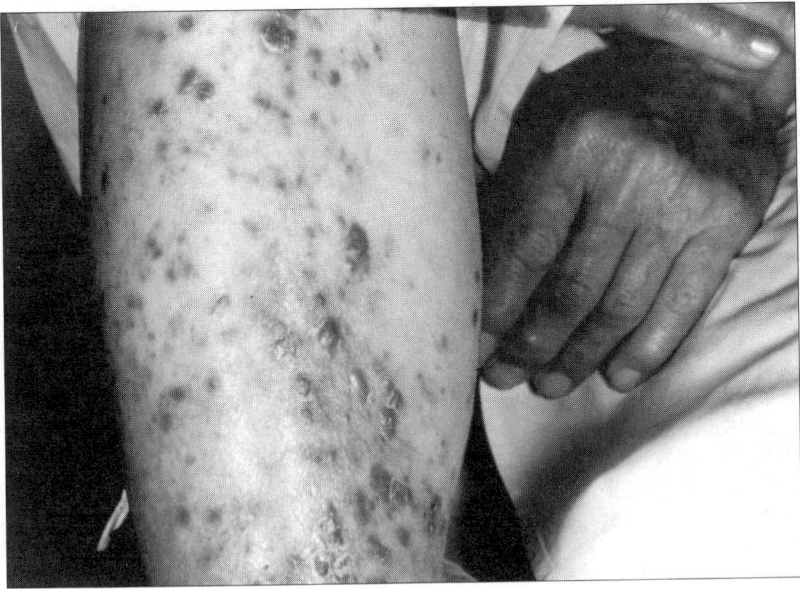

Kaposi's Sarcoma. This submucosal tumor may be found in up to 10% to 15% of HIV-infected individuals. In the alimentary tract, Kaposi's Sarcoma typically occurs as bulky gingival or palatal lesions, or gastrointestinal lesions resulting in difficulty with chewing, swallowing and obstruction to flow, respectively. Rarely, it is a cause of gastrointestinal bleeding.

❑❑ **A 19 year-old man presents with massive hematochezia and hemodynamic instability. He has no other health problems but does experience recurrent painless skin lesions as shown in the figure. What is the diagnosis?**

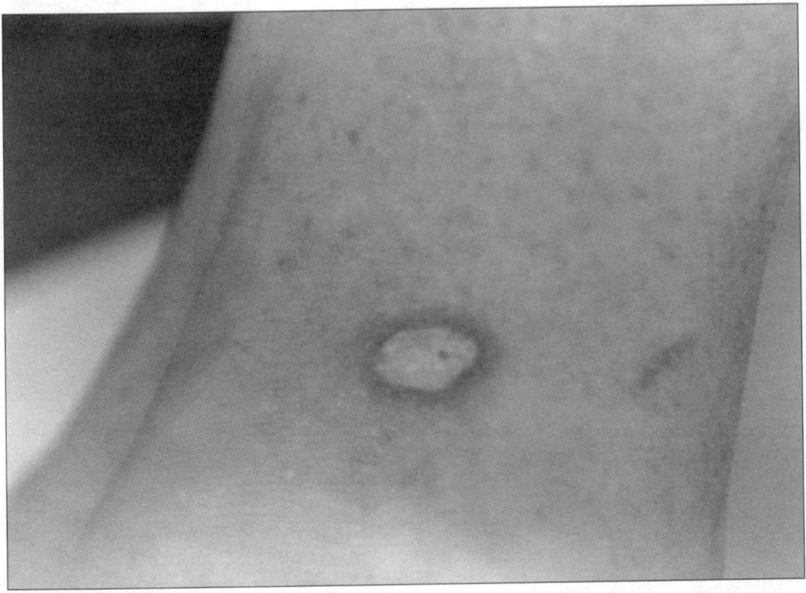

Degos' disease or malignant atrophic papulosis. This is a very rare disorder that affects the skin, gastrointestinal tract and central nervous system. Gut involvement may lead to massive bleeding and death. The pathogenesis of this condition is unknown and there is no effective therapy.

❑❑ **A 54 year-old woman presents with chronic watery diarrhea. Stool tests and a colonoscopy were normal. Random colonic biopsies revealed the findings demonstrated in the figure. What is the most likely diagnosis?**

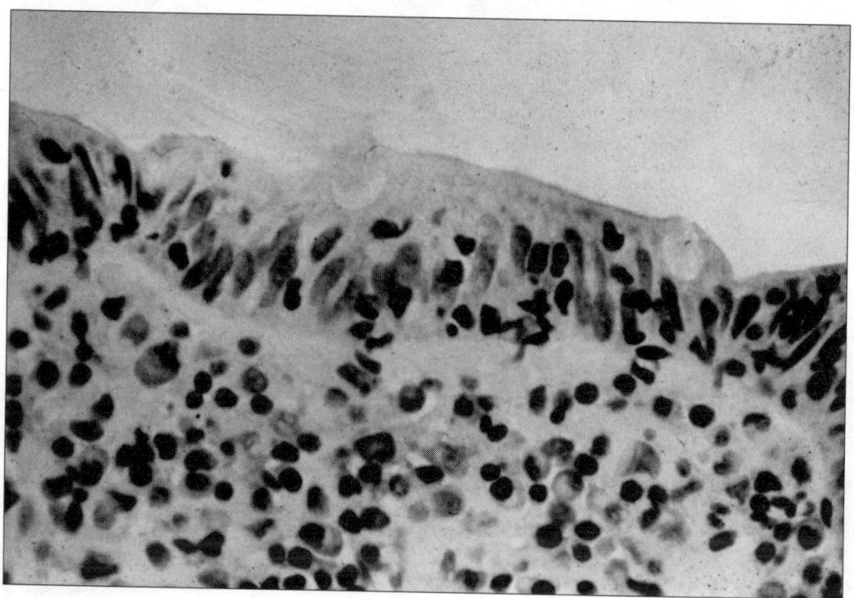

Lymphocytic colitis. An intra-epithelial lymphocytosis is seen with at least 20 lymphocytes per 100 epithelial cells.

❑❑ **What effect does intestinal metaplasia of the gastric mucosa have on the number of *Helicobacter pylori* organisms present?**

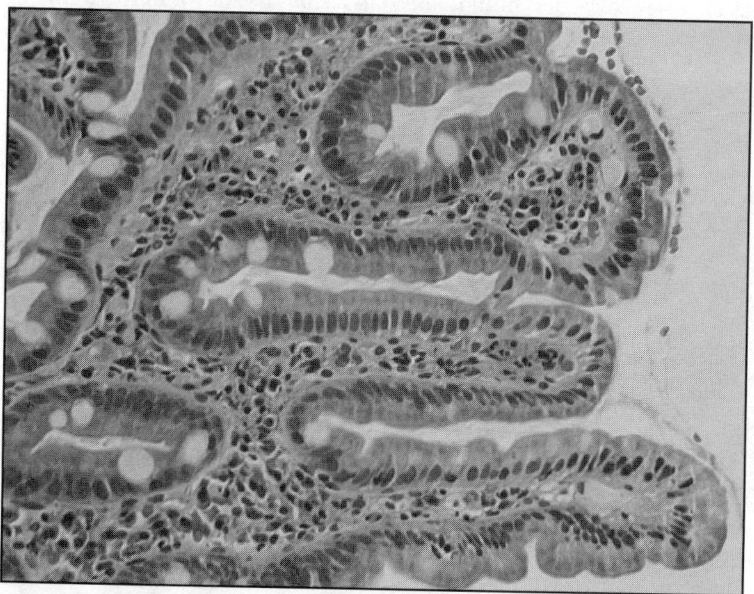

Helicobacter pylori are not typically found in areas of intestinal metaplasia owing to the altered milieu. Note the well developed goblet cells

❑❑ **Endoscopically you see a lesion in the stomach that appears yellow. The biopsy is characterized by an accumulation of foamy histiocytes within the lamina propria. What is the diagnosis?**

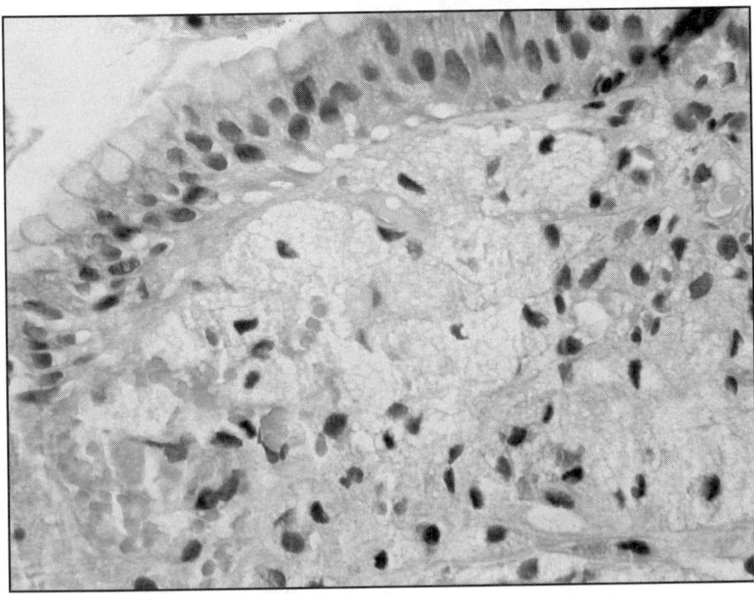

Xanthoma or xanthelasma.

❑❑ **In a background of chronic gastritis, what is the most common gastric polyp that one would expect to find?**

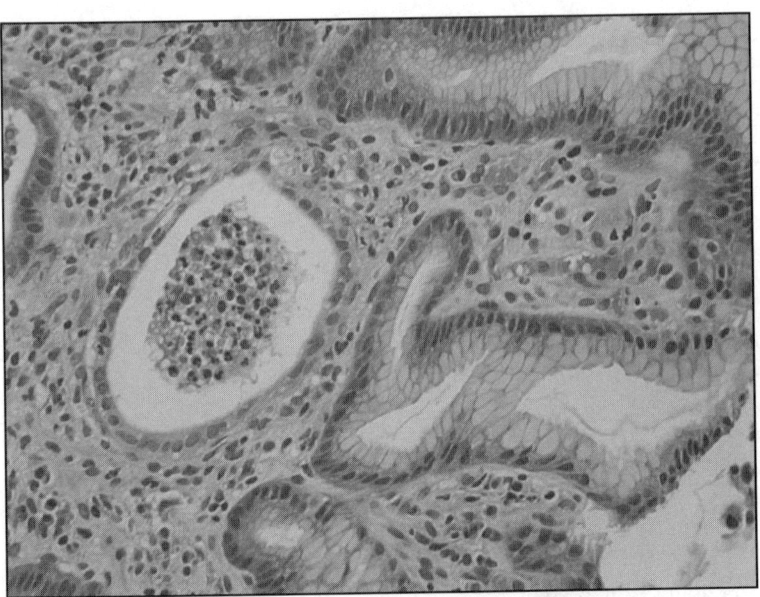

Hyperplastic or regenerative polyp. The figure demonstrates active chronic gastritis with crypt abscess formation?

❑❑ **How does a fundic gland polyp differ histologically from a hyperplastic?**

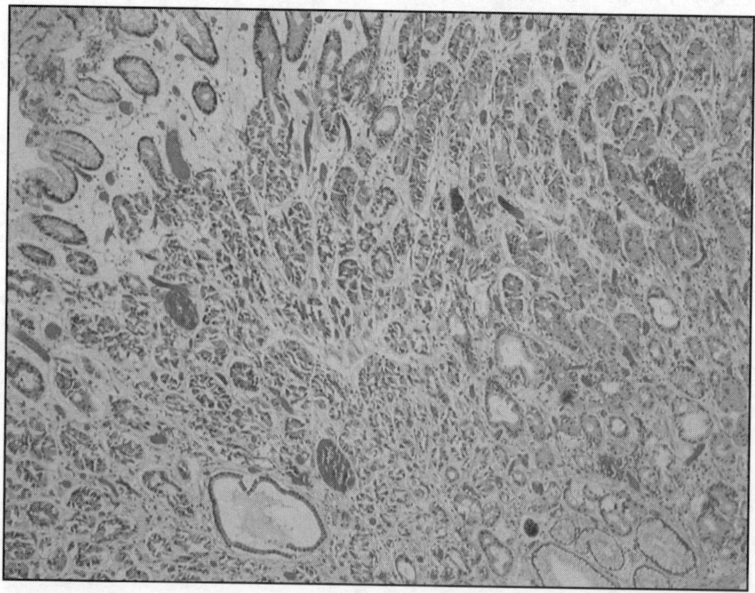

As shown here, fundic gland polyps have fundic epithelial-lined microscysts and shortened foveolae.

❑❑ **With regard to gastrointestinal stromal tumors, what two features are the most important predictors of tumor behavior?**

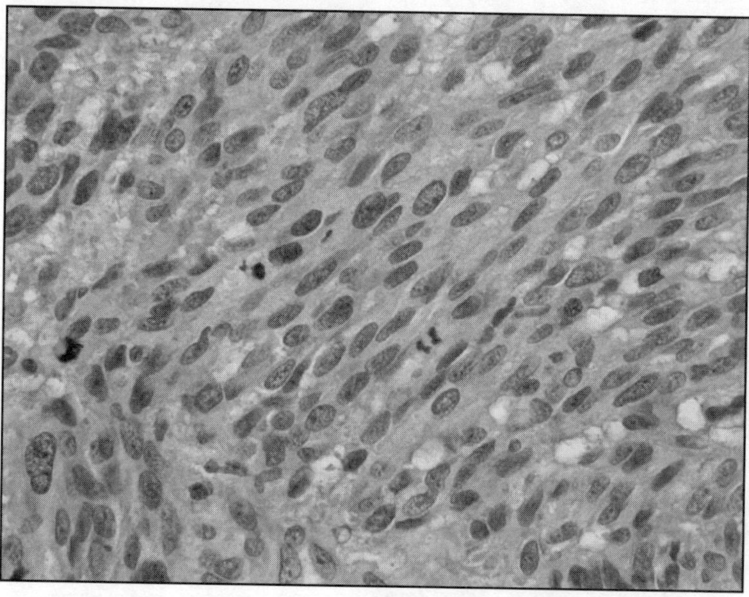

Size and mitotic rate. Note the several mitoses in the figure.

❏❏ **A recently hospitalized man presents to your office complaining of voluminous diarrhea. Stool tests are negative. A colonic biopsy is shown in the figure. What is your diagnosis?**

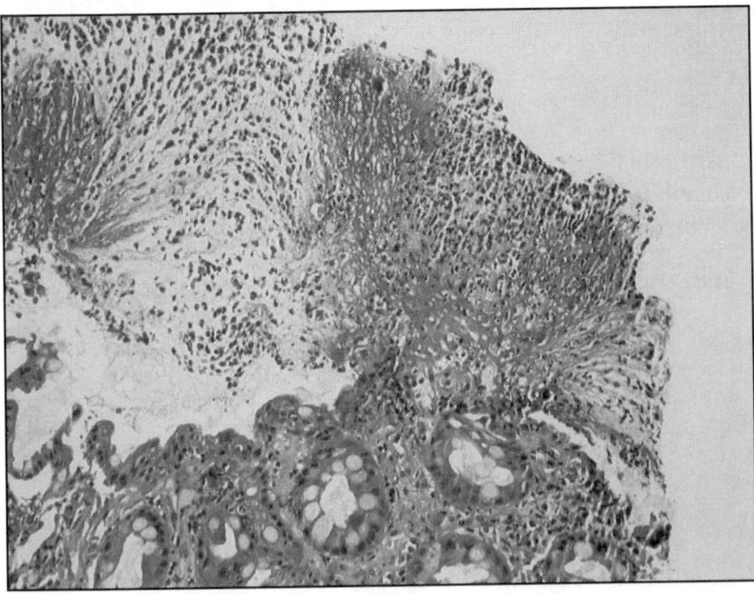

This is the classic low power appearance of pseudomembranous colitis. The biopsy shows the characteristic eosinophilic fibrinous surface debris with a "mushroom" appearance.

❏❏ **What arbitrary thickness must the subepithelial collagen band reach or exceed to qualify for the diagnosis of collagenous colitis?**

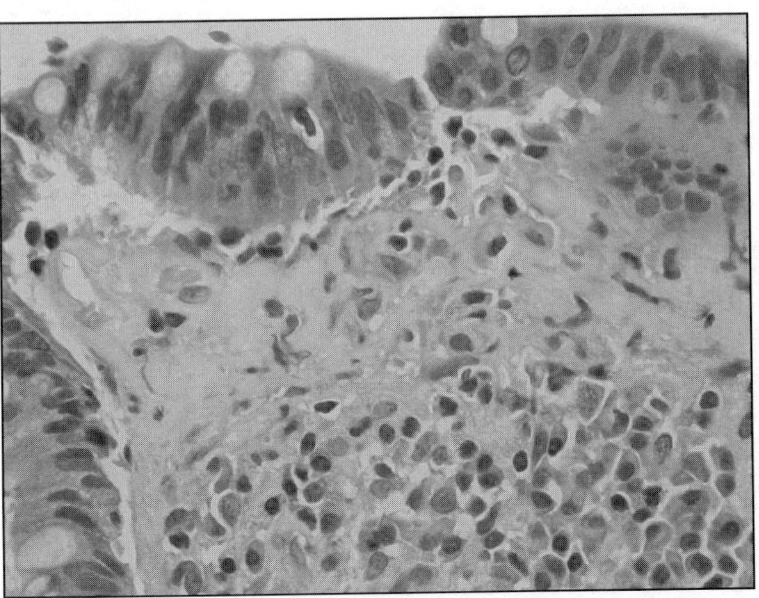

The normal subepithelial collagen band measures up to 7 microns and, in collagenous colitis, it reaches 10 microns or greater. This condition is much more common in elderly women.

❑❑ **What is the risk of malignant transformation in the polyp shown in the photomicrograph below?**

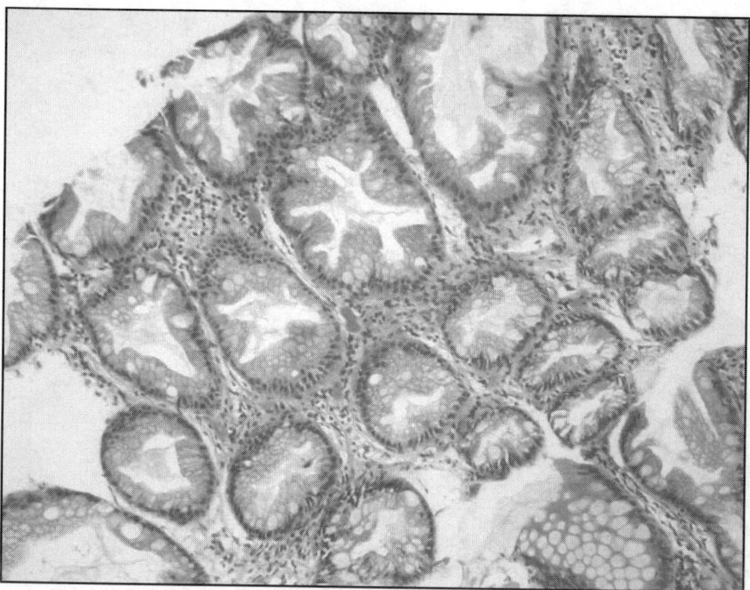

None. This is a benign, non-neoplastic hyperplastic polyp as evidenced by the surface and crypt epithelium with serrated glandular lumina and abundant mucin.

❑❑ **What type of adenomatous polyp has the highest incidence of subsequent development of carcinoma?**

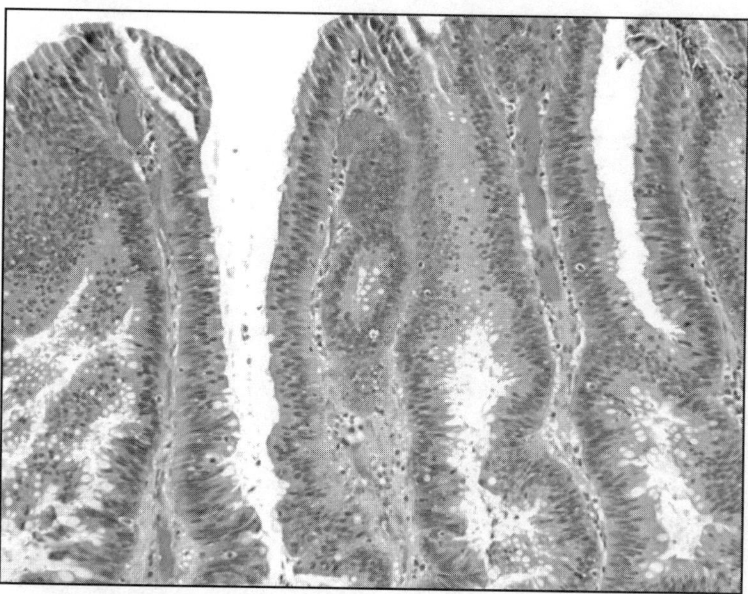

Sessille villous adenomas over 1 to 2 cm in diameter are most likely to develop into an adenocarcinoma. The polyp shown is a tubulovillous adenoma owing to its mixture of villous and tubular architecture.

❑❑ **What type of collagen is deposited to an excessive degree in cases of cirrhosis and what cell is its source?**

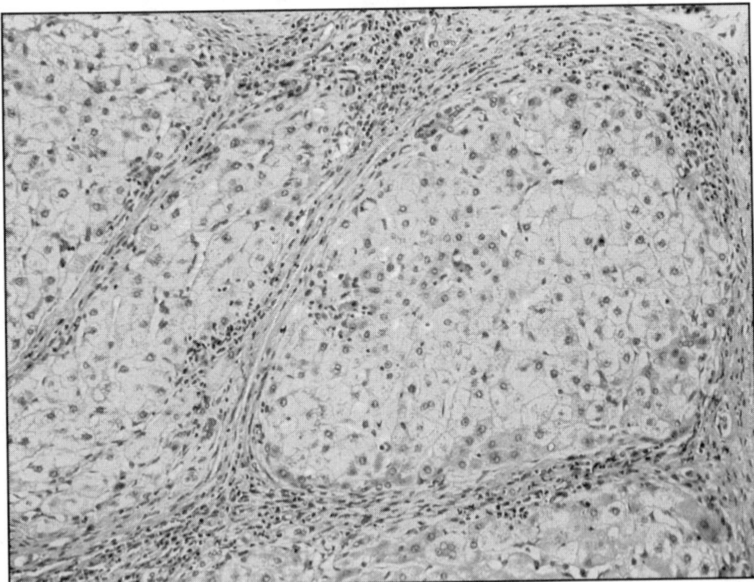

Collagen of types I and III produced by the Ito cell.

❑❑ **A 46 year-old man presents with jaundice, right upper quadrant abdominal pain and fevers. A liver biopsy was eventually performed and is shown below. What is the most likely diagnosis?**

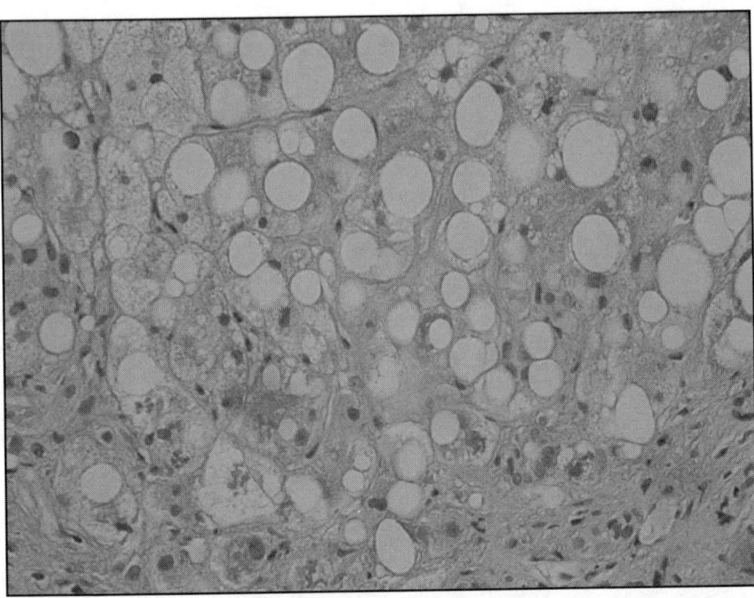

Alcoholic hepatitis. Typical features of alcoholic hepatitis include Mallory's hyaline, which is an eosinophilic inclusion within hepatocytes that stains with ubiquitin, neutrophils surrounding individual degenerating hepatocytes, sclerosing hyaline necrosis and steatosis, predominantly macrovesicular.

❑❑ **T/F: Mallory bodies or Mallory's hyaline are pathognomonic for alcoholic hepatitis.**

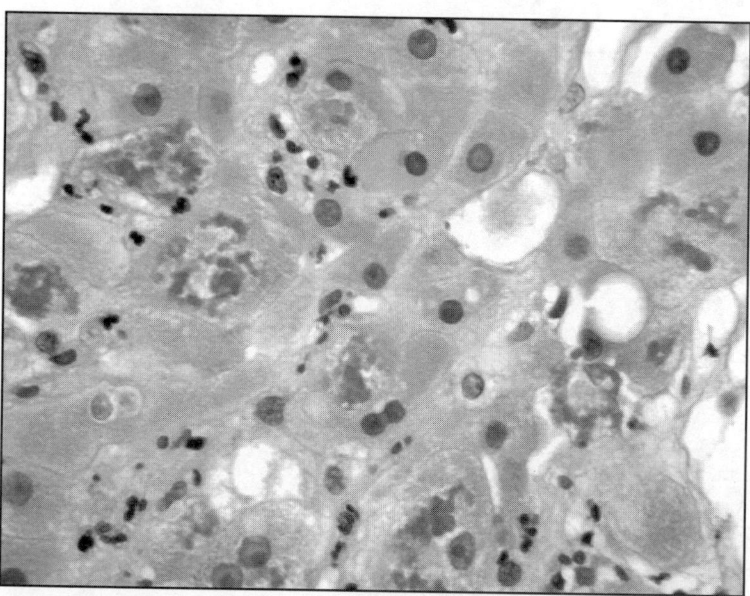

False. Few things in pathology are pathognomonic. Mallory bodies can be seen in many diseases including Wilson's, primary biliary cirrhosis and amiodarone toxicity.

❑❑ **The liver biopsy specimen shown in the figure below is most suggestive of what type of hepatitis?**

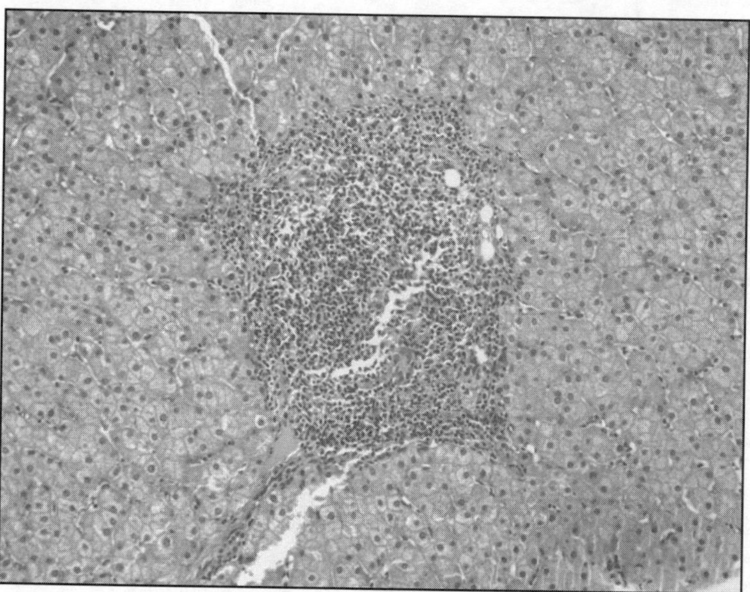

Hepatitis C. The presence of a portal area with a lymphoid aggregate or a follicle with a germinal center in a liver specimen with other features of chronic hepatitis is most suggestive of chronic hepatitis C.

❏❏ **What is the most characteristic inflammatory cell seen in the infiltrate of a chronic hepatitis of an autoimmune nature?**

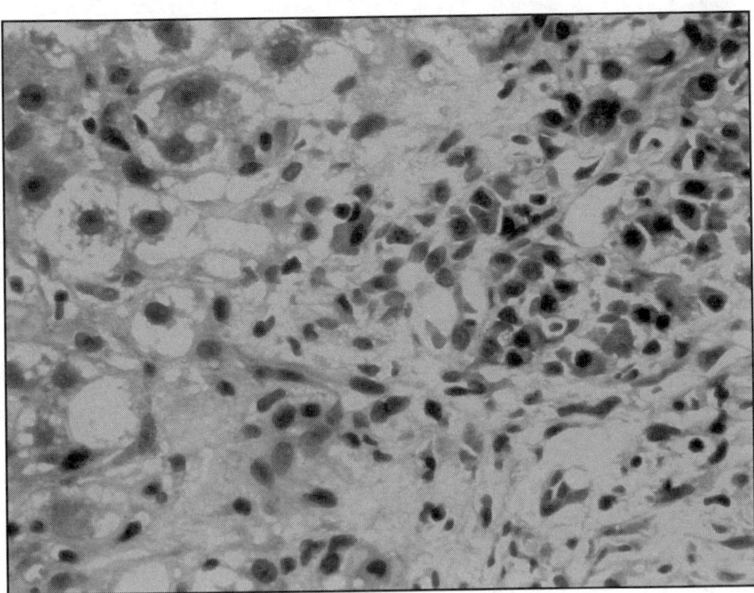

Plasma cell.

❏❏ **The findings present in the figure below are most suggestive of which type of viral hepatitis?**

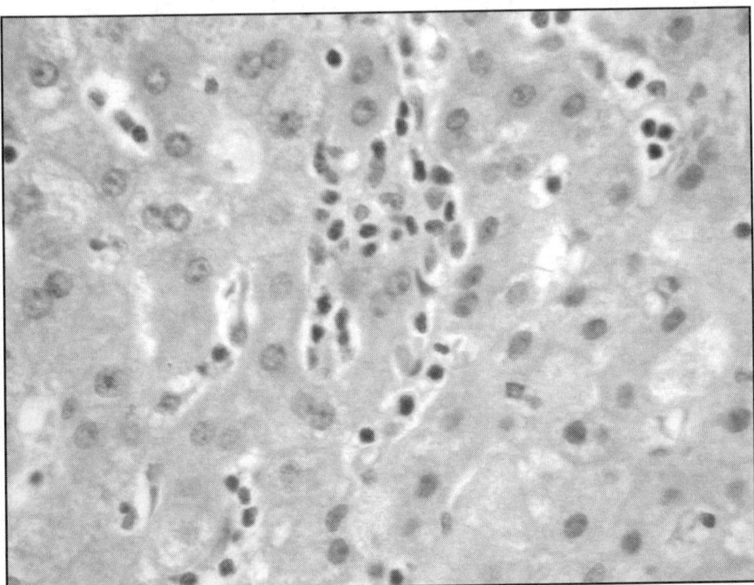

Epstein-Barr virus or infectious mononucleosis-associated hepatitis. Lymphocytes in the hepatic sinusoids which line up in a single file pattern and associated scattered plasma cells are characteristic findings.

❑❑ **In the liver biopsy shown, what is the most likely etiology of these changes?**

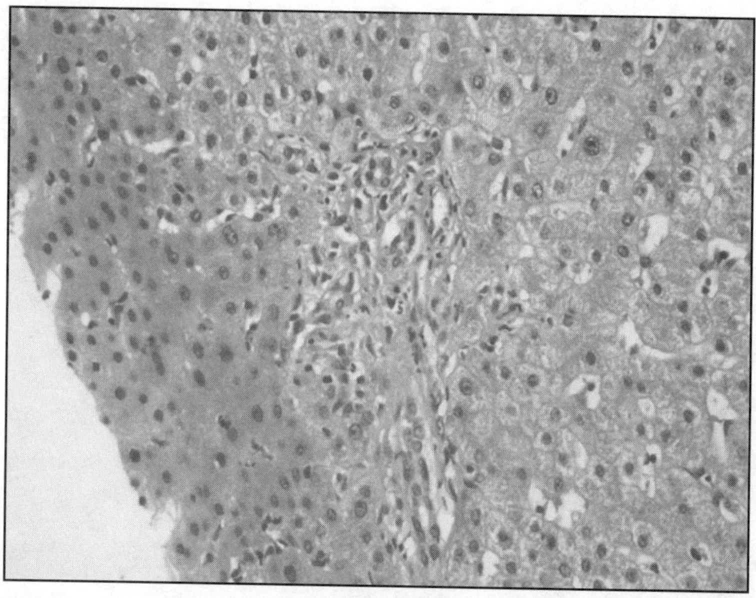

Biliary tract obstruction. Typical findings include bile plugs, portal edema, neutrophils and bile duct proliferation in association with portal expansion by collagen.

❑❑ **A 45 year-old female presents with fatigue and pruritus. Laboratory testing is notable only for a mildly elevated alkaline phophatase. A liver biopsy is performed. What is the diagnosis?**

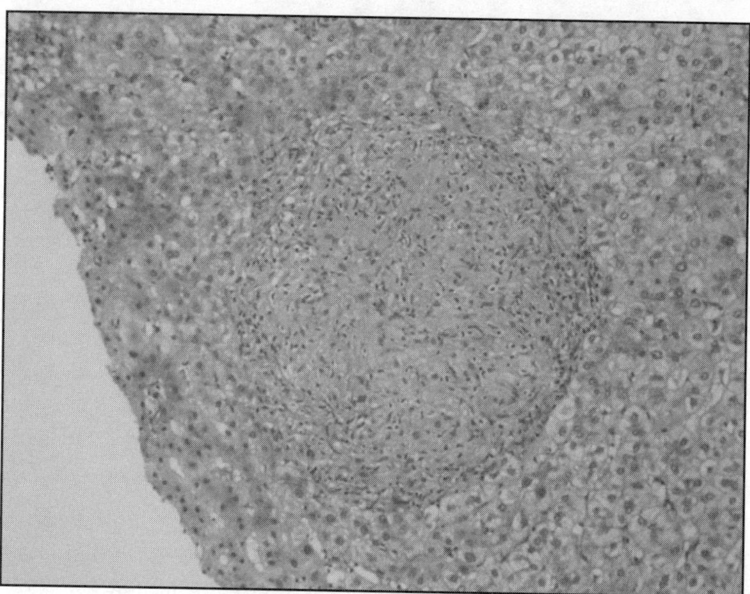

Primary biliary cirrhosis. The biopsy demonstrates a portal granuloma. This woman's antimitochondrial antibodies were markedly elevated.

❑❑ **What diagnosis is most likely and what stain(s) would you use to confirm or disprove it?**

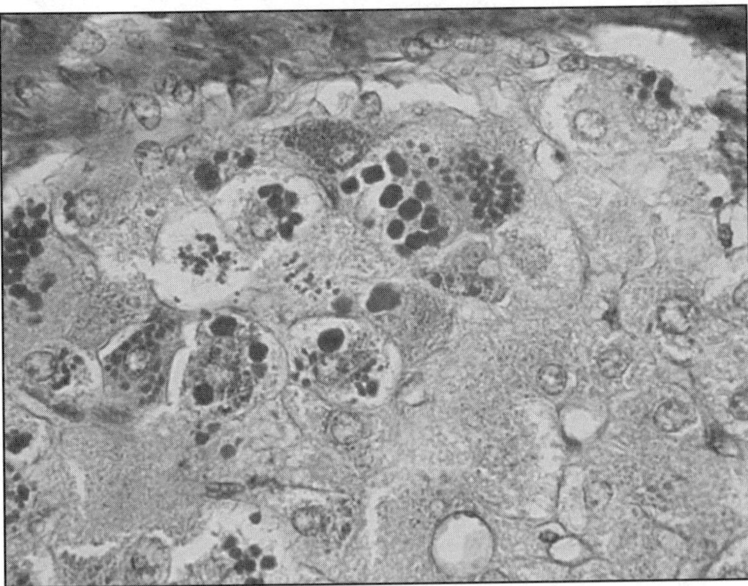

Alpha₁-antitrypsin deficiency (A1AD). This biopsy shows eosinophilic globules within periportal hepatocytes. If it is A1AD, the globules will be PAS-positive and resist diastase digestion. Hence, a PAS and a PAS with diastase should be ordered. There is also an immunohistochemical stain for alpha₁-antitrypsin that would also expected to be positive in a case of A1AD.

❑❑ **Which lymphocytes, B or T cell, are responsible for attacking the bile duct shown in this case of acute (cellular) rejection of a liver allograft?**

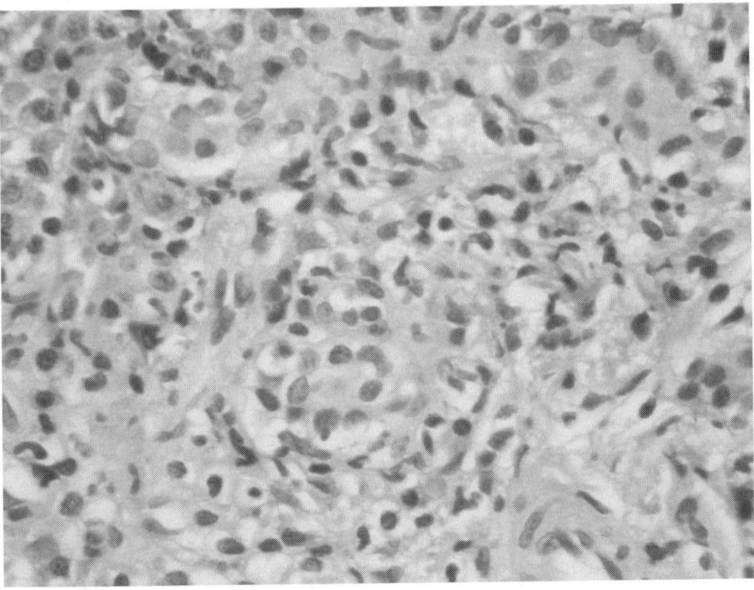

T lymphocytes.

❑❑ What typical histopathologic features seen in Budd-Chiari syndrome and veno-occlusive disease (VOD) are demonstrated in the figures ((a) Venoocclusive disease b) Budd-Chiari syndrome)?

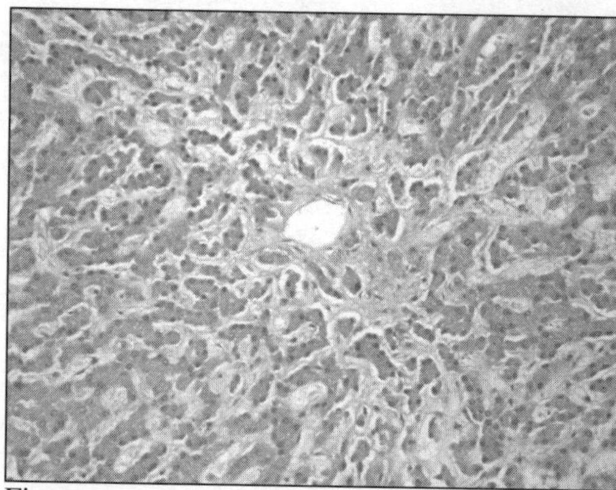

Figure a

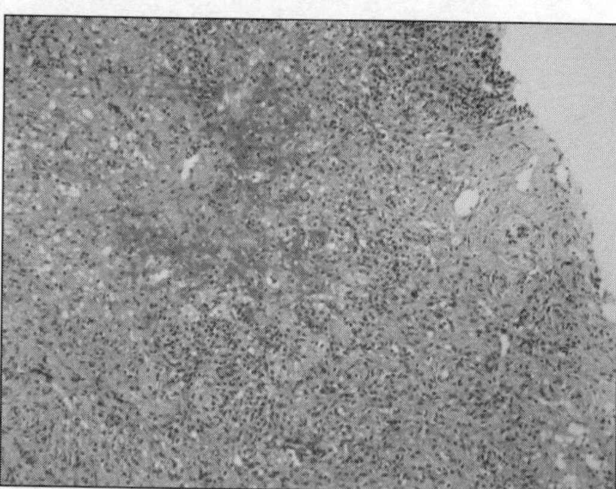

Figure b

Budd-Chiari is characterized by centrilobular congestion with associated hepatocellular drop out or necrosis. In contrast, VOD is characterized by subendothelial sclerosis of the terminal hepatic venules and intercalated veins with associated "atrophy" of the hepatocytes in the lobules.

❑❑ What is the most common benign tumor of the liver?

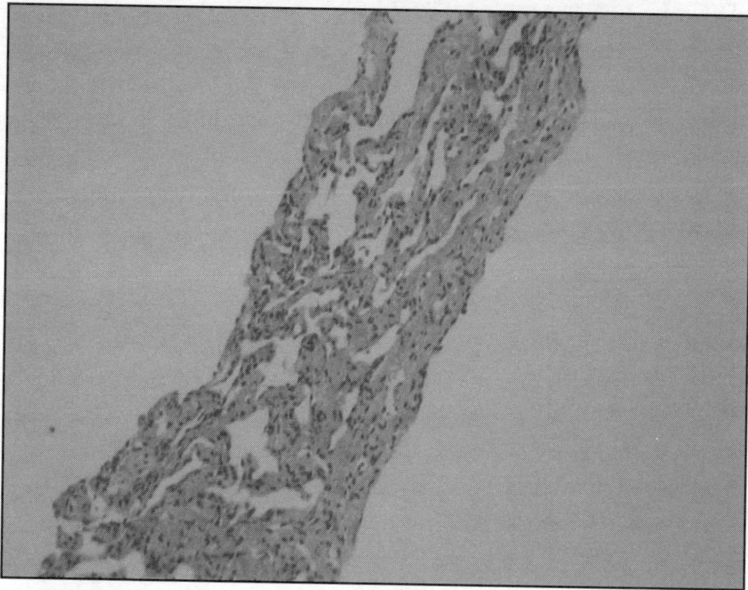

Hemangioma.

❒❒ **What is the most common mesenchymal tumor of the liver in infancy?**

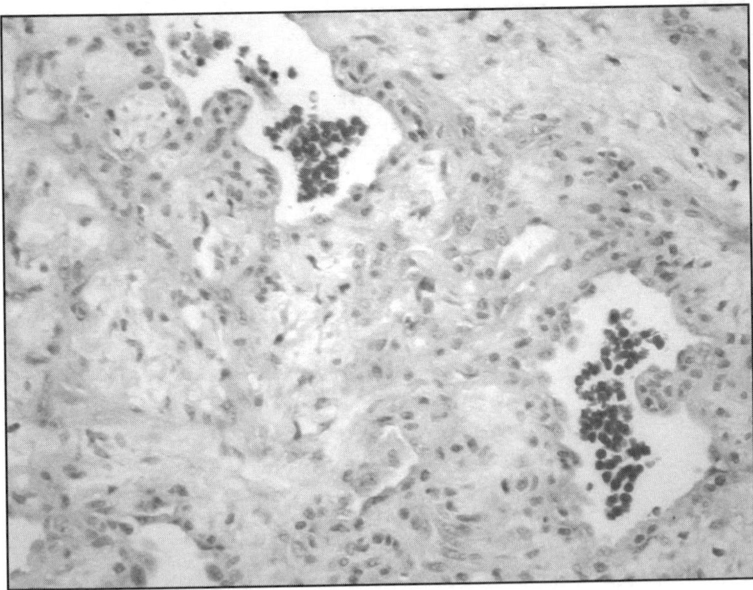

Infantile hemangioendothelioma.

❒❒ **Which histologic type of hepatocellular carcinoma (HCC) occurs in young adults or adolescents, is not associated with cirrhosis, has a better prognosis and is not associated with an elevated serum alpha-fetoprotein?**

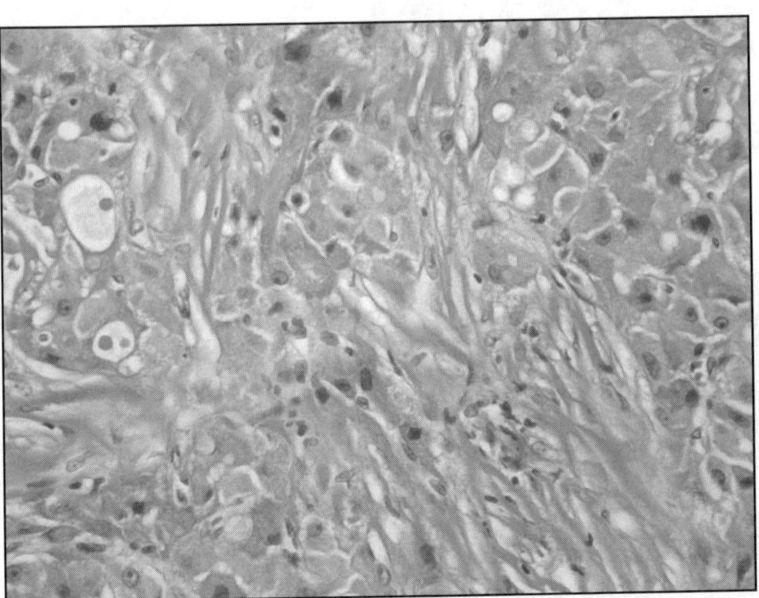

Fibrolamellar HCC. Interestingly, in contrast to many of the other things we have discussed, it is more common in the left lobe of the liver. It is also not associated with hepatitis B or alcohol abuse as most HCC is. Note the histology shown above demonstrating the thick fibrous bands within the tumor.

❑❑ **Describe the typical patient and tumor location in a patient with hepatoblastoma?**

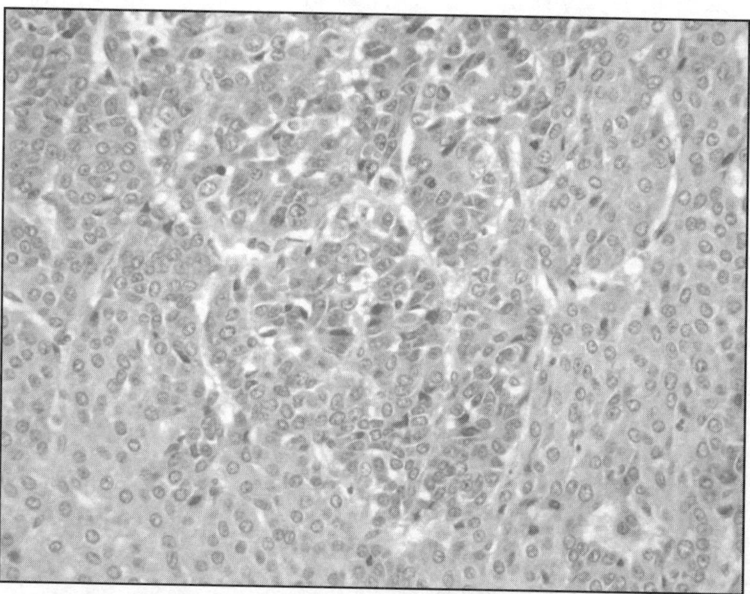

A 2 year-old male with a well-circumscribed mass in the right lobe of the liver and an elevated serum alpha fetoprotein (90% of cases).

❑❑ **What are the typical histologic features of acute allograft rejection in the liver?**

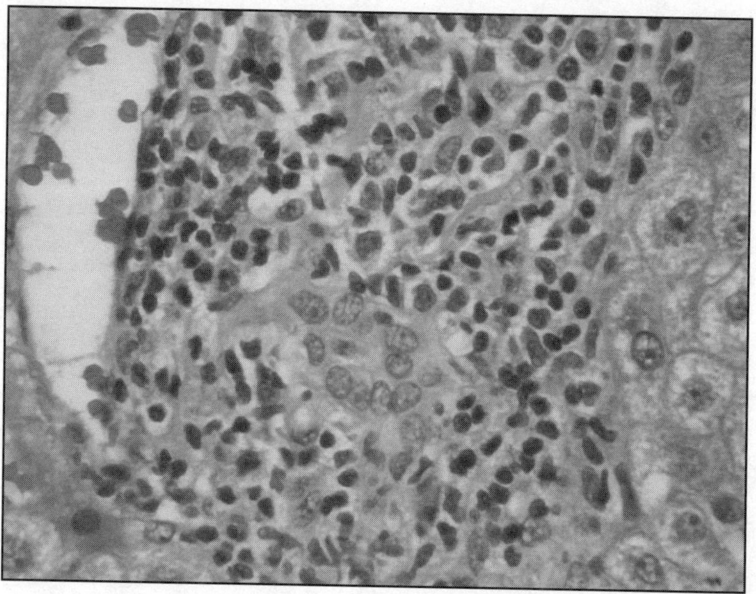

Acute rejection is characterized by a portal infiltrate composed of T-lymphocytes and eosinophils which are generally centered around the bile ducts and portal vein. The ducts show damage (nuclear loss or vacuolated cytoplasm) and often focal infiltration by the lymphocytes. Endotheliitis is usually present involving the portal vein and characterized by subendothelial inflammatory cells causing prominence of the endothelial cells.

❐❐ What etiologic agent is most likely responsible for the hepatitis demonstrated in the figure?

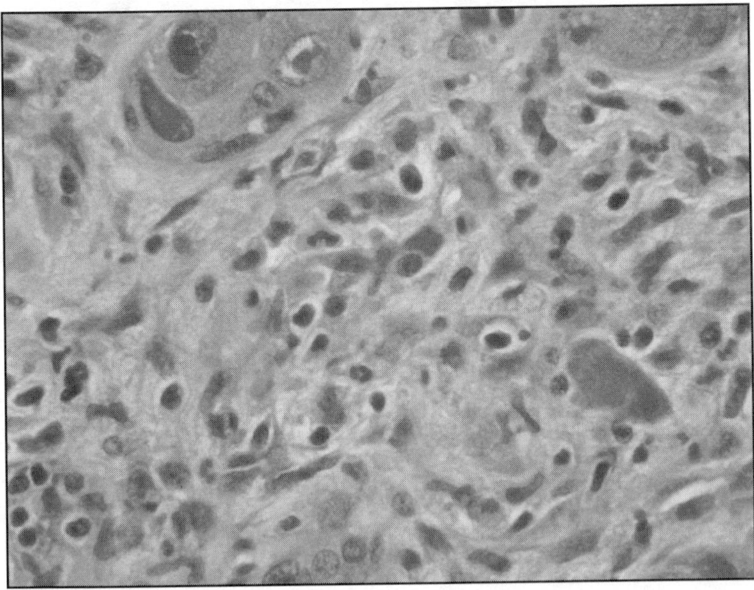

Cytomegalovirus. CMV hepatitis is characterized by hepatocytes which contain both intranuclear and intracytoplasmic viral inclusions.

BIBLIOGRAPHY

BOOKS/ARTICLES

Allan R, Rhodes J, Hanauer S, Keighley M, Alexander-Williams J, Fasio V. *Inflammatory Bowel Diseases*. New York: Churchill Livingstone; 1997.

American Gastroenterological Association Technical Review on the Evaluation and Management of Chronic Diarrhea. *Gastroenterology* 1999;116:1464-1486.

Becker AE, Grinspoon SK, Kilbanaski A, Herzog DB. Current Concepts: Eating Disorders. *N Eng J Med* 1999;340:1092-1098.

Bell R. *Digestive Tract Surgery*. Philadelphia: Lippincott-Raven; 1996.

Bennett JC. *Cecil Textbook of Medicine*. 20th ed. Philadelphia: WB Saunders Co.; 1996.

Bircher J. *Oxford Textbook of Clinical Hepatology*. 2nd ed. New York: Oxford University Press; 1999.

Boley SJ, DiBiase A, Brandt LJ, et al. Lower intestinal bleeding in the elderly. *Am J Surg* 1979;137:57.

Bonacini M. Pancreatic involvement in human immunodeficiency virus infection. *J Clin Gastroenterol* 1991;13:58-64.

Bott S, Prakash C, McCallum RW. Medication-induced esophageal injury: survey of the literature. *Am J Gastroenterol* 1987; 82:758-763.

Brandt LJ. *Clinical Practice of Gastroenterology*. 1st ed. Philadelphia:Current Medicine Inc.; 1999.

Byrne WJ. Foreign bodies, bezoars and caustic ingestion. *Gastroenterol Clin North Am* 1994; 44:99-119.

Castell DO, Richter JE. *The Esophagus*. 3rd ed. Philadelphia:Lippincott Williams & Wilkins; 1999.

Chandrasoma P. *Gastrointestinal Pathology*. Stamford, CT: Appleton and Lange; 1999.

Chang EB, Sitrin MD, Black DD. *Gastroenterology, Hepatobiliary, and Nutritional Physiology*. Philadelphia: Lippincott-Raven; 1996.

Chung SS, Lau JYW, Sung JJY, et al. A randomized comparison between adrenaline injection alone and adrenaline injection plus heat probe treatment for actively bleeding ulcers. *Br Med J* 1997;314:1307-1311.

Clain A. *Hamilton Bailey's Demonstrations of Physical Signs in Clinical Surgery*. 17th ed. Bristol, England: IOP Publishing Ltd; 1986.

Cohn JA, Friedman KJ, Noon PG, et al. Relation between mutations of the cystic fibrosis gene and idiopathic pancreatitis. *N Engl J Med* 1998;339:653-658.

Colton T. *Statistics in Medicine*. Boston: Little, Brown and Company; 1974.

Cullen JJ, Kelly KA. Gastric motor physiology and pathophysiology. *Surg Clin N Am* 1993 73:1145-1160.

Dawson-Saunders B, Trapp RG. *Basic and Clinical Biostatistics*. 2nd ed. Norwalk: Appleton and Lange; 1994.

Diamant NE, Kamm MA, Wald A, Whitehead WE. AGA technical review on anorectal testing techniques. *Gastroenterology* 1999;116:735-60.

Dassopoulos T, Ehrenpreis ED. Acute Pancreatitis in Human Immunodeficiency Virus-Infected Patients: A Review. *The American Journal of Medicine* 1999; 107:78-84.

DuPont HL and the Practice Parameters Committee of the American College of Gastroenterology. Guidelines on Acute Infectious Diarrhea in Adults. *Am J Gastroenterol* 1997;92:1962-1975.

Eagon JC, Kelly KA. Postgastrectomy syndromes. *Surg Clin N Am* 1992;72:445-465.

Ehrenpreis ED. Small intestinal manifestations of HIV infection. *Internat J STD and AIDS* 1995;6:149-155.

Fasano A, Hokama Y.Russell R, et al. Diarrhea in ciguatera fish poisoning: preliminary evaluation of pathophysiological mechanisms. *Gastroenterology* 1991;100:471-476.

Feldman M, Scharschmidt BF, Sleisenger MH. *Sleisenger & Fordtran's Gastrointestinal and Liver Disease*. 6th ed. Philadelphia: W.B. Saunders; 1998.

Foley JF, Vose JM, Armitage JO (eds). *Current Therapy in Oncology*. 2nd ed. Orlando: W.B. Saunders; 1999.

Freedberg IM, Eisen AZ, Wolff K, et al. *Fitzpatrick's Dermatology in General Medicine*. 5th ed. New York: McGraw-Hill; 1999.

Gastroenterology and Hepatology. *Medical Knowledge Self-Assessment Program*. 2nd ed. American College of Physicians; 1997.

Go VLW, Dimagno EP. *The Pancreas: Biology, Pathology and Disease*. 2nd ed. New York: Raven Press; 1993.

Gordon ME. The dark side of bon appetit- (Diagnostic Challenges Series). *Travel Medicine News* 1995;2:16-18.

Gracey M and Burke V. *Pediatric Gastroenterology and Hepatology*. Boston: Blackwell Scientific Publications; 1993.

Greenfield L, et al. *Surgery: Scientific Principles and Practice*. 2nd ed. Philadelphia: Lippincott-Raven; 1997.

Grunfeld C, Pang M, Shimizu L, et al. Resting energy expenditure, caloric intake and short term weight change in human immunodeficiency virus infection and the acquired immunodeficiency syndrome. *Am J Clin Nutr* 1992;55:455-460.

Gupta PK, Fleischer D. Endoscopic hemostasis in nonvariceal bleeding. *Endoscopy* 1994;26:48-54.

Herwaldt B, Ackers ML and the Cyclospora Working Group. An outbreak in 1996 of cyclosporiasis associated with imported raspberries. *N Engl J Med* 1997;336:1548-1556.

Hulley SB, Cummings SR. *Designing Clinical Research. An Epidemiologic Approach*. Baltimore: Williams & Wilkins; 1988.

Jekel JF, Elmore JG, Katz KL. *Epidemiology, Biostatistics and Preventive Medicine*. Philadelphia: WB Saunders Co.; 1996.

Kahrilas PJ. Gastroesophageal reflux disease. *JAMA* 1996;276:983-988.

Kaplowitz N. *Liver and Biliary Diseases*. 2nd ed. Baltimore: Williams & Wilkins; 1996.

Karimgani I, Porter KA, Langevin RE, Banks PPA. Prognostic factors in sterile pancreatic necrosis. *Gastroenterology* 1992;103:1636-1640.

Kikendall JW. Caustic ingestion injuries. *Gastroenterol Clin North Am* 1991;20:847-857.

Krawitt EL, Wiesner RH, Nishioka M. *Autoimmune Liver Disease.* 2nd ed. Amersterdam: Elsevier; 1998.

Laine L, Peterson WL. Bleeding peptic ulcer. *N Eng J Med* 1994;331:717-727.

Lau JYW, Sung JJY, Lam YH. Endoscopic retreatment compared with surgery in patient with recurrent bleeding after initial endoscopic control of bleeding ulcers. *N Eng J Med* 1999;340:751-756.

LaRusso NF. *Gastroenterology and Hepatology.* 1st ed. Philadelphia: Current Medicine Inc.; 1997.

Lee WM. Medical progress: acute liver failure. *N Engl J Med* 1993;329:1862-1872.

Lieber CS. Biochemical and molecular basis of alcohol-induced injury to liver and other tests. *N Engl J Med* 1988;319:1639-1650.

Loeb PM, Eisenstein AM. *Caustic Injury to the Upper Gastrointestinal Tract.* 6th ed. Philadelphia: W.B. Saunders Company; 1998.

MacSween R, Anthony P, Scheuer P, Burt A, Portmann B. *Pathology of the Liver.* 3rd ed. New York: Churchill Livingstone; 1994.

Mandell GL, Bennett JE, Dolin R. *Mandell, Douglas and Bennett's Principles and Practice of Infectious Diseases.* 4th ed. New York: Churchill Livingstone; 1995.

Marshall JK, Irvine EJ. Lymphocytic and collagenous colitis: medical management. *Current Treatment Options in Gastroenterology* 1999;2:127-133.

McNally PR. *GI/Liver Secrets.* Baltimore: Mosby; 1996.

Mead PS, Slutsker L, Dietz V, McCaig LF, Bresee JS, Shapiro C, et al. Food-related illness and death in the United States. *Emerg Infect Dis* 1999;5:607-625.

Moody FG, Carey LC, Jones RS, Kelly KA, Nahrwold DL, Skinner DB. *Surgical Treatment of Digestive Disease.* Chicago: Yearbook Medical Publishers Inc; 1986.

Morales TG, Sampliner RE. Barrett's Esophagus: Update on Screening, Surveillance and Treatment. *Arch Int Med* 1999;159:1411-1416.

Morson B, Dawson I, Day D, Jass J, Price A, Williams G. *Morson and Dawson's Gastrointestinal Pathology.* 3rd ed. Oxford: Blackwell Scientific Publications; 1990.

National Institutes of Health. Therapeutic endoscopy and bleeding ulcers-NIH Consensus Conference. *JAMA* 1989;262:1369-1372.

Noble J, et al. *Textbook of Primary Care Medicine.* 2nd ed. Baltimore: Mosby; 1996.

Nataro JP, Kaper JB. Diarrheagenic *Escherichia coli. Clinical Microbiology Reviews* 1998;11:142-201.

O'Connor PG, Schottenfeld RS. Patients with Alcohol Problems. *N Engl J Med* 1998; 338: 592-602.

Okuda K, Tabor E . *Liver Cancer.* New York: Churchill Livingstone; 1997.

Pederzoli P, Bassi C, Vesenteni S, Campedelli A. A randomized multicenter clinical trial of antibiotic prophylaxis of septic complications in acute necrotizing pancreatitis with imipenem. *Surg Gynecol Obstet* 1993;176:480-483.

Pospai D, Rene' E, Fiasse R, et al. Crohn's disease stable remission after human immunodeficiency virus infection. *Dig Dis Sci* 1998;43:412-419.

Richter JE. Extraesophageal presentations of gastroeophageal reflux disease. *Semin Gastro Dis* 1997;8:75-89.

Roberts I. Disorders of the pancreas in children. *Gastroenterol Clin N Am* 1990;19:958-969.

Rombeau JL, Rolandelli RH. *Clinical Nutrition: Enteral and Tube Feeding*. Philadelphia: WB Saunders Co.; 1997.

Rosenbaum M, Leibel RL, Hirsch J. Medical Progress: Obesity. *N Eng J Med* 1997;337:396-407.

Rothschild, MA, Berk, PD, Williams R. Fulminant Hepatic Failure. *Sem Liv Dis* 1996;4:341-454.

Rowe NM, Kahn FB, Acinapura AJ, Cunningham JN, Jr. Nonsurgical Pneumoperitoneum: A Case Report and Review. *Am Surgeon* 1998;64:313-322.

Rudolf AM, et al. *Pediatrics*. 20th ed. Baltimore: Appleton and Lange; 1996.

Sabiston DC. *Textbook of Surgery*. 13th ed. Philadelphia: WB Saunders Co; 1986.

Sampliner RE and The Practice Parameters Committee of the American College of Gastroenterology. Practice guidelines on the diagnosis, surveillance, and therapy of Barrett's esophagus. *Am J Gastroenterol* 1998;93:1028-1032.

Scheuer PJ, Lefkowitch JH. *Liver Biopsy Interpretation*. 5th ed. Philadelphia: WB Saunders Co; 1994.

Schiodt FV, Atillasoy E, Shakil AO, et al. Etiology and outcome for 295 patients with acute liver failure in the United States. *Liver Transplantation and Surgery* 1999;5:29-34.

Schiff ER, Sorrell MF, Maddrey WC. *Schiff's Diseases of the Liver*. 8th ed. Philadelphia: Lippincott – Raven; 1998.

Schwartz MW. *Clinical Handbook of Pedatrics*. 2nd ed. Baltimore: Williams & Wilkins; 1999.

Sharpstone D, Gazzard B. Gastrointestinal manifestations of HIV infection. *Lancet* 1996;348:379-383.

Sherlock S, et al. *Diseases of the Liver and Biliary System*. 9th ed. London: Oxford-Blackwell Scientific; 1993.

Sontag SJ. Rolling review: Gastroesophageal reflux disease. *Aliment Pharmacol Ther* 1993; 7:293-312.

Spiro HM. *Clinical Gastroenterology*. 4th ed. New York: McGraw-Hill Inc.; 1993.

Suchy J. *Liver Diseases in Children*. St. Louis: Mosby-Year Book; 1994.

Tanner S. *Pediatric Hepatology*. Edinburgh: Churchill Livingstone; 1989.

Tavill AS. Clinical Implications of the Hemochromatosis Gene (editorial). *N Engl J Med* 1999;341:755.

Thung SN, Gerber MA. *Differential Diagnosis in Pathology: Liver Disorders*. New York: Igaku-Shoin; 1995.

Torres AJ, Landa JI, Moreno-Azceita M, Argüello JM, Silecchia G, Castro J, et al. Somatostatin in the management of gastrointestinal fistulas. *Arch Surg* 1992;127:977-1000.

Vasudeva R. Gastrointestinal and hepatic complications in bone marrow transplant recipients. *Current Opinion in Critical Care* 1997;3:132-137.

Webb WA. Management of Foreign Bodies of the Upper Gastrointestinal Tract: Update. *Gastrointest Endosc* 1995;41:39-51.

Whitehead WE, Wald A, Diamant NE, Enck P, Pemberton JH, Rao SSC. Functional disorders of the anus and rectum. *Gut* 1999;45(suppl II):II55-II59.

Yamada T, Alpers D, Laine L, Owyang C, Powell D. *Textbook of Gastroenterology*. 3rd ed. Philadelphia: Lippincott Williams & Wilkins; 1999.

Zakim D, Boyer TD. *Hepatology: A Textbook of Liver Disease*. 3rd ed. Philadelphia: WB Saunders Co.; 1996.

Zetterman RK. Long-term management of the liver transplant patient. *Sem Liv Dis* 1995;15:123-180.